AF352071

TUMORS AND TUMORLIKE LESIONS OF SOFT TISSUE

CONTEMPORARY ISSUES
IN SURGICAL PATHOLOGY
VOLUME 18

SERIES EDITOR

Lawrence M. Roth, M.D.

Professor of Pathology
Director, Division of Surgical Pathology
Indiana University School of Medicine
Indianapolis, Indiana

Previously Published

TUMORS AND TUMORLIKE LESIONS OF SOFT TISSUE

Edited by

Vito Ninfo, M.D.
Professor of Anatomic Pathology
Director, Institute of Anatomic Pathology
University of Padua, School of Medicine
Padua, Italy

E.B. Chung, M.D., M.Sc., Ph.D.
Professor
Department of Pathology
Howard University College of Medicine
Director of Surgical Pathology
Howard University Hospital
Washington, D.C.

Andrea O. Cavazzana, M.D.
Institute of Anatomic Pathology
University of Padua, School of Medicine
III° Servizio Anatomia Patologica USL 21
Padua, Italy

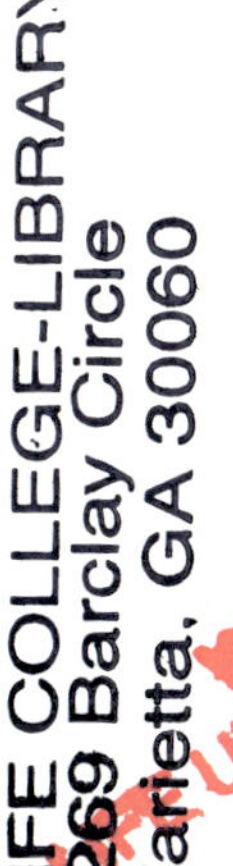
LIFE COLLEGE-LIBRARY
1269 Barclay Circle
Marietta, GA 30060

WITHDRAWN
LIFE UNIVERSITY LIBRARY

Churchill Livingstone
New York, Edinburgh, London, Melbourne, Tokyo

Library of Congress Cataloging-in-Publication Data
Tumors and tumorlike lesions of soft tissue / edited by Vito Ninfo,
    E.B. Chung.
        p cm. — (contemporary issues in surgical pathology : v. 18)
        Includes bibliographical references and index.
        ISBN 0-443-08672-9
        1. Soft tissue tumors—Diagnosis. 2. Pathology, Surgical.
    I. Ninfo, Vito. II. Chung, E.B. III. Series.
        [DNLM: 1. Soft Tissue Neoplasms. W1 C0769MS v. 18 / WD 375 T925]
    RC280.S66T86 1991
    616.99'2—dc20
    DNLM/DLC
    for Library of Congress   91–10915
                                                                        CIP

© **Churchill Livingstone Inc. 1991**

All rights reserved. No part of this publication may be reproduced, stored in a retrieval system, or transmitted in any form or by any means, electronic, mechanical, photocopying, recording, or otherwise, without prior permission of the publisher (Churchill Livingstone Inc., 650 Avenue of the Americas, New York, NY 10011).

Distributed in the United Kingdom by Churchill Livingstone, Robert Stevenson House, 1–3 Baxter's Place, Leith Walk, Edinburgh EH1 3AF, and by associated companies, branches, and representatives throughout the world.

Accurate indications, adverse reactions, and dosage schedules for drugs are provided in this book, but it is possible that they may change. The reader is urged to review the package information data of the manufacturers of the medications mentioned.

The Publishers have made every effort to trace the copyright holders for borrowed material. If they have inadvertently overlooked any, they will be pleased to make the necessary arrangements at the first opportunity.

Acquisitions Editor: *Robert A. Hurley*
Copy Editor: *Christina Joslin*
Production Designer: *Angela Cirnigliaro*
Production Supervisor: *Jeanine Furino*

Printed in the United States of America

First published in 1991   7 6 5 4 3 2 1

Contributors

Lennart Angervall, M.D. Ph.D
Professor, Department of Pathology II, University of Göteborg; Sahlgrenska Hospital, Göteborg, Sweden

Andrea O. Cavazzana, M.D.
Institute of Anatomic Pathology, University of Padua, School of Medicine, III° Servizio Anatomia Patologica USL 21, Padua, Italy; Member, Research Group of Pediatric Solid Tumors for the Italian Rhabdomyosarcoma and Neuroblastoma Research Program

E.B. Chung, M.D., M.Sc., Ph.D.
Professor, Department of Pathology, Howard University College of Medicine; Director of Surgical Pathology, Howard University Hospital, Washington, D.C.

Ambrogio S. Fassina, M.D.
Associate Professor, Institute of Anatomic Pathology, University of Padua, School of Medicine, Padua, Italy

Dieter Harms, M.D.
Professor, Institute of Pathology, University of Kiel, Kiel, Federal Republic of Germany

Lars-Gunnar Kindblom, M.D., Ph.D.
Associate Professor, Department of Pathology II, University of Göteborg; Sahlgrenska Hospital, Göteborg, Sweden

Vito Ninfo, M.D.
Professor of Anatomic Pathology and Director, Institute of Anatomic Pathology, University of Padua, School of Medicine, Padua, Italy

Dietmar Schmidt, M.D.
Associate Professor of Pathology, Institute of Pathology, University of Kiel, Kiel, Federal Republic of Germany

James M. Woodruff, M.D.
Associate Professor, Department of Pathology, Cornell University Medical College; Attending Pathologist, Memorial Sloan-Kettering Cancer Center, New York, New York

Preface

The task of editing a book on soft tissue tumors is both challenging and extremely difficult. For many years, soft tissue pathology has been considered the underdog of surgical pathology. Thanks primarily to the pioneering work of A.P. Stout, later associated with R. Lattes, this field underwent a period of rebirth. In the time that followed, many experts contributed to the growth of knowledge, but it was mainly due to the unremitting dedication of F.M. Enzinger that pathologists became aware of the numerous, sometimes enigmatic and fascinating aspects of these lesions. In fact, his book, written in collaboration with S. Weiss, is not only a defacto authority on soft tissue tumors, but it also represents a formidable milestone for others to reach.

The application of techniques such as immunocytochemistry, molecular biology, cytogenetics, and tissue culture provides new information and provocative redefinitions of old models almost daily. This is a rapidly expanding process that demands constant time and energy to remain current. Considering the limited time available in everyday practice, we felt the necessity for a quick, concise reference tool and a handy companion to the microscope.

An outstanding group of experts from the United States and Europe helped us attain this goal by sharing with us their invaluable knowledge and expertise. We hope that we have provided the fundamental criteria for diagnosis, whether it be clinical, morphologic, immunocytochemical, or whatever other unconvential criteria may apply to a particular case.

Finally, we wish to express our sincere gratitude to all those who have made equally significant contributions to the realization of this book: technicians, photographers, secretaries, and proofreaders. Special thanks also go to Robert Hurley for his effort in organizing the intercontinental concert and to Ambrogio S. Fassina for his inexhaustible drive, without which the final score would not likely have been appreciated.

Vito Ninfo, M.D.
E.B. Chung, M.D., M.Sc., Ph.D.
Andrea O. Cavazzana, M.D.

Contents

1

An Approach to Soft Tissue Tumors and Their Current Classification

Vito Ninfo and E. B. Chung

Soft tissue tumors encompass a vast heterogeneous group of lesions that range from tumorlike proliferations to true neoplasms. They include all tumors of nonepithelial extraskeletal tissues except those of hematopoietic and reticuloendothelial origin and glial tissue. Traditionally they also include tumors of peripheral nervous tissue.

Soft tissue tumors are relatively uncommon, accounting for about 0.8 percent of all malignancies.[1] However, their incidence is difficult to ascertain with accuracy. Age-adjusted studies suggest that malignant lesions have an incidence of approximately 2 new cases/year/ 100,000 population.[2, 3] In view of the fact that benign tumors outnumber malignant cases by 100:1,[4] it is reasonable to assume that a pathologist working in a general hospital serving a community of 100,000 will encounter about 200 cases of soft tissue tumor a year. The relative frequency of these tumors is not randomly distributed in all age groups since malignant mesenchymal tumors are more frequent in the elderly. It is estimated that in patients aged 80 years or over the incidence is 8/100,000.[5]

The median age at diagnosis for soft tissue sarcomas is about 43 years,[6, 7] and more than half of the cases are located in the extremities.[6, 7] A slight male preponderance is recorded in the larger series,[5–8] with a male: female ratio of approximately 1.3:1. Malignant fibrous histiocytoma, liposarcoma, and leiomyosarcoma are the most common histotypes encountered.[5–8]

DIAGNOSTIC APPROACH

The evaluation of clinical data (i.e., age, sex, site and location, duration of symptoms, etc.) is the first step in establishing a correct diagnosis of a soft tissue tumor.

Some tumors occur in selected age groups more frequently than others (Table 1-1); for example, embryonal and alveolar rhabdomyosarcomas are almost exclusively found in children, whereas liposarcoma is exceedingly rare in the pediatric age group, being primarily observed in elderly people. Size and depth of a lesion are also important features in distinguishing benign from malignant tumors. A large, deeply seated mass is more likely to be malignant compared with a small, superficially located lesion, although musculoaponeurotic fibromatosis and intramuscularly located lipoma, angioma, and myxoma are notable exceptions to this common rule.

These tumors have no specific symptoms whether superficial or deep seated, the latter often being detected when they displace or otherwise affect nearby organs. Pain, a rare symptom, is characteristically associated with glomus tumor, intramuscular hemangioma, and pseudomalignant osseous tumor of soft tissue.[9] Paresthesias and motor dysfunctions are usually related by patients with nerve sheath tumors.

A rapid growth of a tumor mass, although a worrisome feature, is not necessarily indicative of malignancy. Reactive lesions such as myositis

Table 1-1. Distribution of Sarcomas by Age

< 15 Years	15 to 40 Years	> 40 Years
Rhabdomyosarcoma	Synovial sarcoma	MFH
Fibrosarcoma	MPNST	Liposarcoma
PNET	Epithelioid sarcoma	Leiomyosarcoma
	Clear cell sarcoma	Angiosarcoma
	Alveolar soft part sarcoma	
	Extraosseus Ewing's sarcoma	

PNET, primitive neuroectodermal tumors; MPNST, malignant peripheral nerve sheath tumors; MFH, malignant fibrous histiocytoma.

ossificans and nodular fasciitis usually develop within a few weeks in young individuals. However, a sudden growth of a pre-existing longstanding mass is frequently observed in degenerating benign lesions (e.g., in malignant nerve sheath tumor arising in a neurofibroma). On the other hand, an indolent clinical course does not necessarily rule-out a malignancy. Clear cell sarcoma and epithelioid sarcoma may present as longstanding, slowly growing masses.

The gross appearance of the lesion might add further information regarding its nature and histogenesis, although soft tissue tumors often share many macroscopic features. An encapsulated fusiform mass involving a major nerve is the typical appearance one would anticipate for a peripheral nerve sheath tumor, whereas a brown or yellowish nodular neoplasm attached to a tendon strongly suggests a giant cell tumor of the tendon sheath. The final diagnosis, however, must rest upon the microscopic examination of the specimen.

RECOGNITION OF SOFT TISSUE TUMORS

In 1967 Stout and Lattes[10] wrote in the Introduction to the second edition of their fascicle:

". . . all (soft tissue) neoplasms develop from two primitive sources: the mesoderm and the neuroectodermal tissues of the peripheral nervous system. . . . If the various tumors developing from these tissues reproduced their prototypic tissues in pure form, even though in various stages of differentiation, recognition would be relatively simple. Unfortunately this is not always the case. . . ."

Soft tissue tumors can thus be recognized by virtue of their ability to reproduce cellular aspects and architectural patterns similar to the tissue from which they developed. These features are, indeed, morphologic expressions of the functional commitment of the primitive mesenchymal or neuroectodermal cells toward a more differentiated phenotype. The eosinophilic fibrillary cytoplasm that characterizes muscle cells is due to the active synthesis and polymerization of myosin and actin filaments. Likewise, the presence of spindle structures resembling tactile corpuscles in a spindle cell neoplasm is an expression of schwannian differentiation. Individual characteristics are apparent in the majority of cases of soft tissue tumor on routine hematoxylin and eosin (H&E)-stained slides, although they may be absent or less apparent in different parts of the same tumor. A careful and adequate sampling of the specimen is, therefore, of utmost importance.

In some cases special stains, such as the Periodic Acid-Schiff (PAS), Masson's trichrome, and reticulin stains, may be necessary for the adequate interpretation of the tumor. The presence of demonstrable intracytoplasmic glycogen together with fuchsinophilic longitudinal fibrils is helpful in distinguishing myogenous from nerve sheath tumors. Similarly, highly characteristic growth patterns are better outlined with the reticulin stain. A perivascular arrangement of reticulin fibers that encircle individual cells is a distinctive feature of hemangiopericytoma. Likewise, the biphasic pattern of a synovial sarcoma is highlighted and unmasked by the reticulin stain.

Nevertheless, 8 to 15 percent of soft tissue sarcomas cannot be recognized on the basis of their light microscopic features.[5–8] Other approaches are then required to improve our diagnostic accuracy. Despite the sampling limitations, electron microscopic studies provide important additional information on the subcellular structure of many soft tissue tumors. In most cases, spindle cell tumors can be reliably differentiated on the basis of their ultrastructural features. A cytoplasmic collection of thin actin filaments with focal densities along their course and numerous micropinocytotic vescicles are highly characteristic of a smooth muscle lesion.[11] Spindle cells showing transitional features of both smooth muscle cells and fibroblasts, occasionally unsheathed by basal lamina-like material, are readily identified as myofibroblasts.[12] Long intertwining cellular processes surrounded by a distinct basal lamina and mesaxons or pseudomesaxons are hallmarks of the schwannian origin of a spindle cell tumor.[13]

Furthermore, ultrastructural analysis has made an important contribution to the differential diagnosis among undifferentiated small round cell tumors such as extraskeletal Ewing's sarcoma, poorly differentiated rhabdomyosarcoma, and primitive sarcomas. These tumors may be indistinguishable by conventional light microscopic criteria alone, however, each can be recognized by its ultrastructural characteristics.[14, 15]

Our knowledge of cellular differentiation and functions has been greatly expanded over the past two decades with the identification of a large number of antigens in both normal and neoplastic tissues. Specific cellular products and extracellular material can be easily identified through the application of immunocytochemical methods. These methods have been now widely applied by pathologists as useful diagnostic tools to solve difficult cases. Although a detailed discussion of immunocytochemical methods and their application is beyond the scope of this chapter, here we are compelled to describe some relevant pitfalls.

There is a significant overlapping in immunocytochemical findings among different soft tissue tumors. Therefore, no *single* marker alone can reliably and reproducibly be used to substantiate the presumptive diagnosis. Markers such as neuron-specific enolase and S-100 protein, initially thought to be specific for tumors of a neuroectodermal lineage, are now found to have a broader expression in different cell types, such as skeletal muscle cells[16, 17] and chondrocytes.[18] Moreover a positive reaction to a single marker cannot necessarily support one histotype over another. Desmin, a well-known muscle marker, has been shown to be positive in other cell types, such as glial cells[19] and myofibroblasts.[20] On the other hand, a negative reaction to a marker does not preclude the diagnosis. About one-half of the cases of malignant schwannoma fail to demonstrate S-100 protein,[21] and factor VIII-associated antigen is seldom positive in malignant tumors of endothelial origin.[22]

Furthermore, the preservation of the antigenicity depends largely on the type of fixative used; intermediate filaments are generally better preserved in alcohol than formalin fixatives, and a preliminary enzymatic digestion is often required to reveal them in formalin-fixed, paraffin embedded material.[23] Great caution must, therefore, be used when interpreting the immunocytochemical findings, which can lead to a mistaken diagnosis if considered independently from the histopathologic aspects and the appropriate clinical setting.

Other nonconventional techniques can shed a light on the differential diagnosis. Tumors lacking diagnostic features in vivo can undergo spontaneous differentiation in vitro. Short-term tissue culture, first attempted in 1887,[24] can be successfully applied as an additional diagnostic tool[25, 26] in selected cases.

Table 1-2. Chromosomal Changes in Sarcoma

Tumor	Chromosomal Abnormality
Synovial sarcoma	t(x;18)(p11.2;q11.2)
Peripheral neuroepithelioma	t(11;22)(q24;q12)
Neuroblastoma	del (1)(p32 p36)
Myxoid liposarcoma	t(12;16)(q13;p11)
Embryonal rhabdomyosarcoma	Loss of heterozygosity chromosome 11
Alveolar rhabdomyosarcoma	t(2;13)(q37;q14)
Extraskeletal myxoid chondrosarcoma	t(9;15;22)(q31;q25;q122)

Finally, an alternative approach to differential diagnosis in soft tissue tumors is also offered by the genetic analysis of tumor specimens. Numerous chromosomal abnormalities have been consistently reported in various soft tissue tumors such as peripheral neuroepithelioma,[27] neuroblastoma,[28] synovial sarcoma,[29] and myxoid liposarcoma,[30] and they are being proposed as specific tumor markers (Table 1-2).

Identifying the Tumor as Benign or Malignant

Determination of whether a tumor is benign or malignant can be extremely difficult, even for the most experienced pathologist. Great care should be exercised when applying the general morphologic criteria of malignancy, such as nuclear atypia, mitoses, and infiltrative growth, when diagnosing a soft tissue lesion. There is a group of lesions, collectively known as *pseudosarcomas,* whose histologic aspects closely mimic true sarcomas (Table 1-3). Nodular fasciitis, a common benign reactive lesion, is often misdiagnosed as sarcoma because of its high mitotic rate and infiltrative growth pattern. Nuclear and cellular atypia are frequently observed in longstanding benign nerve sheath tumors (ancient neurilemmoma),[31] whereas bizarre pleomorphic giant cells are occasionally encountered in atypical lipoma[32] and fibroma of the skin.[33] A highly cellular "tumor" occurring after a surgical maneuver in the genitourinary tract can closely simulate a leiomyosarcoma.[34] On the other hand, fully malignant tumors can have a deceptively bland appearance. Well-differentiated (lipomalike) liposarcomas can easily be misinterpreted as ordinary lipomas and myxoid liposarcomas can be misdiagnosed as benign myxomas.

Moreover, there are tumors whose malignant potential is not always clearly predictable on morphologic bases; terms such as *atypical* or *aggressive* have been often used to indicate these borderline tumors.[35, 36]

Summary

In summary, a correct diagnosis will emerge primarily from a combination of clinical and histopathologic findings. The latter may be supplemented and verified by the immunocytochemical and/or electronmicroscopic studies. A panel of selected antibodies should be preferentially applied in order to confirm the diagnosis. Ultrastructural studies complemented by immunocytochemical analysis thus allow us to considerably narrow the number of diagnostic possibilities and increase our diagnostic precision.

CLASSIFICATION

Earlier classifications were largely descriptive and based more on morphologic than histogenetic criteria. Hence soft tissue tumors can be

Table 1-3. Benign Lesions Simulating Sarcomas

Benign Lesion	Simulated Sarcoma
Nodular fasciitis	MFH, fibrosarcoma
Proliferative fasciitis and myositis	MFH, RMS, fibrosarcoma
Myositis ossificans	Extraskeletal osteosarcoma
Atypical fibrous polyps	MFH, embryonal RMS
Xantogranulomatous inflammatory processes	MFH, liposarcoma
Intravascular papillary endothelial hyperplasia	Angiosarcoma
Infantile fibromatosis	Fibrosarcoma, liposarcoma, embryonal RMS
Lipoblastoma	Liposarcoma
Spindle cell lipoma	Liposarcoma, fibrosarcoma
Pleomorphic lipoma	Liposarcoma, MFH
Epithelioid leiomyoma	Round cell liposarcoma, carcinoma
Epithelioid hemangioma	Angiosarcoma, carcinoma
Ancient schwannoma	MPNST, MFH
Cellular schwannoma	MPNST
Myxoma	Myxoid liposarcoma

MFH, malignant fibrous histiocytoma; RMS, rhabdomyosarcoma; MPNST, malignant peripheral nerve sheath tumor.

simply divided into four main categories: round cell, spindle cell, epithelioid and pleomorphic sarcomas (Table 1-4). Obviously this simplistic classification precludes any correlation with either histogenetic or clinical parameters.

Stout[37] in 1957 outlined a scheme for a new comprehensive classification based on the cell origin of the tumors. The tumors were identified and classified according to their ability to reproduce cellular and architectural patterns characteristic of their normal counterpart. This methodologic approach remained unchanged in the subsequent, updated edition of the original classification.[10]

In 1969 the World Health Organization (WHO)[38] recommended a classification of soft tissue tumors based on histologic typing and clinical findings. It was further emphasized that a close collaboration between pathologists and clinicians was imperative for establishing the correct diagnosis and a vigorous therapy at early stage.

The recognition of different histotypes and accurate diagnosis of soft tissue tumors have improved considerably with the availability and widespread use of new techniques such as immunocytochemistry, electron microscopy, and tissue culture. Tumors previously classified under the "uncertain histogenesis" category, such as adenomatoid tumor of the genital tract[39] or Kaposi's sarcoma,[40] have been properly assigned and more than 50 new entities have been added to the original WHO classification. An exhaustive updated classification of soft tissue tumors according to currently accepted histogenetic criteria is reported by Enzinger and Weiss in their outstanding book.[41]

If ancillary techniques such as electron microscopy and immunohistochemistry provided important information regarding the origin of many "uncertain" entities, they also underlined the difficulties and the drawbacks of classifications based on histogenetic criteria alone. It has recently been shown that markers of epithelial

Table 1-4. Descriptive Classification of Soft Tissue Tumors

Spindle cell sarcomas	Epithelioid sarcomas
Fibrosarcoma	Synovial sarcoma
Leiomyosarcoma	MPNST
Synovial sarcoma (fibrous monophasic)	Epithelioid sarcoma
MPNST	Clear cell sarcoma
Angiosarcoma	Angiosarcoma
	Alveolar soft part sarcoma
	MFH
	Epithelioid leiomyosarcoma
Round cell sarcomas	Pleomorphic sarcomas
Rhabdomyosarcoma	Rhabdomyosarcoma
PNET	MFH
Extraosseus Ewing's sarcoma	liposarcoma
Extrarenal rhabdoid tumor	MPNST
Extraosseus mesenchymal chondrosarcoma	Dedifferentiated sarcomas

MPNST, malignant peripheral nerve sheath tumor; MFH, malignant fibrous histiocytoma; PNET, primitive neuroectodermal tumors.

origin, such as keratins, are also expressed in mesenchymal tumors, such as leiomyoma,[42] rhabdomyosarcoma,[17] and malignant fibrous histiocytoma.[43] Furthermore, specific tumor markers rarely are homogeneously expressed in all tumor cells, reflecting variable degrees of tumor differentiation.[44] Different cell types and multiple differentiations can occur in soft tissue tumors. Malignant mesenchymoma is composed of a collection of different phenotypes, including osteoblasts, chondroblasts, fibroblasts, and lipoblasts.[45] Dermatofibrosarcomas protuberans can occasionally display fibrosarcomatous changes,[46] and a malignant fibrous histiocytoma pattern is commonly observed in dedifferentiated sarcomas.[47] The genomic instability of tumor cells and/or epigenetic factors can partially explain this variability of histologic features and functional aspects.[48] Therefore, it can be arduous and sometimes impossible to classify some tumors on the basis of strict histogenetic criteria.

On the other hand, a simple diagnosis of sarcoma or malignant mesenchymal tumor is no longer considered acceptable for the effective clinical management of the patient. Accordingly, the proper surgery and adjuvant chemotherapy have produced notable improvement in long-term survival,[49, 50] but their efficacy depends greatly on an accurate histologic typing and grading of malignancy. Therefore, malignant soft tissue tumors can be classified into three or four prognostically different groups (grades of malignancy) according to several parameters.[51–55] Histologic subtype and tumor differentiation, necrosis, size, and mitotic activity are the most important parameters to be considered both in evaluating malignancy and predicting the final outcome of patients.[51–53, 55] The 5-year survival rates for patients with low-grade sarcomas range from 100 to 69 percent, whereas only 40 to 0 percent of patients with high-grade sarcomas are alive at 5 years.[51, 52, 54, 55]

Flow-cytometry measurement of the tumor DNA content has recently been proposed as a valuable adjunct to the clinical and histopathologic assessment of cancers.[56] An abnormal (aneuploid) DNA content in human tumors is generally known to be a poor prognostic factor,[57, 58] with few notable exceptions. Diploid neuroblastomas apparently pursue a worse clinical course than aneuploid tumors.[59] A correlation between ploidy and grading has recently been reported in other soft tissue tumors. According to Kreicberg and co-workers,[60] both benign tumors and low-grade sarcomas were diploid, whereas high-grade malignant tumors were associated with an aneuploid DNA content. Nonetheless, 4 out of 26 cases of malignant fibrous histiocytoma (grades III to IV) examined were diploid. This finding seems to suggest an independent role of DNA measurement in assessing the degree of malignancy in soft tissue sarcomas.

SUMMARY

In summary, soft tissue tumors represent one of the most challenging fields of clinical oncology from the standpoint of understanding the individual characteristics, effective management, and predicting prognosis. Therefore, as more reliable methods of investigation become available, revision of present diagnostic criteria will be necessary.

REFERENCES

1. American Cancer Society: Cancer Facts and Figures-1988. American Cancer Society, New York, 1988, p. 8
2. Cutler SJ, Young IL: Third National Cancer Survey. Incidence Data. National Cancer Institute Monograph, 1975
3. Cancer in Ontario 1988. Screening for cancer. O.C.E., 1989
4. Rydholm A, Berg NO: Size, site and clinical incidence of lipoma. Acta Orthop Scand 54:929, 1983
5. Rydholm A, Berg NO, Gullberg B, et al: Epidemiology of soft-tissue sarcoma in the locomotor system. Acta Pathol Microbiol Immunol Scand (Sect A) 92:363, 1984
6. Russel WO, Cohen J, Enzinger F, et al: A clinical and pathological staging system for soft tissue sarcomas. Cancer 40:1562, 1977
7. Trojani M, Contesso G, Coindre JM, et al: Soft-tissue sarcomas of adults: study of pathological variables and definition of histopathological grading system. Int J Cancer 33:37, 1984
8 Mettlin C, Priore R, Rao U, et al: Results of the National Soft-Tissue Sarcoma Registry. J Surg Oncol 19:224, 1982
9. Angervall L, Stener B. Stener I, et al: Pseudo-malignant osseous tumor of soft tissue. A clinical, radiological and pathological study of five cases. J Bone Joint Surg 51B:654, 1969
10. Stout AP, Lattes R: Tumors of the soft tissues. p. 12. In Atlas of Tumor Pathology, Second Series. Armed Forces Institute of Pathology, Washington, DC, 1967
11. Morales AR, Fine G, Pardo V, Horn RC: The ultrastructure of smooth muscle tumors with a consideration of the possible relationship of glomoangioma, hemangiopericytomas and cardiac mixomas. Pathol Annu 10:65,92, 1975
12. Ghadially FN: Diagnostic electron microscopy of tumors. Second Ed. Butterworths, London, 1985
13. Erlandson RA, Woodruff SM: Peripheral nerve sheath tumor. Cancer 49:273, 1982
14. Dickman PS, Triche TJ: Extraosseus Ewing's sarcoma versus primitive rhabdomyosarcoma: diagnostic criteria and clinical correlation. Hum Pathol 17:881, 1986
15. Erlandson RA: The ultrastructural distinction between rhabdomyosarcoma and other undifferentiated "sarcomas." Ultrastruct Pathol 11:83, 1987
16. Tsokos M, Linoilla RI, Chandra RS, Triche TJ: Neuron-specific-enolase in the diagnosis of neuroblastoma and other small round cell tumors in children. Hum Pathol 15:575, 1984
17. Coindre SM, De Moscarel A, Trojani M, et al: Immunohistochemical study of rhabdomyosarcoma. Unexpected staining with S-100 protein and cytokeratin. J Pathol 155:127, 1988
18. Stefansson K, Wellmann R, Moore BW, Arnason BGW: S-100 protein in human chondrocytes. Nature 295:63, 1982
19. Dahl D, Bignami A: Immunohistological localization of desmin, the muscle type 100 A filament protein, in rat astrocytes and Müller glia. J Histochem Cytochem 80:207, 1982
20. Wargotz ES, Weiss SW, Norris HJ: Myofibro-

blastoma of the breast. Am J Surg Pathol 11:493, 1987

21. Weiss SW, Langloss S, Enzinger FM: Value of S-100 protein in the diagnosis of soft tissue tumors with particular reference to benign and malignant Schwann cell tumors. Lab Invest 49:299, 1983

22. Schested M, Hon-Jensen K: Factor VIII-related antigen as an endothelial cell marker in benign a malignant disease. Virchows Arch [A] 371:217, 1981

23. Miettinen M, Lehto VP, Virtanen L: Antibodies to intermediate filament protein in the diagnosis and classification of human tumors. Ultrastruct Pathol 7:83, 1984

24. Arnold S: Ueber Theilungsvorgange an den Wonderzellen, ihre progressiven und retrogressiven metamorphosen. Arch Mikr Anat 30:205, 1887

25. Murray MR, Stout AP: Distinctive characteristics of the sympathicoblastoma cultivated in vitro: a method for prompt diagnosis. Am J Pathol 23:429, 1947

26. Navarro-Fos S, Cavazzana AO, Noguera R, et al: Valor de las tecnicas de cultivos celulares y biologia molecular en el diagnostico diferential de los sarcomas de celulas redondas de la infancia y adolescencia. Oncologia 9:133, 1988

27. Thiele CS, Wang Peng J, Kao Shan CS, et al: Translocation of c-sis protooncogene in peripheral neuroepithelioma. Cancer Genet Cytogenet 24:119, 1987

28. Brodeur GM, Green AA, Hayes FA, et al: Cytogenetic features of human neuroblastomas and cell lines. Cancer Res 41:2256, 1981

29. Turc-Carel C, Dal Cin P, Limon J, et al: Translocation X;18 in synovial sarcoma. Cancer Genet Cytogenet 23:93, 1986

30. Turc-Carel C, Limon J, Dal Cin P, et al: Cytogenetic studies of adipose tissue tumor. II. Recurrent reciprocal translocation t(12;16) (q13;p11) in myxoid liposarcomas. Cancer Genet Cytogenet 23:291, 1986

31. Ackerman LV, Taylor FH: Neurogenous tumors within the thorax. A clinicopathological evaluation of forty-eight cases. Cancer 4:669, 1951

32. Kindblom LG, Angervall L, Svendsen P: Liposarcoma. A clinico-pathologic, radiographic and prognostic study. Acta Pathol Microbiol Scand, 253(suppl):1, 1975

33. Kamino H, Yu-Yun Lee J, Berke A: Pleomorphic fibroma of the skin: a benign neoplasm with cytologic atypia. A clinicopathologic study of eight cases. Am J Surg Pathol, 13:107, 1989

34. Proppe KH, Scully RE, Rosai J: Postoperative spindle cell nodules of genitourinary tract resembling sarcomas: a report of eight cases. Am J Surg Pathol 8:101, 1984

35. Kempson RL, Mc Gavran MN: Atypical fibroxantomas of the skin. Cancer 17:1463, 1964

36. Steefer TA, Rosaj J: Aggressive angiomyxoma of the female pelvis and perineum. Report of nine cases of a distinctive type of gynecologic soft tissue neoplasm. Am J Surg Pathol 7:463, 1983

37. Stout AP: Tumors of Soft Tissue. Atlas of Tumor Pathology. First Series, Fascicle 1, Armed Forces Institute of Pathology, Washington, DC, 1957

38. Enzinger FM, Lattes R, Torloni R: Histological typing of soft tissue tumors. International Histological Classification of Tumors, No. 3. World Health Organization, Geneva, 1969

39. Said SW, Nash G, Lee M: Immunoperoxidase localization of keratin proteins, carcinoembryonic antigen and Factor VIII in adenomatoid tumors. Evidence of mesothelial derivation. Hum Pathol 13:1106, 1982

40. Guarda LG, Silvia EG, Ordonez HG, et al: Factor VIII in Kaposi's sarcoma. Am J Clin Pathol 76:197, 1981

41. Enzinger FM, Weiss SW: Soft Tissue Tumors. CV Mosby, St. Louis, 1988

42. Norton AJ, Thomas JA, Isaacson PG: Cytokeratin-specific monoclonal antibodies are reactive with tumors of smooth muscle derivation. An immunocytochemical and biochemical study using antibodies to intermediate filament cytoskeletal proteins. Histopathology 11:487, 1987

43. Weiss SW, Bratthauer GL, Morris PA: Postirradiation malignant fibrous histiocytoma expressing cytokeratin. Am J Surg Pathol 12:554, 1988

44. Schmidt D, Reimann D, Treuner J, Harms D: Cellular differentiation and prognosis in embryonal rhabdomyosarcoma. A report from Cooperative Soft Tissue Sarcoma Study 1981 (CWS 81). Virchows Arch [A] 409:183, 1986

45. Stout AP: Mesenchymoma, the mixed tumor of mesenchymal derivates. Am Surg 127:278, 1948

46. Ding J, Hashimoto H, Enjoji M: Dermatofibrosarcoma protuberans with fibrosarcomatous areas. Cancer 64:721, 1989

47. Brooks JJ: The significance of double phenotypic

patterns and markers in human sarcomas. A new model of mesenchymal differentiation Am J Pathol 125:113, 1986

48. Henson DE: Heterogeneity in tumors. Arch Pathol Lab Med 106:597, 1982

49. Yang JC, Rosemberger SA: Surgery for adult patients with soft tissue sarcomas. Semin Oncol 16:289, 1989

50. Elias AD, Antman KH: Adjuvant chemotherapy for soft tissue sarcoma: an approach in search of an effective regimen. Semin Oncol 16:305, 1989

51. Myhre-Jensen O, Kaae S, Hjollund Madsen E, Sneppen O: Histopathological grading in soft-tissue tumors. Relation to survival in 261 surgically treated patients. Acta Pathol Microbiol Immunol Scand (Sect A) 91:145, 1983

52. Trojani M, Contesso G, Coindre JM, et al: Soft tissue sarcomas of adults: study of pathological prognostic variables and definition of a histopathological grading system. Int J Cancer 33:37, 1983

53. Costa J, Wesley RA, Glatstein E, Rosenberg SA: The grading of soft tissue sarcomas. Results of a clinicopathologic correlation in a series of 163 cases. Cancer 53:530, 1984

54. Markhede G, Angervall L, Stener B: A multivariate analysis of the prognosis after surgical treatment of malignant soft-tissue tumors. Cancer 49:1721, 1982

55. Mandard AM, Petiot JF, Marnay J, et al: Prognostic factors in soft tissue sarcomas. A multivariate analysis of 109 cases. Cancer 63:1437, 1989

56. Dressler LG, Bartow S: DNA flow cytometry in solid tumors: practical aspects and clinical applications. Semin Diagnost Pathol 6:55, 1989

57. Barlogie B, Raber MN, Schumann J, et al: Flow cytometry in clinical cancer research. Cancer Res 43:3982, 1983

58. Friedlander ML, Hedley DW, Taylor IW: Clinical and biological significance of aneuploidy in human tumors. J Clin Pathol 37:961, 1984

59. Gansler T, Chatten J, Varello M, et al: Flow cytometric analysis of neuroblastoma. Correlation with histology and clinical outcome. Cancer 58:2453, 1986

60. Kreicberg A, Tribukait B, Willems J, et al: DNA flow analysis of soft tissue tumors. Cancer 59:128, 1987

2

Fibrous and Fibrohistiocytic Tumors and Tumorlike Lesions

E. B. Chung, Andrea O. Cavazzana, Ambrogio S. Fassina, Vito Ninfo

Despite the large number of anatomic-clinical entities commonly listed under the heading fibrous and fibrohistiocytic, and the variety of histological aspects that may be observed, these tumors are essentially composed of fibroblasts, histiocytelike cells, and myofibroblasts.

In reference to the *myofibroblasts,* we feel compelled to provide brief explanatory notes about this peculiar phenotype. The term myofibroblast was first coined by Majno et al.[1] and refers to a specialized mesenchymal cell with distinctive ultrastructural features that are intermediate between typical fibroblasts and smooth muscle cells. In fact, myofibroblasts show fibroblastic traits, such as a prominent rough endoplasmic reticulum and Golgi apparatus, and smooth muscle cell characteristics, such as bundles of filaments with focal densities parallel to their course, subplasmalemmal densities, and occasionally well developed basal lamina. The immunocytochemical profile of myofibroblasts confirms their double fibroblastic and muscular nature, as revealed by the coexpression of different types of cytoskeleton proteins, such as vimentin/alpha-smooth muscle actin and vimentin/alpha-smooth muscle actin/desmin.[2, 3]

Myofibroblasts are commonly found in granulation tissue[1, 3] and in the desmoplastic reaction to many carcinomas,[4, 5] as well as in many fibroblastic and fibrohistiocytic lesions, such as those in adult and infantile fibromatoses,[6, 7, 8] nodular fasciitis,[9] proliferative fasciitis,[10] benign fibrous histiocytoma,[11] and juvenile fibroxanthoma.[12] Moreover, tumors such as myofibromatosis and myofibroblastoma are almost exclusively composed of myofibroblasts.[13, 14]

While the term myofibroblast summarizes the unique morphological aspect of these cells, it does not shed any light on their fibroblastic,[15] myogenic,[16] or histiocytic[12] origins, all of which have been previously proposed. At present, it seems reasonable to consider the myofibroblast as a functional and transitory phase of fibroblast modulation in response to different kinds of exogeneous or endogeneous stimuli.[3, 15, 17]

FIBROUS TUMORS AND TUMORLIKE LESIONS

Based on the biologic behavior and age affected, fibrous lesions are usually classified into four groups: (1) benign fibroblastic proliferations, (2) fibromatoses, (3) fibrous tumors of infancy and childhood, and (4) fibrosarcomas (Table 2-1).

Benign Fibroblastic Proliferations

While the diagnostic difficulties posed by some of these lesions, such as cutaneous fibroma, are essentially nil, some others, such as nodular fasciitis, proliferative fasciitis, and proliferative myositis, due to their rapid growth, exuberant histomorphologic appearance, and relatively obscure clinical course, are at times mistaken for sarcomas; therefore, they are desig-

Table 2-1. Histologic Classification of Fibrous Tumors and Tumorlike Lesions[a]

Benign	Malignant
Fibroblastic proliferation	
Fibroma	**Adult-type fibrosarcoma**
Nodular fasciitis	**Congenital and infantile fibrosarcoma**
Proliferative fasciitis	
Proliferative myositis	
Fibroma of tendon sheath	
Elastofibroma	
Nasopharyngeal angiofibroma	
Keloid	
Fibromatoses	
Superficial (fascial)	
Palmar fibromatosis	
Plantar fibromatosis	
Penile fibromatosis	
Knuckle pads	
Deep (musculoaponeurotic)	
Abdominal and intra-abdominal fibromatoses	
Extra-abdominal fibromatosis	
Fibrous Tumors of Infancy and Childhood	
Fibrous hamartoma of infancy	
Infantile digital fibromatosis	
Infantile myofibromatosis: solitary and	
multicentric types	
Juvenile hyaline fibromatosis	
Gingival fibromatosis	
Fibromatosis colli	
Infantile (desmoid-type) fibromatosis	
Calcifying aponeurotic fibroma	
Giant cell fibroblastoma	

[a] Boldface material denotes material discussed in text.

nated as *pseudosarcomatous lesions of soft tissue.*[18, 19]

Nodular Fasciitis

Following the original description by Konwaler et al.[20] in 1955, much has been written about nodular fasciitis, which is now readily recognized by most pathologists. Further histologic subtypes of nodular fasciitis were recently identified, namely cranial fasciitis and intravascular fasciitis, and deserve special attention, as they still may pose diagnostic dilemmas.

Cranial Fasciitis. This lesion, first reported by Lauer and Enzinger[21] in 1980, is thought to be closely related to periosteal fasciitis.[22] This rare lesion most likely arises from a deep fascial layer of the scalp or periosteum, and occurs almost exclusively in infants and young children with an average age at diagnosis of 18 months. The clinical presentation is one of a readily observable, rapidly growing mass. Cranial fasciitis features a distinct skull involvement with erosion. In the majority of cases, radiographs of the skull underlying the soft tissue mass reveal a lytic defect in the outer table, often accompanied by a sclerotic rim, giving an appearance of a saucer with preservation of the inner table (saucerlike erosion).[21] Grossly the mass is usually well circumscribed and grayish-white, and rubbery and firm in texture. The cut surface may show focal gelatinous or cystic areas, and occasionally a gritty sensation is felt when the mass is cut.

As in ordinary nodular fasciitis, there is a

spectrum of histomorphology. Most of the lesions are made up of loosely or haphazardly arranged spindle-shaped to stellate fibroblasts set in a myxoid matrix often accompanied by foci of hemorrhage and mononuclear cell infiltrates (Figs. 2-1 and 2-2). In some areas, the fibroblasts are arranged in a vague storiform pattern, whereas in others they tend to form broadly sweeping fascicles or a whorled pattern. Mitotic figures are common, and values range from 1 to 5 per 10 high-power fields. Multinucleated giant cells are also occasionally noted. Foci of reactive bone formation are observed in about two-thirds of the cases.[23]

Differential Diagnosis. In view of their anatomic location, meningioma at times may enter the differential diagnosis. However, neither whorls of meningothelial cells nor psammoma bodies are seen in cranial fasciitis. Whorls of plump spindle-shaped cells resembling myofibroblasts may raise the possibility of infantile myofibromatosis, while a focal vague storiform pattern may cause some confusion with fibrous histiocytoma. Nonetheless, areas exhibiting confusing features are invariably associated with more typical fasciitislike zones elsewhere in the lesions.

More collagenized areas may be mistaken for fibromatosis. Infantile (desmoid-type) fibromatosis, however, tends to show a more uniform growth pattern and a greater amount of interstitial collagen. As immature-appearing fibroblasts and mitotic figures may be present, cranial fasciitis may also be confused with infantile fibrosarcoma, which, however, is more cellular, with neoplastic cells arranged in distinct fascicles. Moreover, both fibromatosis and fibrosarcoma tend to infiltrate the surrounding structures, recur locally, and in the case of infantile fibrosarcoma, even metastasize.

Intravascular Fasciitis. This lesion, a rare variant of nodular fasciitis, was initially reported by Patchefsky and Enzinger[24] in 1981. These painless slow growing masses are most commonly found in the upper extremities, particularly the hands, head, and neck, which account for 70 percent of the cases. The lesion typically involves small or medium-sized veins and mus-

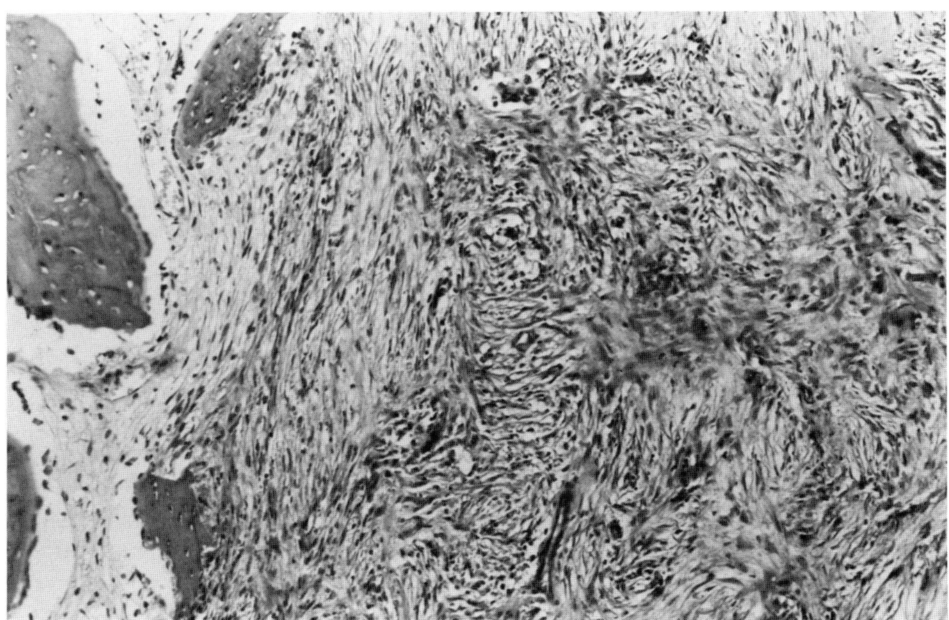

Fig. 2-1. Cranial fasciitis exhibiting proliferating fibroblasts that are arranged in a vague storiform or intertwining fascicular pattern. Spicules of woven bone are shown at the left. (H&E, × 125.)

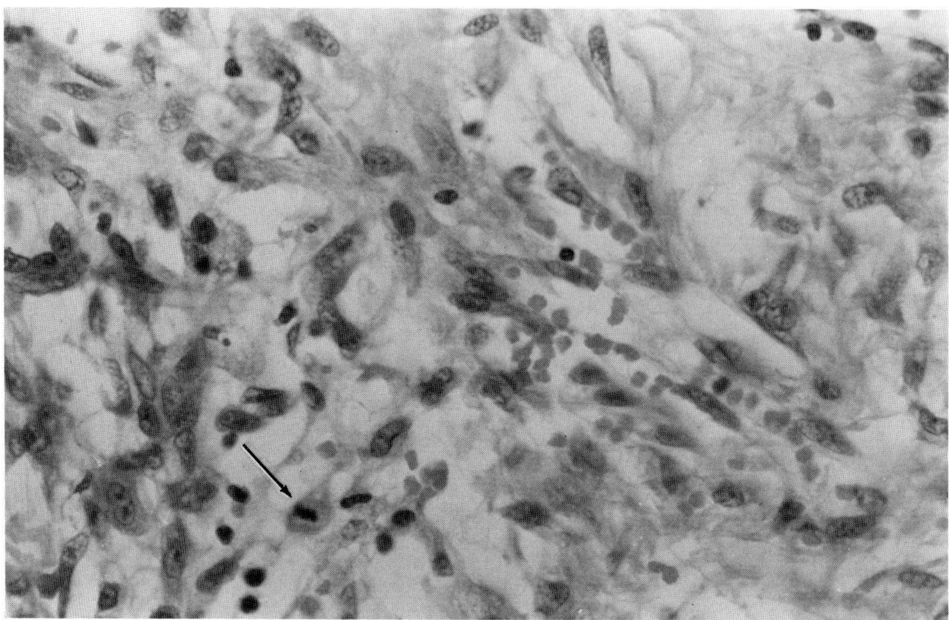

Fig. 2-2. High-power view of cranial fasciitis showing loosely arranged feathery fibroblasts associated with interstitial hemorrhage and scattered mononuclear inflammatory cells set in a myxoid background. Note the mitotic figure (arrow) and the histomorphologic similarity to an ordinary modular fasciitis. (H&E, × 500.)

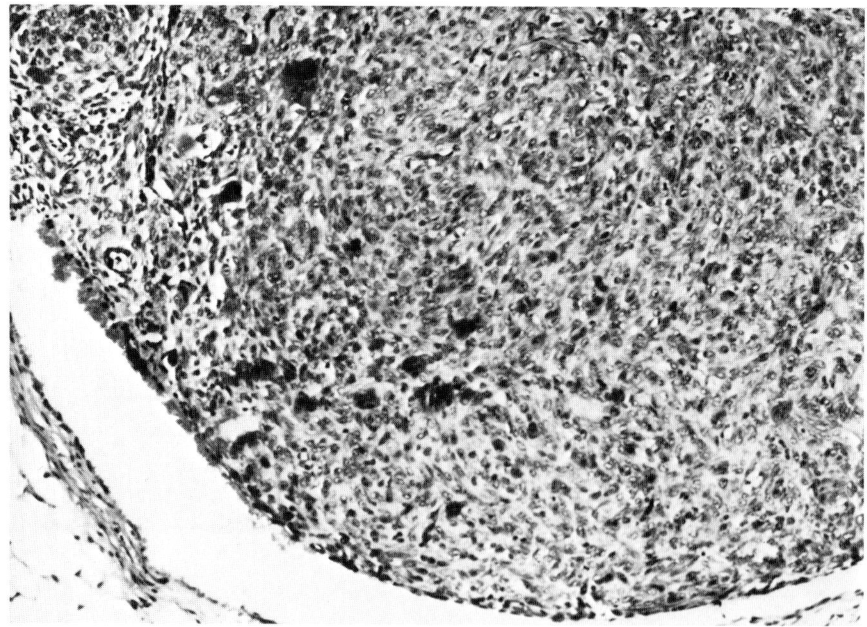

Fig. 2-3. Intravascular fasciitis, cellular variant, displaying intravascular fibroblastic proliferation, accompanied by scattered multinucleated giant cells. (H&E, × 125.)

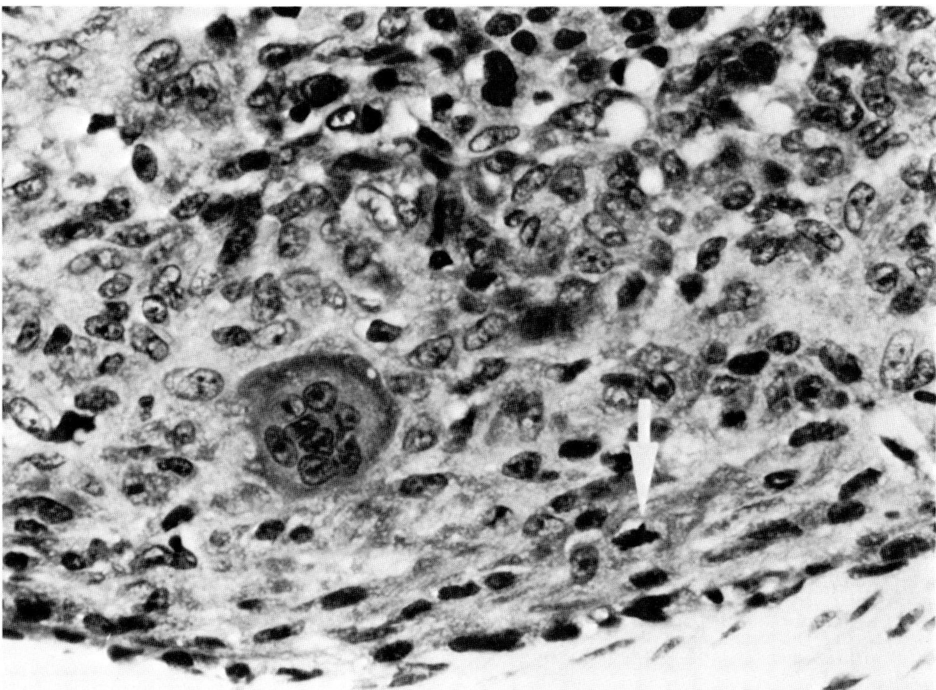

Fig. 2-4. High-power view of the same tumor shown in Fig. 2-3. Note the multinucleated giant cell and mitotic figure (arrow). (H&E, × 500.)

cular arteries, giving an erroneous impression of vascular invasion by malignant growth. Intravascular fasciitis occurs more commonly in children (47 percent occurring in children under age 15) and in young adults.[24] In nearly 25 percent of the cases, gross evidence of vascular involvement may be discernible. Most of the lesions are superficially located, involving the subcutaneous tissue adjacent to tendons, and only occasionally arise in deep soft tissues. Scalp lesions may be associated with periosteal involvement.

Microscopically the characteristic feature is a multinodular or serpentine growth pattern, intimately associated with blood vessels. When large-caliber vessels are involved, polypoid intraluminal growth may be appreciated. In some cases, the vascular component is relatively unapparent without step sections or special stains for elastic and muscle fibers. Elsewhere, the more familiar diagnostic features of nodular fasciitis are noted, although multinucleated giant cells are more readily found in this variant (Figs. 2-3 and 2-4).

Differential Diagnosis. Like ordinary nodular fasciitis, these lesions may be confused with fibrosarcoma, leiomyosarcoma, hemangiopericytoma, and the giant cell variant of malignant fibrous histiocytoma, but with vascular invasion. The demonstration of vascular elastic fibers and smooth muscle surrounding or incorporated into nodular lesions displaying various histologic patterns of nodular fasciitis should lead to the correct diagnosis of intravascular fasciitis.

Prognosis. There is no evidence that either intravascular or cranial fasciitis behaves differently from ordinary nodular fasciitis. Although these lesions rarely recur locally (despite the intravascular growth), there has been no documentation of metastasis.[24]

Proliferative Fasciitis

Proliferative fasciitis is a pseudosarcomatous process that involves the fascia and interlobular

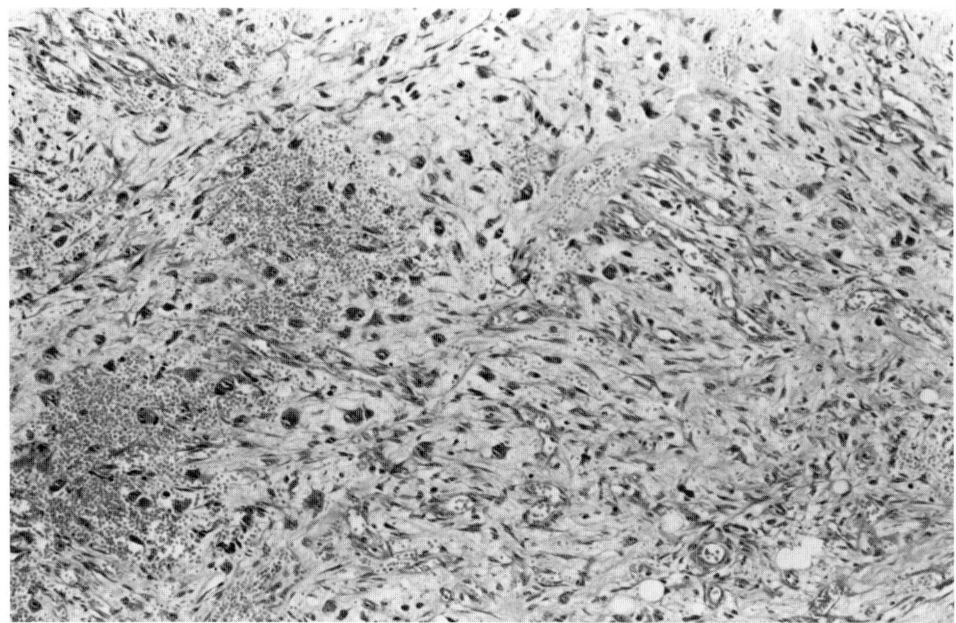

Fig. 2-5. Proliferative fasciitis displaying large cells possessing abundant basophilic cytoplasm that mimic ganglion cells. Note the associated hemorrhage and the richly myxoid matrix. (H&E, × 125.)

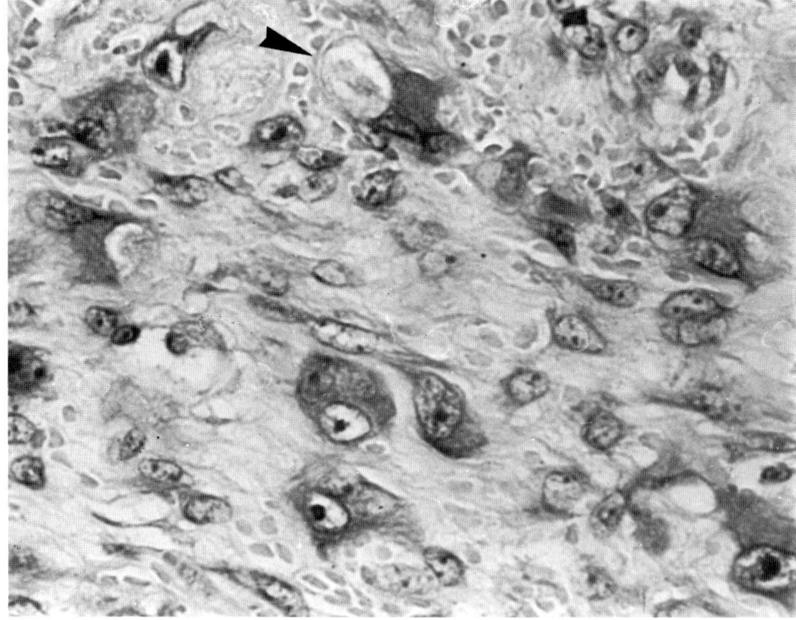

Fig. 2-6. Proliferative fasciitis with characteristic mononuclear giant cells, one of which displays an intracytoplasmic inclusion of engulfed collagen debris (arrow). (H&E, × 500.)

fibrous septa of subcutaneous fat.[25] It is essentially the subcutaneous and fascial counterpart of proliferative myositis[26] and affects adults almost exclusively, with a median age of 54 years.[27, 28] The majority of lesions occur in the extremities, particularly the forearm and thigh, where they manifest as firm, palpable, and rapidly growing nodules.[25, 26] The lesions are usually poorly circumscribed, situated primarily in the superficial fascia, and often extend along the fibrous septa separating the lobules of adipose tissue. The lesions infiltrate in a wedgelike manner into the underlying striated muscle, making distinction from proliferative myositis difficult.

Histologically the characteristic features are a mixture of large basophilic giant cells and fibroblastlike spindle cells in a background of a more or less prominent myxoid matrix and collagenous tissue (Fig. 2-5); the myxoid matrix is more prominent in earlier lesions. While the ''giant'' cells may bear a close resemblance to mature ganglion cells or at times simulate rhabdomyoblasts, their cytoplasm is more basophilic and fibrillar rather than granular, and one or two large vesicular nuclei with prominent nucleoli are present; no intracellular myofibrils or cross striations are seen. Giant cells occasionally possess intracytoplasmic inclusions with collagenlike staining characteristics (Fig. 2-6). From time to time, cells display large acidophilic nucleoli surrounded by a clear zone, giving the impression of viral inclusions. In older lesions, these cells are often surrounded by bundles of mature hyalinized collagen that may mimic neoplastic osteoid. Ultrastructurally these giant cells were shown to be modified fibroblasts.[27]

Differential Diagnosis. As in other pseudosarcomatous processes, the diffuse infiltrative growth, cellularity, and immature appearance of the proliferated cells may lead to confusion with a sarcoma. In particular, the presence of large, basophilic giant cells resembling ganglioneuroblasts and rhabdomyoblasts may be interpreted as ganglioneuroblastoma and rhabdomyosarcoma, respectively. However, the small size of the lesion, its superficial location, and the absence of desmin or myoglobin expression

by the tumor cells should lead to the correct diagnosis. Furthermore, both ganglioneuroblastoma and rhabdomyosarcoma are essentially tumors of children and young adults, whereas these lesions usually occur in patients older than 40 years of age.

Prognosis. Proliferative fasciitis is a self-limiting reactive process that is invariably resolved by simple local excision.

Fibroma of the Tendon Sheath

Fibroma of the tendon sheath is believed to represent a quasineoplastic reactive fibrosing process of the tendon sheath.[29] The exact nature of the tumor is not clear; however, there appear to be two phases of development, namely the initial transient cellular phase, which resembles either nodular fasciitis or fibrous histiocytoma, and the late collagenous phase, which is typical and diagnostic of this entity. This lesion is most commonly found in adults in the third to fifth decade of life, with a median age of 31 years. Men are more commonly affected than women, with a ratio of 2:1.

Nearly all of the tumors originate in the extremities, occurring in the volar aspects of the fingers and palms of the hands. They are usually attached to a tendon or tendon sheath, and in general are well circumscribed and lobulated. These lesions are small, from 1 to 2 cm in their greatest diameter, but they may reach sizes up to 5.5 cm. They are firm and rubbery and at times a cartilaginous appearance is noted as well as occasional areas of mucoid or cystic change.

Microscopically these distinctly lobulated lesions are intimately associated with tendinous tissue. The nodules are composed of haphazardly arranged fibroblasts embedded within a dense and often hyalinized collagenous matrix that contains dilated but slitlike spaces resembling entrapped tenosynovial clefts (Fig. 2-7). In the more cellular variants, the tumor is largely made up of spindle cells that tend to be arranged in fascicles, and sometimes are accompanied by a myxoid matrix, extravasated erythrocytes,

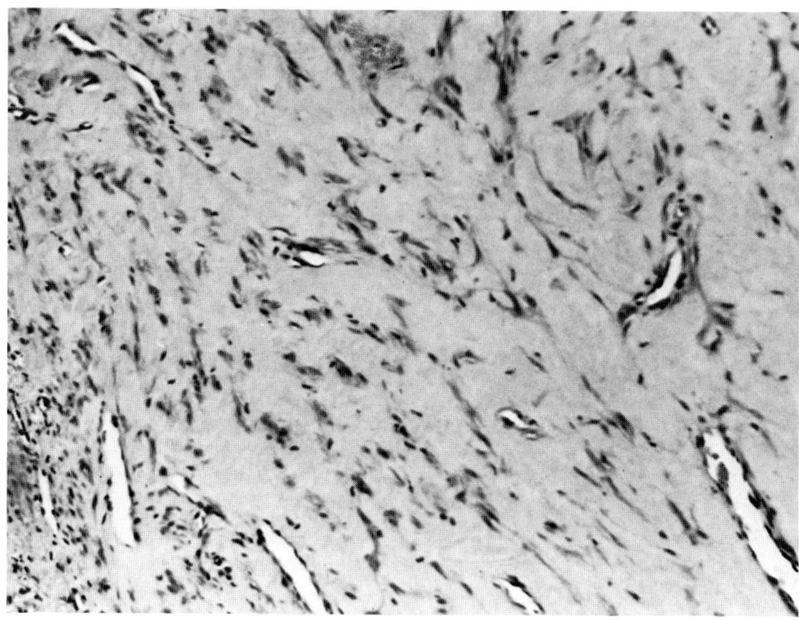

Fig. 2-7. Fibroma of tendon sheath showing haphazardly arranged fibroblasts embedded within a dense collagenous matrix containing dilated vessels and narrow slitlike spaces. (H&E, × 125.)

and a sprinkling of mononuclear cells. Elsewhere in the cellular areas, the spindle cells assume a vague, focal cartwheel or storiform pattern, as in fibrous histiocytoma. These cellular areas, however, always blend in more typical collagenized hypocellular areas. A few multinucleated giant cells are found occasionally, but no xanthoma cells or siderophages, as in giant cell tumors of tendon sheath.

Ultrastructurally the lesion consists of a mixture of myofibroblasts and fibroblasts.[30, 31] Unlike giant cell tumors of the tendon sheath,[32] the cells of fibroma of the tendon sheath do not show features of synoviocytic differentiation.[31] Furthermore, immunostaining has identified the characteristic slitlike spaces as vascular rather than synovial spaces.[33]

Differential Diagnosis. Recognition of a typical case of fibroma of the tendon sheath should not be too difficult. However, the more cellular variants may simulate either a nodular fasciitis or a fibrous histiocytoma. The cellular portions, though, are invariably associated with dense hypocellular fibrocollagenous areas characteristic of fibroma of the tendon sheath. Infre-

quently these variants have been mistaken for sarcoma,[33] including fibrosarcoma, synovial sarcoma, and malignant schwannoma.[29]

Prognosis. Fibroma of the tendon sheath is a benign process that recurs in 24 percent of the cases. All are treated effectively by local excision, or re-excision of the lesion. Complete removal of the entire tumor is necessary to prevent local recurrence.[34]

Elastofibroma

Elastofibroma is a rare, tumorlike lesion of fibroelastic tissue that was first described by Järvi and Saxén[35] at the Twelfth Congress of Scandinavian Pathologists in 1959 and was subsequently reported in 1961 under the term *elastofibroma dorsi*. It is believed to result from the excessive formation of collagen and abnormal elastic fibers (abnormal elastogenesis) secondary to repeated microtraumas between the scapula and chest wall.[36]

The lesion manifests as a slowly growing mass occurring more frequently in adult women older than 55 years of age.[37] Although its classic location is the inferior tip of the scapula,[36] cases involving the deltoid region,[38] the ischial tuberosity,[39] and the greater trochanter[40] have been reported.

Microscopically the lesion is unencapsulated and consists of dense collagenous fibrous tissue associated with some fibroblasts, foci of myxoid change, aggregates of eosinophilic, broad, wavy fibers, and beaded petaloid globules, and groups of mature fat cells (Fig. 2-8). The entrapped adipose tissue is more prominent at the periphery. Masson and Gomori trichrome stains reveal dense collagenous tissue containing numerous red-staining fibers, some with beaded or serrated edges that are better seen on Weigert or Verhoeff elastic stains as randomly arranged elastic fibers (Fig. 2-9). Elastic stains show elongated fibers with a branching and serpiginous course, and occasionally a dense central core.

Ultrastructural and biochemical studies have led to different conclusions regarding the origin and nature of the spindle cells in elastofibroma. These cells were recently shown to possess fibroblastic[41] rather than myofibroblastic[42, 43] characteristics. Moreover, elastin in these lesions appears to have different biochemical properties and amino acid composition compared with normal controls.[41] These findings, therefore, seem to add a "neoplastic" connotation to the original degenerative hypothesis.

Differential Diagnosis. Once familiarized with this lesion, its histologic diagnosis should not be too difficult, although elastofibroma may be clinically confused with fibromatosis or fibrosarcoma.[44]

Prognosis. Elastofibroma is a benign condition with no propensity to recur; malignant transformation has not yet been described.

FIBROMATOSES

The term *fibromatosis* was first proposed by Stout in 1954[45] to define a group of fibrous proliferations, other than fibroma, exuberant

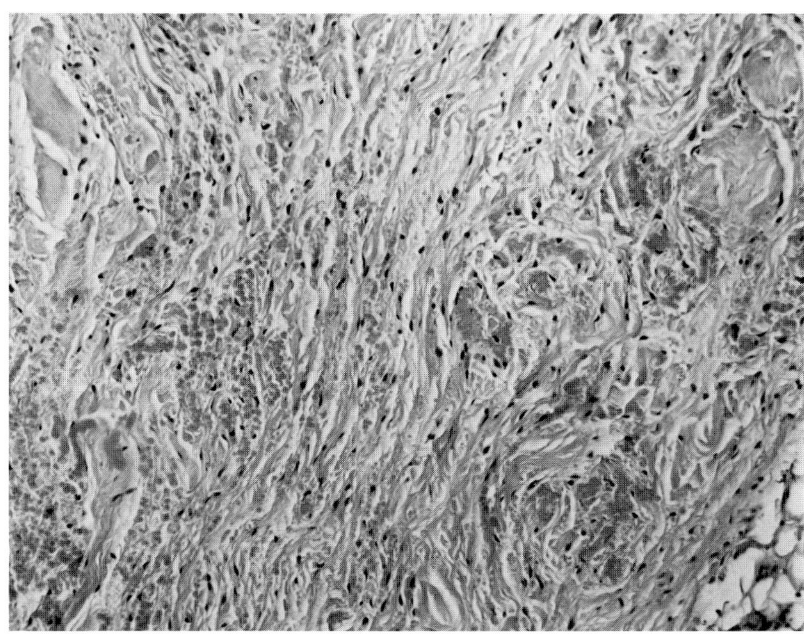

Fig. 2-8. Elastofibroma consisting of a mixture of intertwining swollen collagen and beaded elastic fibers associated with fibroblasts. (H&E, × 125.)

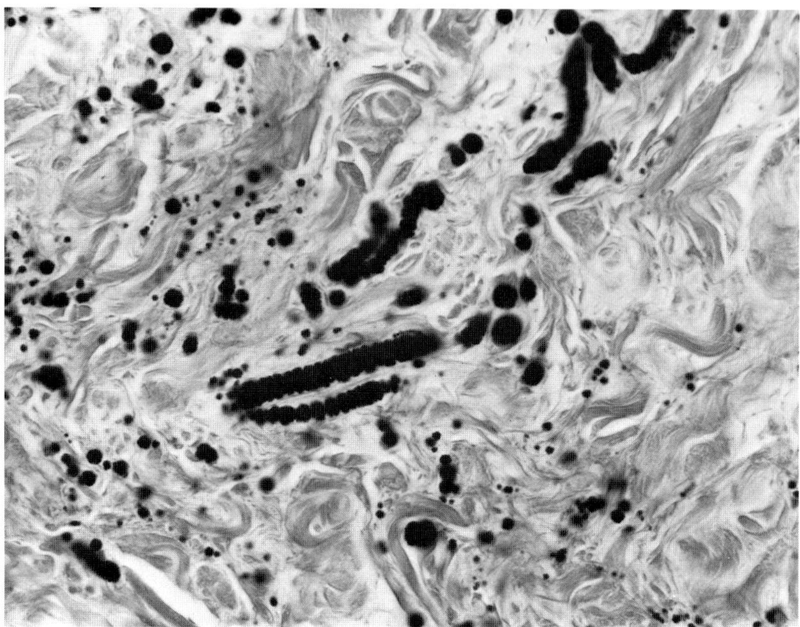

Fig. 2-9. Elastofibroma revealing elongated elastic fibers and beaded globules of elastin. (Verhoeff van Gieson, × 500.)

scar tissue, keloid, and fibrosarcoma, which included reactive and degenerative lesions, such as nodular fasciitis and elastofibroma, and some other proliferations almost exclusively found in infancy and childhood. Originally described in the first edition of *Fascicles* (Armed Forces Institute of Pathology)[46] and later kept in the revised edition, this group of lesions remained substantially unchanged in the *International Histological Classification of Tumors* (World Health Organization) as well.[48] Nevertheless, fibromatoses as originally conceived underwent a thorough revision, so that the term fibromatosis is currently applied to tumorous proliferations of unknown etiology, characterized by ill-defined and infiltrating margins and composed of extensive fascicles or bundles of fibroblasts in different stages of maturation embedded in a rich collagenous stroma.

While these lesions are most commonly found in adults,[49] they have also been described in infants and adolescents.[45] These proliferations take origin from the superficial or deep fascial planes, or the connective tissue of large muscles, and have thus been accordingly classified as *superficial* and *deep* (musculoaponeurotic) fibromatoses. Superficial fibromatoses comprise a number of lesions known as palmar fibromatosis (Dupuytren's contracture), plantar fibromatosis (Ledderhoses' disease), penile fibromatosis (Peyronie's disease), and knuckle pads; among these, palmar fibromatosis is by far the most common. They are well-recognized and their assessment poses no particular problem.

Deep fibromatoses, also known as *desmoid tumors* for the frequent occurrence of a highly collagenized stroma, deserve special attention in view of their alarming clinical presentation, as well as the diagnostic problems they still pose. Little is known about the pathogenesis of these fibrous lesions; it is thought that an inherited connective tissue defect may play an important role in their development, while the patient's hormonal status and level of estrogen receptors seem to influence the growth rate.[50, 51] The estimated incidence of these relatively infrequent lesions is 2 to 4 new cases per million inhabitants per annum.[52, 53] An incidence peak occurs in the second and third decades of life.[52] With the exclusion of abdominal desmoid tumors that occur almost exclusively in parous women, both sexes are equally affected.[52]

Unlike the superficial forms, deep fibromatoses often show rapid massive growth (greatest diameter up to 45 cm,[54] infiltration of surrounding tissues, and a high tendency to recur. These lesions are further classified as abdominal, intra-abdominal, and extra-abdominal fibromatoses, and recently a fourth type arising within the mammary parenchyma was added to the list.[55, 56] Abdominal fibromatosis is a well-defined entity that tends to occur in fertile women during or following pregnancy; however, it has also been observed in men and children.[52, 57, 58] The small bowel mesentery is the most commonly involved site in intra-abdominal fibromatosis,[59, 60, 61] while shoulder, chest wall, back, and extremities are the predilected sites in extra-abdominal fibromatosis.[62, 63] The tumors are generally solitary, but multicentric lesions have also been described.[52, 61, 64] Up to 13 percent of the reported cases of intra-abdominal fibromatosis are associated with multiple colonic adenomas (Gardner syndrome), while up to 80 percent of the patients with deep fibromatoses present demonstrable minor bone anomalies.[50]

Microscopically desmoid tumors are poorly circumscribed, and infiltrate the surrounding tissues in a tentacular fashion, despite an occasional, apparently well-demarcated appearance at gross inspection. The lesion is composed of slender, uniform, spindle-shaped cells arranged in broad bundles, and embedded in variable amounts of collagenous stroma (Fig. 2-10). An increased cellularity coupled with atrophic and multinucleated muscle cells is occasionally observed at the periphery. Myxoid changes occur in more than 50 percent of the intra-abdominal tumors; keloidal collagen fibers are also found, more frequently in male patients.[54] Mitoses are usually rare, while atypical or hyperchromatic nuclei are notably absent (Fig. 2-11).

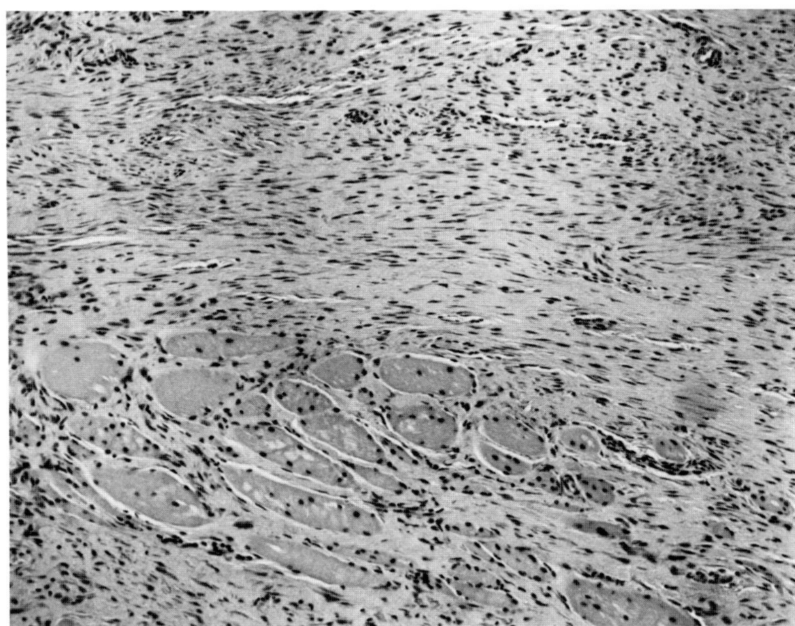

Fig. 2-10. Extra-abdominal fibromatosis exhibiting slender fibroblasts having uniform spindle-shaped nuclei associated with abundant collagen. Note the infiltrative growth pattern. (H&E, × 125.)

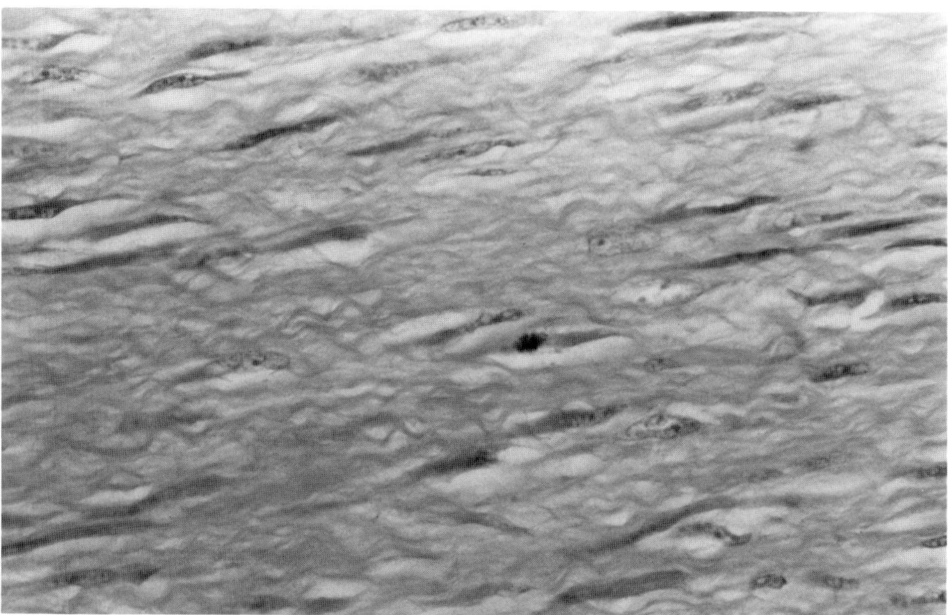

Fig. 2-11. High-power view demonstrating minute nucleoli and rather indistinct cytoplasm of the elongated fibroblasts. A mitotic figure is seen in the center. (H&E, × 500.)

Differential Diagnosis

Despite the bland cytological features, the presence of hypercellular areas, increased mitotic figures, and poor tumor demarcation may lead to an erroneous diagnosis. Indeed, in reviewing 130 cases Burke and colleagues found that more than 60 percent were incorrectly classified.[61] Fibrosarcoma, smooth muscle tumors, nerve sheath tumors, and reactive fibroblastic proliferations must be considered in the differential diagnoses. Fibrosarcomas are more cellular tumors with less collagenous stroma and higher mitotic rates. The presence of one or more mitotic figures per high-power field should always arouse the suspicion of malignancy. Myxoid liposarcoma and nerve sheath tumors, such as neurofibroma or neurilemoma, may enter the assessment of intra-abdominal fibromatoses. The absence of atypical lipoblasts, and negative immunostaining for S-100 protein in fibromatoses will clarify the diagnosis. Mammary fibromatoses should also be distinguished from myofibroblastoma.[14] Myofibroblastoma, probably a histogenetically related breast lesion,

is more frequent in the male breast, and is well demarcated from the surrounding mammary parenchyma; glandular lobules or ducts are not, in fact, entrapped in the lesion. The lack of inflammation, fat necrosis, and hemorrhage distinguish fibromatoses from exuberant reactive fibrosis.

Prognosis

Due to their infiltrative growth pattern, deep fibromatoses have a high tendency to recur despite wide, margin-free excisions; nevertheless, they never metastasize. Recurrence rates vary according to the anatomic sites, and range from 57 percent in the shoulder girdle[62] to 21[56] and 16[61] percent in breast and intra-abdominal lesions respectively. Patients with Gardner syndrome have a high morbidity rate, and a higher risk of recurrence (rates are close to 100 percent) than sporadic cases.[54, 61] A death rate of about 6 percent, mostly due to intestinal obstruction or short-bowel syndrome, has been reported.[61] Due to the reported high recurrence rate for incompletely removed lesions (up to 90 percent of cases), a wide excision is the treatment of choice.[65, 66]

FIBROUS TUMORS OF INFANCY AND CHILDHOOD

Fibrous proliferations, which are peculiar to infancy and childhood and have no well-recognized morphologic counterpart in adult life, are uncommon. Because of their unusual microscopic features, however, they pose special diagnostic problems. In these lesions, exuberant cellularity, high mitotic index, infiltrative growth pattern, and poor differentiation do not invariably indicate aggressive clinical behavior and yet, innocent-appearing conditions may recur repeatedly. Moreover, fibromatoses affecting infants and children present a more variable picture and differ considerably from those in adults in their histologic appearance. Therefore, the definition as well as the classification of fibromatoses occurring in childhood are not clear-cut, and some are still poorly delineated by pathologists. Since 1954, when Stout published his original series on ''juvenile fibromatosis'' that included a heterogeneous group of fibrous tumors, many of these fibrous proliferations have been recognized and categorized as specific entities[23] (see Table 2-1).

Fibrous Hamartoma of Infancy

In 1956 Reye[67] reported this lesion under the heading of ''subdermal fibromatous tumors of infancy.'' Because of its organoid growth pattern of superfluous tissue, in 1965 Enzinger[68] suggested the term fibrous hamartoma of infancy and this gained wide acceptance as a distinct entity. The lesion occurs during the first year of life and in about 20 percent of the cases is present at birth. Boys are more frequently affected, with a male to female ratio of more than 2:1.[68] The lesions are found most commonly in the lower dermis or subcutis of the axilla and upper arm, and less commonly in

the thigh, inguinal region, shoulder, back, and forearm. Grossly the tumorous lesions are poorly circumscribed and the cut surfaces display a mottled appearance owing to an admixture of firm, glistening gray-white tissue and irregular islands of yellow fat.

The histomorphologic findings are strikingly uniform except for variations in the relative proportions of the principal tissue components. The three tissue components characteristic of these lesions are (1) well-defined fibrous tissue trabeculae, (2) loosely textured whorls of immature mesenchymal cells set in a myxoid matrix, and (3) interspersed mature fat (Fig. 2-12). The fibrous tissue trabeculae are composed of mature collagen intermixed with well-oriented spindle-shaped fibroblasts that may be accompanied by occasional elastic fibers. Mitotic figures are infrequently found and when present, are usually seen around blood vessels. In some cases, the loosely textured mesenchymal tissue gradually blends in the more mature fibrous tissue trabeculae, reminiscent of infantile fibromatosis (Fig. 2-13). In others, there may be curly wire-like bundles of fibrocollagenous tissue mimicking neurofibroma, although proliferation of nerve fibers is not appreciated. In some lesions, considerable vascularity with numerous capillaries may give an angiomatoid appearance, as originally emphasized by Reye.[67] Ultrastructurally myofibroblasts intermingled with more typical fibroblastlike cells are commonly observed.[69, 70]

Differential Diagnosis. Once familiar with the characteristic histologic features, the pathologist should not encounter any difficulty in making the correct diagnosis. Despite its repetitive histomorphologic pattern, however, the lesion may be mistaken for infantile fibromatosis, especially when an unusual degree of hyalinization is present. Although infantile fibromatosis may encroach upon the subcutaneous tissue in a similar trabecular manner, these tumors arise primarily in the muscle rather than in the subcutis and lack the organoid pattern of fibrous hamartoma.[68]

Because of its cellularity and the immature quality of the myxoid tissue elements, the lesion may be taken for infantile fibrosarcoma. When

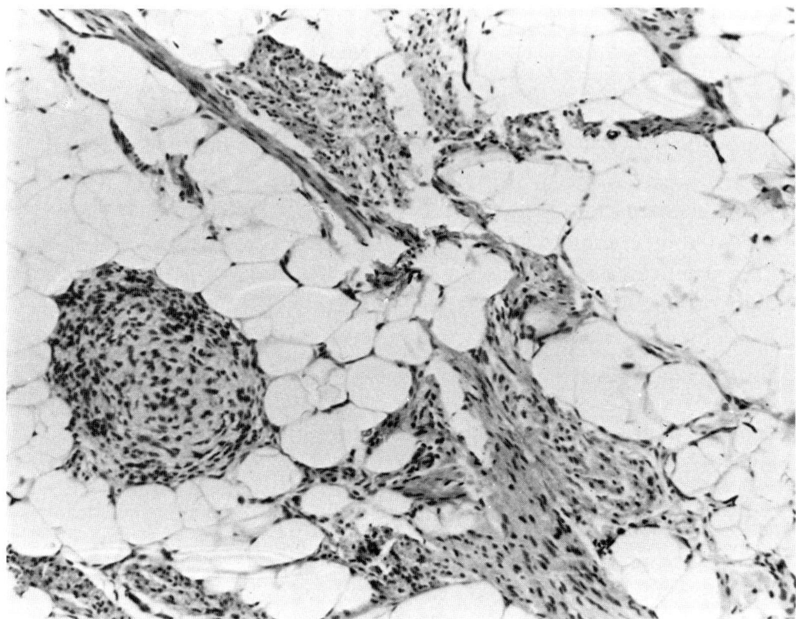

Fig. 2-12. Fibrous hamartoma of infancy consisting of a mixture of dense fibrous tissue trabeculae, whorls of immature mesenchymal cells, and lobules of mature adipose tissue. (H&E, × 125.)

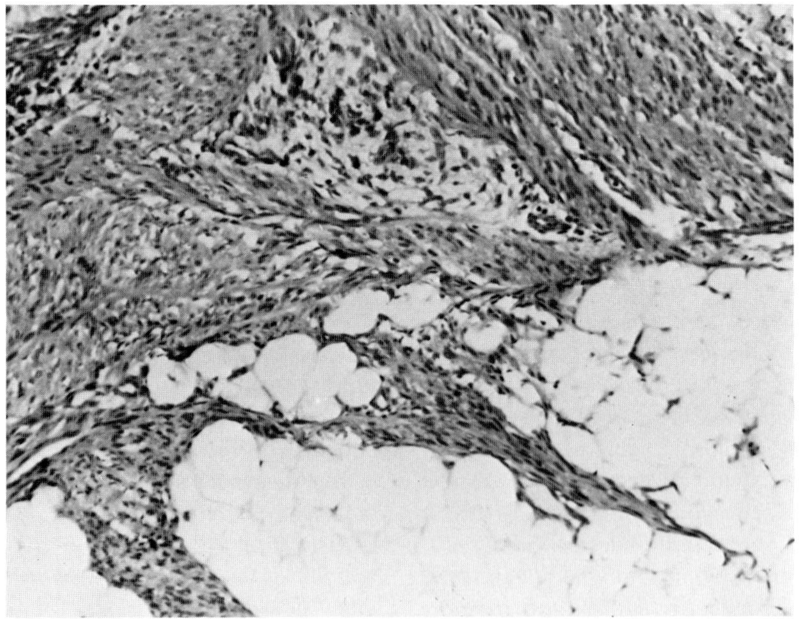

Fig. 2-13. Fibrous hamartoma of infancy showing loosely textured mesenchymal tissue that appears to blend gradually with broad fascicles of more mature fibrous tissue reminiscent of infantile fibromatosis. (H&E, × 125.)

some of the three characteristic components are replaced by short, thick curly bundles of collagen, the histologic appearance may mimic leiomyoma or neurofibroma. Neither smooth muscle fibers nor an increased number of neurites are found in these lesions.

Prognosis. Fibrous hamartomas of infancy are nearly always cured by complete local excision, although a recurrence rate of about 10 to 16 percent has been reported.[68]

Infantile Digital Fibromatosis

Infantile digital fibromatosis is a distinct entity almost exclusively involving the fingers and toes,[71, 72] and is characterized by the presence of intracytoplasmic inclusion bodies within proliferating fibroblasts. Tumor nodules are usually small and initial lesions often measure less than 1.0 cm in their greatest diameter.[73] With the exception of the thumbs and great toes, nearly all the lesions are located on the digits; extradigital lesions involving hands, feet, arms, and legs have also been described.[74, 75, 76] The tumors may be single or multiple and often affect more than one digit of the same hand or foot.[77] In some cases, the lesion may extend downward to attach to the periosteum, although the underlying bone is usually not involved.[78] Functional impairment or joint deformities have been observed, even though the tumor regressed spontaneously.[79] The overwhelming majority of cases (94 percent) is observed during the first year of life,[57] and in about one-third of cases the lesion is present at birth. Histomorphologically similar lesions in adults have been described[74, 76] in extradigital locations; therefore, the more descriptive term of *inclusion body fibromatosis* has been suggested for this entity.[74]

Histologically infantile digital fibromatosis consists of interlacing fascicles of fibroblasts closely associated with a dense collagenous stroma similar to the desmoid type of infantile fibromatosis. The lesions are ill-defined and may extend from the papillary dermis into the deep corium or subcutis, surrounding or replacing skin appendages. The fascicles of fibroblasts often appear to run perpendicular to the overly-

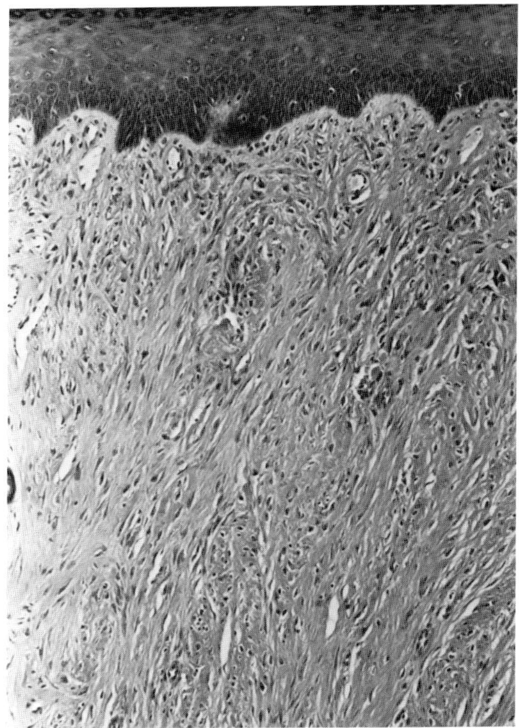

Fig. 2-14. Infantile digital fibromatosis involving the skin of the right fourth toe of a 12-month-old girl. (H&E, × 125.)

ing epidermis (Fig. 2-14). Mitotic figures are usually rare and nuclear variations are mild. The most striking feature is the presence of the characteristic cytoplasmic inclusions (Fig. 2-15) that may vary in diameter from 1.5 μm[80] to 10 μm.[81] These inclusions are eosinophilic and typically adjacent to the nucleus, which often appears indented and at times surrounded by a clear halo. The number of inclusions varies from case to case and area to area. Indeed, they may be difficult to find, or easily overlooked and confused with extravasated erythrocytes, particularly when the cells are seen in cross-section. Ultrastructurally the inclusions appear round and sharply demarcated, but not membrane-bound. They consist of closely packed electron-dense fine granular and fibrillar material. Whether this material represents abnormal contracted actin filaments[80] is controversial,[81] and the nature of the inclusions still remains obscure.

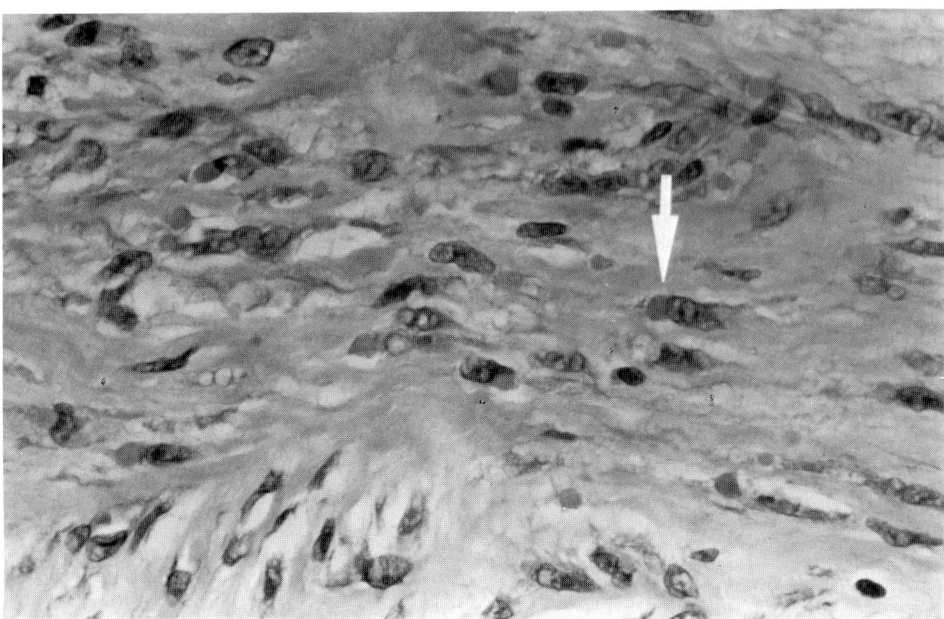

Fig. 2-15. High-power view of the tumor shown in Fig. 2-14. Note the fibroblasts with characteristic intracytoplasmic inclusions (arrow). (H&E, × 500.)

Differential Diagnosis. Because of its multicentric origin and tendency to recur, in the past this lesion was confused with malignant tumors such as neurofibrosarcoma[82] and low grade fibrosarcoma.[72, 83] Histologically it may be mistaken for other benign tumors and tumorlike lesions, namely fibroma, hamartoma, dermatofibroma, and even scar tissue. Infantile digital fibromatosis, however, may be distinguished from these tumors by its distinctive topography as it is almost exclusively limited to the distal extremities. Moreover, this lesion is primarily intradermal and composed of a coarsely woven network of fibroblasts with characteristic intracytoplasmic inclusions, with an absence of a storiform pattern and foam cells.

Prognosis. Although the overall local recurrence rate of these lesions is high, ranging from 60[77] to 75 percent,[49] aggressive clinical behavior or metastatic potential are absent.

Infantile Myofibromatosis: Solitary and Multicentric Types

Congenital generalized fibromatosis, a rare but distinct childhood form of fibromatosis, was first described by Stout[45] in 1954. Since that time, many additional examples have been reported under a number of different names, including congenital multiple fibromatosis, multiple congenital mesenchymal tumors, multiple congenital neoplasms, generalized hamartomatosis, multiple mesenchymal hamartomas, multiple vascular leiomyomas, diffuse congenital fibromatosis, and congenital fibrosarcoma.[84] The term *myofibromatosis* is preferred in view of its histologic resemblance to smooth muscle tissue and to distinguish it from the more locally aggressive infantile fibromatosis of the desmoid type.

These lesions clinically present two major types: solitary and multicentric. In the series described by Chung and Enzinger,[84] 74 percent were solitary and 26 percent were multicentric, although an almost equal distribution of solitary and multicentric forms was more recently reported.[85] In more than half of the cases (54 percent), the lesion is noted at birth or soon thereafter, and in nearly 90 percent of the cases the tumor becomes apparent during the first 2 years of life. On rare occasions, adults may be affected as well.[84, 86] As with other fibrous tumors of infancy, the solitary form is more common in boys (69 percent), but the reverse is true for the multicentric type (63 percent in girls). Occasional cases of the multicentric type display a familial tendency.[84]

In the solitary type, the tumor chiefly affects the soft tissues of the head and neck region (36 percent), followed by the trunk (33 percent), and lower and upper extremities. In the multicentric type, about 30 percent show visceral involvement including the central nervous system, and in 50 percent of these cases, bones are also involved.

The usual presenting symptom is the occurrence of rubbery firm to hard palpable nodules or masses. Superficially located nodules may be freely movable, but those deeply seated appear fixed. When the skin is involved, the lesions sometimes manifest as purplish macules, giving an impression of hemangioma. In about two-thirds of the solitary forms, skeletal muscle is involved. Radiologically, extraosseous lesions may present as soft tissue masses with foci of calcification. When bones are affected, they appear as radiolucent lytic or cystic lesions, at times with sclerotic margins and usually without apparent penetration of the cortex.

Grossly the tumor nodules are usually discrete, well-circumscribed and sometimes "encapsulated," unlike other types of fibromatosis, which are generally ill defined and often "infiltrative." On the average, they measure 2.5 cm in their greatest diameter.

Histologically a zoning phenomenon is usually observed, particularly in large lesions. At the periphery, the tumor consists of an admixture of fibroblastlike spindle cells and plump fusiform cells resembling smooth muscle fibers in different stages of maturation, arranged in short fascicles or bundles that often give a whorled or nodular appearance (Figs. 2-16 and 2-17).

Tumor cells have the staining characteristics of both myoblastic and fibroblastic lesions; namely, they possess occasional PTAH-positive and fuchsinophilic longitudinal fibrils (Fig. 2-18), but at the same time most of these cells are intimately associated with considerable amounts of reticulin or collagen. Unlike true myogenic tumors, however, intracellular glyco-

gen is virtually absent on PAS preparations. Immunocytochemically, the presence of immunoreactive actin, desmin, and vimentin has been reported.[87] Ultrastructurally the tumors are shown to consist of a mixture of fibroblasts and cells having the characteristics of both fibroblasts and smooth muscle fibers (myofibroblasts).[88, 89]

Less differentiated round or polygonal cells, arranged in solid sheets and usually accompanied by a prominent hemangiopericytomalike vascular pattern, are often more centrally located and blend in with the peripheral spindle cell areas. In many cases, the central area of the tumor undergoes coagulative necrosis, but it often still conserves its pericytomalike features. At times the junctional zone is focally calcified and shows deposits of hemosiderin pigment and scattered mononuclear cells and siderophages.

The number of mitotic figures ranges from 0 to 8 per 10 high-power fields, mostly within the central portion of the lesion. In some cases, papillary or polypoid ingrowths of tumor tissue into vascular spaces are observed that give the impression of vascular invasion. Despite the slight cellular pleomorphism, some mitotic figures, and intravascular extension of the growth, there is no evidence that these tumors behave differently from those without these features.[84] Bony and visceral lesions differ little from those affecting soft parts; however, they generally appear less differentiated.

Differential Diagnosis. Solitary forms of infantile myofibromatosis may be mistaken for other types of fibromatosis and nodular fasciitis. In the former, the tumors tend to be less well circumscribed and lack the zoning phenomenon and myofibroblastic characteristics. Likewise, nodular fasciitis can be distinguished from myofibromatosis by its typical location in the fascia or the fibrous septa of the subcutaneous fat, together with pictures of interstitial hemorrhage, myxoid areas, and mononuclear cell infiltrates. Furthermore, these lesions do not show a pericytomalike pattern.

The immature appearance, the high cellularity, and sometimes the increased number of mitotic figures may lead one to interpret this tumor as a sarcoma. Although it may display a pericy-

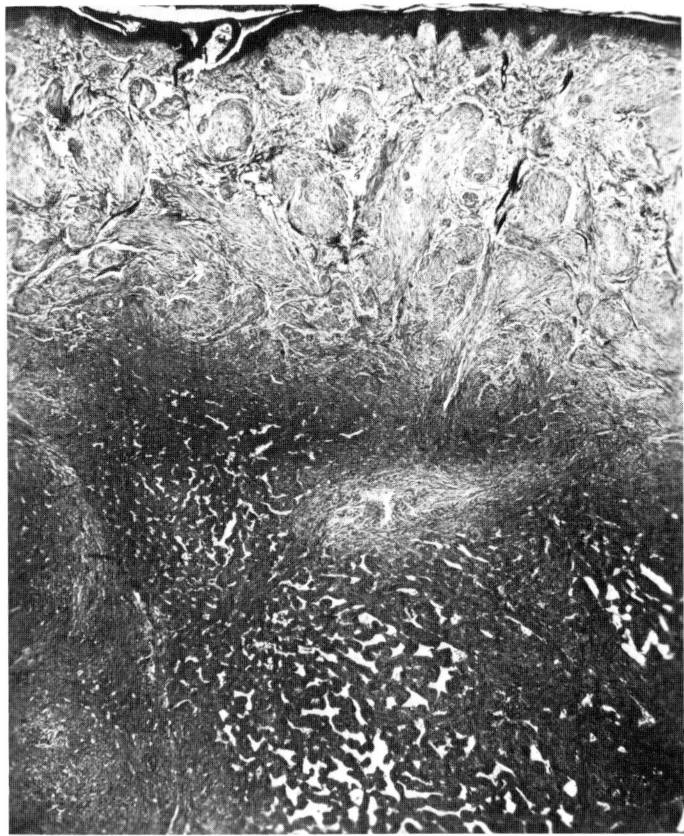

Fig. 2-16. Infantile myofibromatosis showing a zoning phenomenon. Note the peripheral whorls of fusiform cells resembling smooth muscle fibers surrounding a hemangiopericytoma-like area below. (H&E, × 25.)

tomalike pattern, infantile fibrosarcoma differs in its greater cellularity, high mitotic activity, and cellular atypia.[90] Moreover, it has a rather homogeneous cell growth pattern devoid of leiomyomalike areas.

When this lesion manifests with multiple nodules at birth or soon thereafter, it may be confused with other multicentric disease processes, such as neurofibromatosis and juvenile hyaline fibromatosis. In general, neurofibromatosis affects older children and there is a history of familial involvement as well as café-au-lait spots on the skin. Similarly, juvenile hyaline fibromatosis is a very rare hereditary condition. In cellular areas, the tumor cells may be arranged in columns or streaks that are separated by characteristic hyaline amorphous eosinophilic material.[91] Moreover, they do not reveal whorls or a fascicular arrangement of cells resembling smooth muscle fibers or pericytomalike features.

Prognosis. A solitary tumor limited to muscle and the subcutis has an excellent prognosis; however, recurrence rates from 9 to 11 percent have been reported.[91,85] In the case of a multicentric lesion, spontaneous regression may occur in nearly half of the patients unless the visceral organs are involved. The prognosis is less favorable in infants with multiple visceral lesions, and in many of these cases death usually occurs from cardiopulmonary or gastrointestinal problems.

Infantile Fibromatosis

Of all the forms of juvenile fibromatoses, infantile fibromatosis is the most controversial and most difficult to delineate with precision.[57] Infantile fibromatosis displays a considerable histomorphologic variation that ranges from immature mesenchymal lesions, more commonly

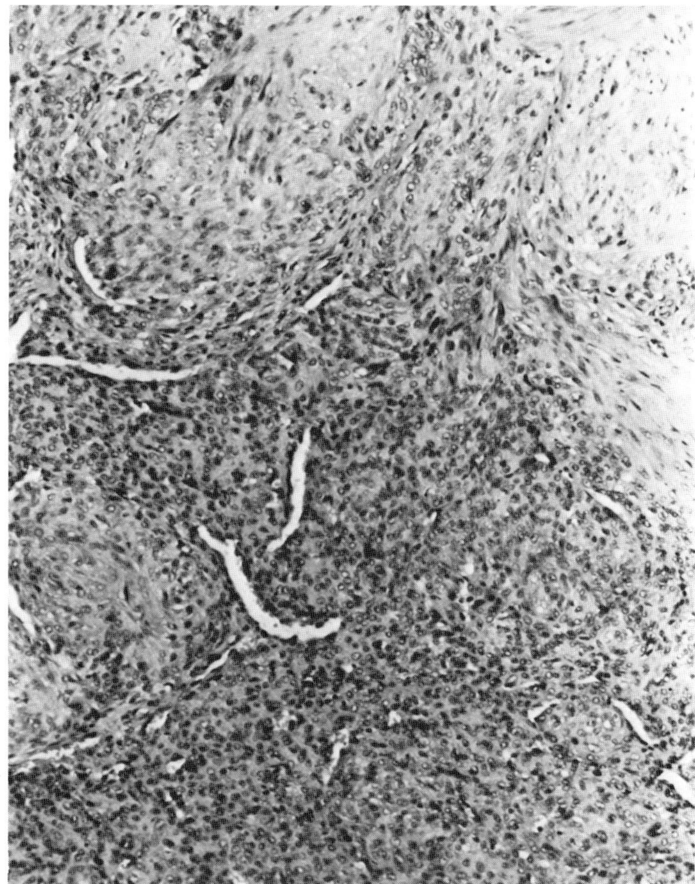

Fig. 2-17. Infantile myofibromatosis displaying a peripheral solid area with whorls or fascicles of smooth musclelike cells, and a more vascular and less differentiated area in the center. (H&E, × 125.)

observed in the first months of life, to mature lesions which occur in older children and closely resemble adult musculoaponeurotic fibromatosis (desmoid tumor). The tumor is relatively uncommon and usually manifests with a painless asymptomatic mass. In the majority of cases, medical advice is sought because recent rapid growth is noted. In 20 to 37 percent of the patients, the lesion is present at birth[49, 92] and occasionally associated with other congenital abnormalities.[92] The tumor originates most commonly in skeletal muscle, at times in the adjoining fascia or aponeurosis, and occasionally in the periosteum. Head and neck, shoulder, arm, and thigh are the common sites of involvement, while bones are rarely involved.[92, 93]

With the exception of lesions occurring in very young children, the microscopic features of infantile fibromatosis roughly parallel those of its adult counterpart (Fig. 2-19). The tumor is composed of mature looking spindle-shaped fibroblasts arranged in fascicles or bundles and embedded in variable amounts of collagen fibers that infiltrate the surrounding tissues (Fig. 2-20). More cellular areas, as well as occasional mitotic figures (up to 1 per 10 high-power fields), may be observed at the periphery of the lesion. Occasionally, areas of ossification are found.[94] More immature proliferations are referred to as "diffuse type" of infantile fibromatosis. These bland-looking lesions are composed of round to oval immature fibroblasts, often associated with considerable amounts of acid mucopolysaccharides, a sprinkling of mononuclear cells, including mast cells, and importantly stromal fatty infiltration (Fig. 2-21).

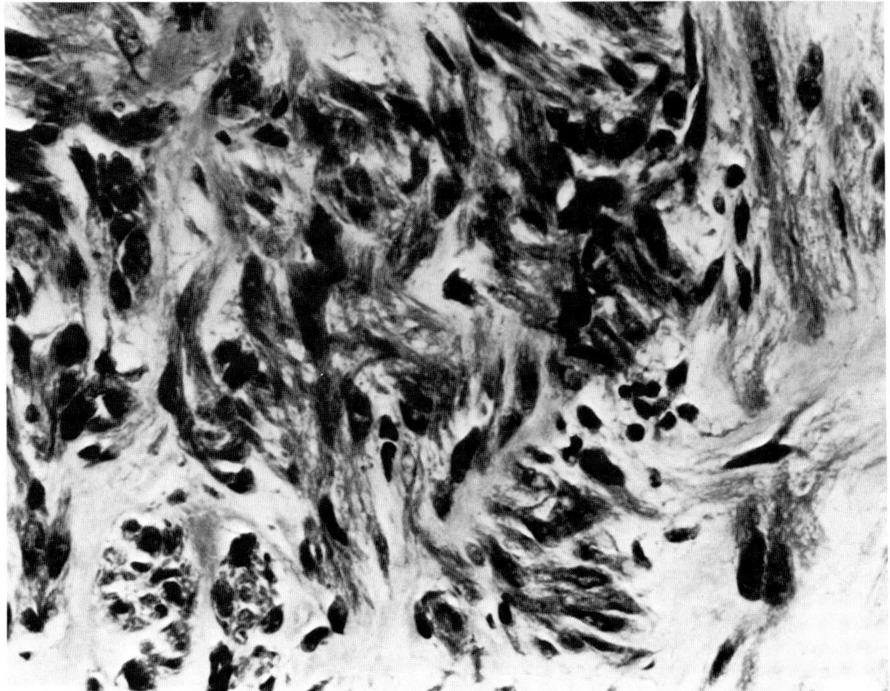

Fig. 2-18. Infantile myofibromatosis. Note the longitudinal fibrils resembling those of smooth muscle fibers. (Masson trichrome, × 500.)

Differential Diagnosis. Due to the large amount of mucopolysaccharides in its stroma, together with immature-appearing adipose tissue replacing the muscle, the immature or diffuse form of infantile fibromatosis may be confused with myxoid or lipomatous tumors. Lipoblastomatosis may be distinguished by the lobular arrangement of the adipose tissue and the orderly appearance of the fibrous septa. Myxoid liposarcomas are extremely rare in children under 5 years of age. Moreover, unlike these two entities, unequivocal lipoblasts are not found.

A more difficult and challenging problem, however, is the separation of the more cellular variants of infantile fibromatosis from infantile fibrosarcoma. Terms used in the past, such as aggressive fibromatosis,[73] differentiated fibrosarcoma,[57] and fibrosarcoma grade I desmoid type,[95] stress the difficulty of the diagnosis. In general, the higher mitotic rate, minor collagen production, and destructive growth reflected by the absence of entrapped fat or muscle fibers favor the diagnosis of infantile fibrosarcoma over infantile fibromatosis.

Prognosis. Although infantile fibromatoses are relatively well circumscribed, they do infiltrate surrounding tissues. Complete resection of the tumor with adequate margins is therefore the treatment of choice. Preoperative chemotherapy has been also successfully employed for unresectable head and neck tumors.[92] Despite wide local resections, recurrences are frequently observed; 14 of 25 patients reported by Ayala and colleagues[92] developed from 1 to 7 recurrences. Neither the anatomic site nor the histomorphologic pattern of the tumor appears to allow an accurate prediction of the clinical course.

Calcifying Aponeurotic Fibroma

Calcifying aponeurotic fibroma, a distinct tumor among juvenile fibromatoses, was first de-

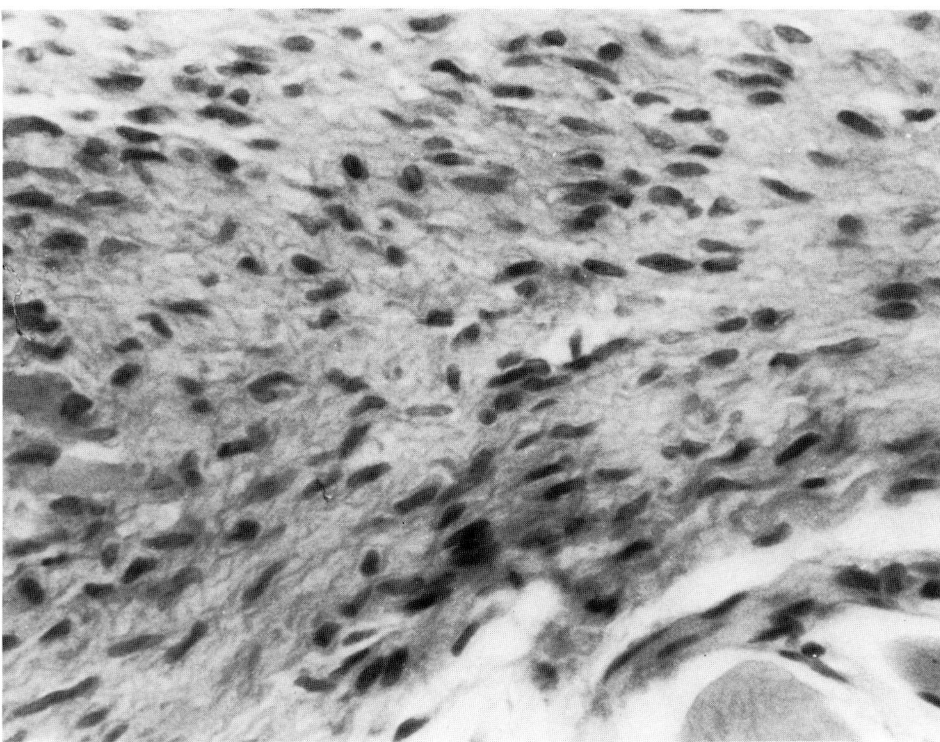

Fig. 2-19. Less cellular variant of infantile fibromatosis mimicking an adult musculoaponeurotic fibromatosis. The tumor was removed from the foot of a 3-month-old boy. (H&E, × 500.)

scribed by Keasbey[96] in 1953 as juvenile apo-neurotic fibroma. Because of its unique histologic features represented by the emergence of focal chondroid differentiation, some workers consider it to be a cartilage analogue of fibromatosis.[97, 98]

The lesion manifests clinically as a slow-growing painless mass in the hands or feet of several months or sometimes years duration. The tumor may affect any age from birth to adulthood. Although cases as old as 64 years have been reported in the literature,[98] the tumor is more frequent in children and adolescents.

The lesions occur most commonly in the hands (64 to 76 percent)[57, 99]; the majority involve the palms and frequently the thenar or hypothenar eminence and fingers. The foot is much less frequently affected. Lesions have also been found elsewhere in the forearm, elbow, thigh, popliteal fossa,[99] supraclavicular regions, and paravertebral fascia of the lumbar region.[100]

Radiographic examination reveals a faint soft tissue mass with characteristic finely stippled calcification.

The histologic appearance of the tumor varies little from case to case and is characterized by a diffuse, often ramifying, type of proliferation of spindle cells with plump, round, or oval-shaped nuclei, and ill-defined cytoplasm embedded in a highly collagenized stroma (Figs. 2-22 and 2-23). In some areas, these cells tend to line up with their nuclei parallel to one another in a palisading fashion, whereas in others, they grow haphazardly or tend to form intersecting fascicles in a vague storiform pattern.[99] Occasionally they may even display a herringbone pattern. Despite the focal cellularity of the lesion, mitotic figures are scarce. Focal calcification is invariably found; however, it varies in density and may even be altogether absent in the initial biopsy, particularly in infants and small children. The calcified areas are often

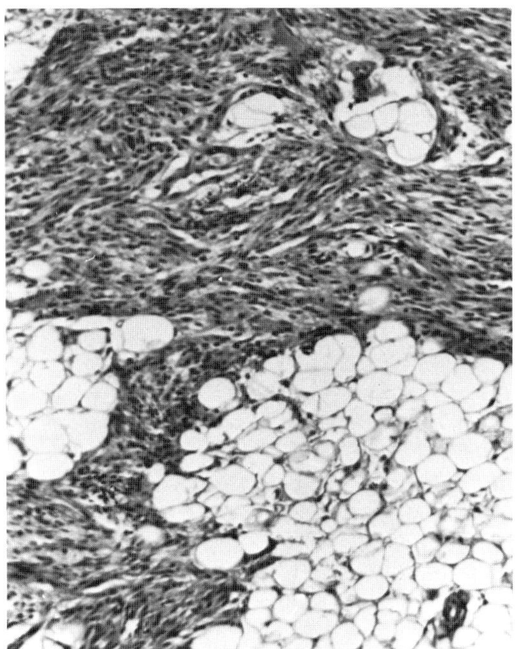

Fig. 2-20. Infantile fibromatosis revealing more mature-appearing spindle cells with collagen production. Note the superficial resemblance to fibrous hamartoma of infancy (H&E, × 500.)

surrounded by compact, well-marked columns of round cells bearing a close resemblance to chondrocytes (Fig. 2-23). Occasionally binucleated forms and multinucleated giant cells of the osteoclastic type may also be present within the compact cellular rim along the calcified areas. Ossification is rarely found. In general, calcification as well as chondroid differentiation is much more pronounced in lesions of older children and adults.[78]

Differential Diagnosis. In infants and small children, when there is still little or no calcification, the distinction from infantile fibromatosis and fibrous hamartoma of infancy may pose problems.[99] However, their association with a dense, hyalinized collagen and the characteristic anatomic location of the calcifying aponeurotic fibroma in the fingers or palm of the hand often lead to a correct diagnosis.

In older children, palmar and plantar fibromatosis may cause some problems, although these lesions are rare in patients under 20 years of age.[99] They can be distinguished by their nodular growth pattern, more abundant collagen pro-

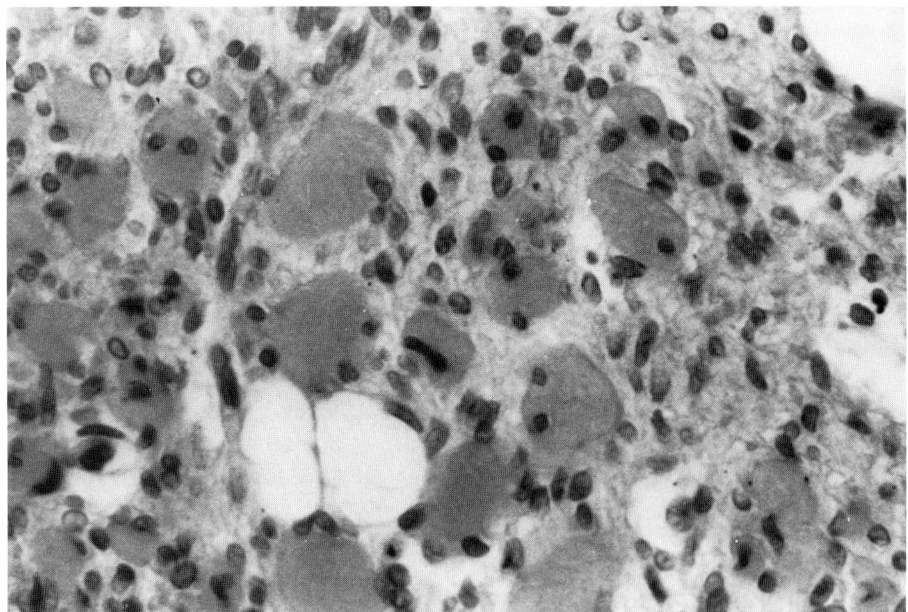

Fig. 2-21. Diffuse variant of infantile fibromatosis showing separation of striated muscle fibers by primitive fibroblasts, accompanied by a sprinkling of mononuclear cells and stromal fatty infiltration. (H&E, × 500.)

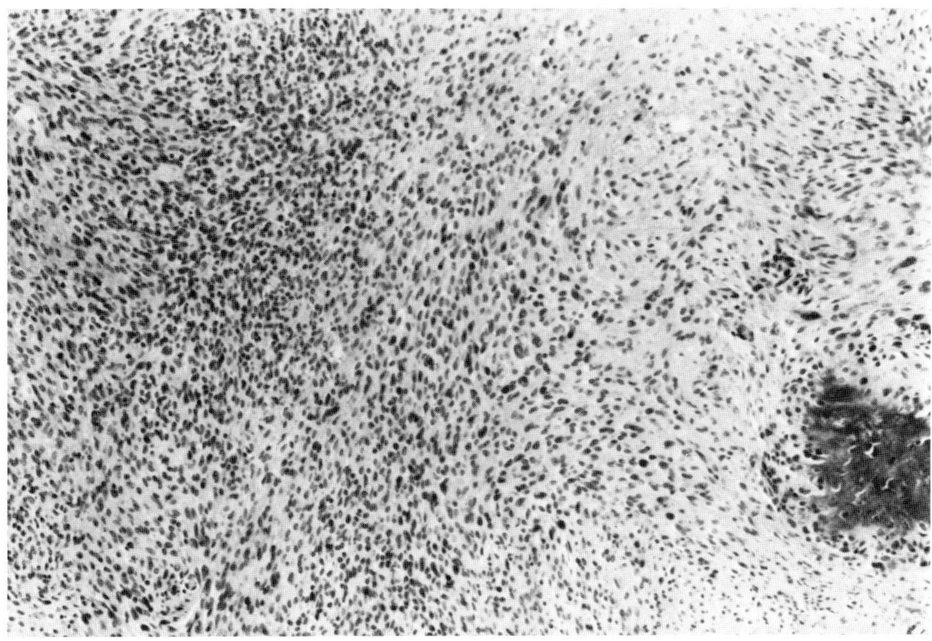

Fig. 2-22. Calcifying aponeurotic fibroma exhibiting diffuse proliferation of plump fibroblasts with focal calcification. (H&E, × 125.)

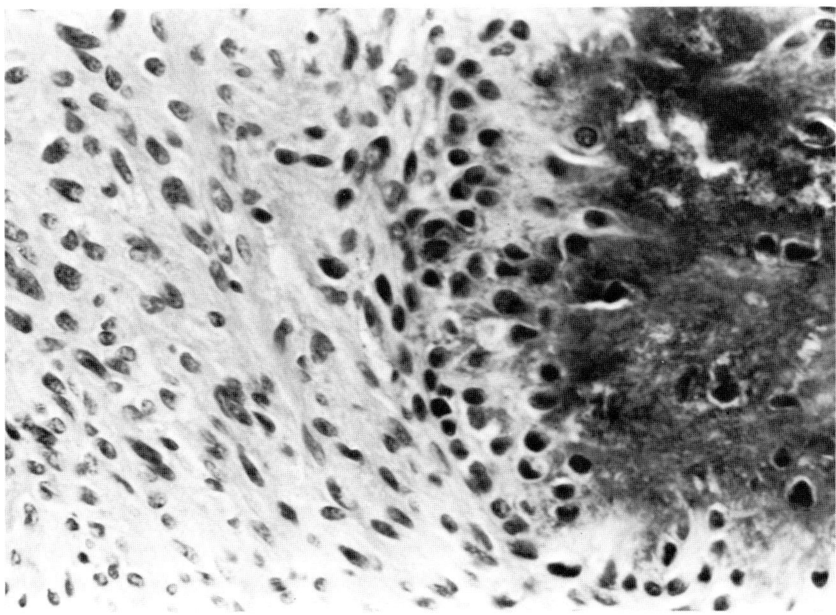

Fig. 2-23. Calcifying aponeurotic fibroma showing cartilaginous metaplasia within an area of calcification. (H&E, × 500.)

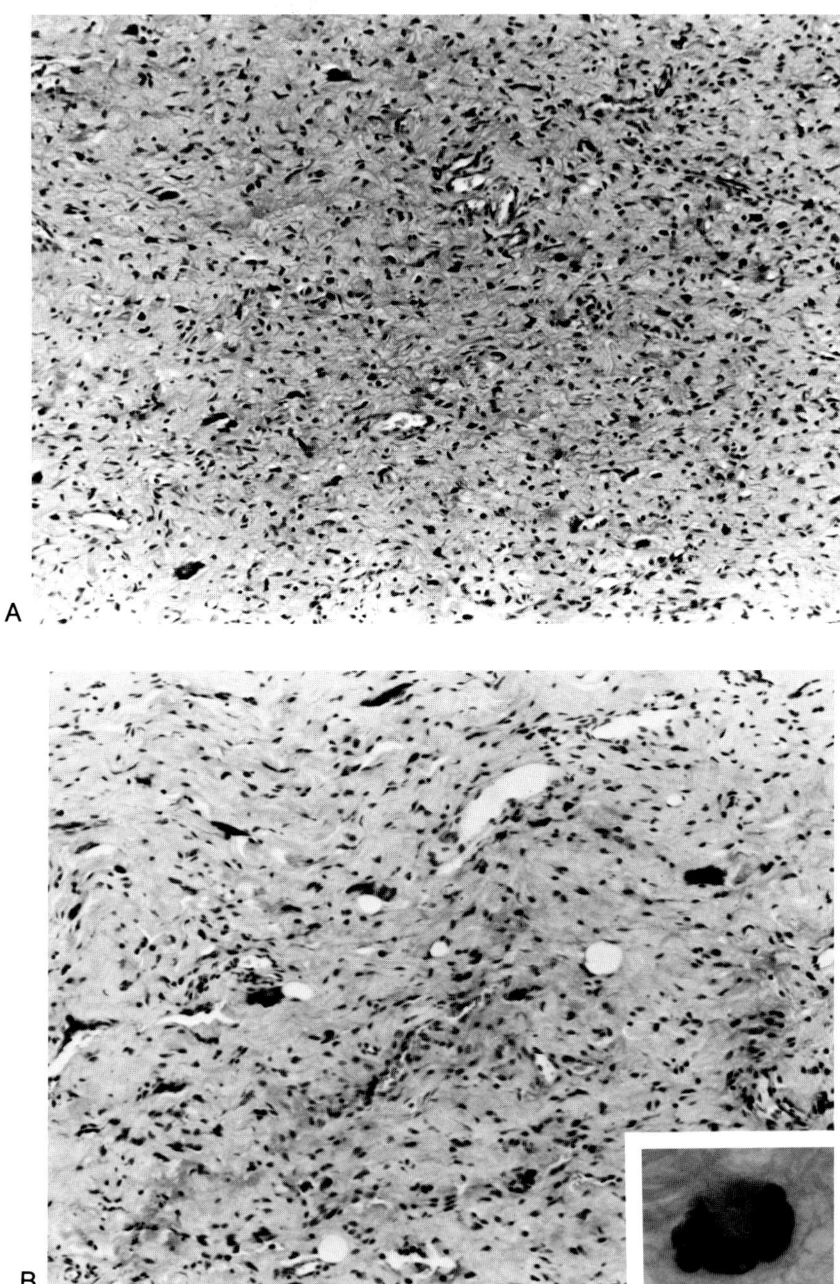

Fig. 2-24. Giant cell fibroblastoma. **(A)** Loosely arranged spindle cells and multinucleated giant cells associated with myxoid stroma. **(B)** A more collagenized area containing clefts or sinusoidal spaces, often lined by pleomorphic cells. (H&E, × 125.) Floretlike cell in inset. (× 500.)

duction, and the absence of calcification or chondroid metaplasia. Similarly, because of the common anatomic location involved, a clear distinction from soft tissue chondromas may be difficult in some cases. However, these are most commonly found in the fingers of patients older than 25 years, well demarcated and lobulated, and composed chiefly of cartilage lacking of areas of fibromatosis.[101] Finally, because of their cellularity with some mitotic figures, infiltrative growth pattern, and propensity to recur after excision, calcifying aponeurotic fibromas have been mistaken for fibrosarcoma.[96, 99]

Prognosis. At least 50 percent of the cases of calcifying aponeurotic fibroma recur. The rate of recurrence is particularly high in children under 5 years of age.[49] With advancing age of the patient the tumor seems to become quiescent or regress spontaneously.[100] Adequate local excision is the recommended treatment. Because the ultimate prognosis is excellent, further surgery to remove residual or recurrent tumor may be unnecessary other than to relieve symptoms.[49, 78]

Giant Cell Fibroblastoma

Giant cell fibroblastoma, a rare distinctive fibrous tumor of childhood, was first described in 1982 by Shmookler and Enzinger,[102] who suggested that the lesion could represent a juvenile variant of dermatofibrosarcoma protuberans. Since then, isolated reports in the literature have brought the total number of documented cases to 38.[23, 103–106] The histogenesis of this tumor is still obscure and fibroblastic,[102] fibrohistiocytic,[104] and vascular[105] origins have been alternatively advanced.

These lesions usually manifest as asymptomatic painless, non-mobile, slowly growing intradermal subcutaneous masses. Like other fibrous tumors of infancy and childhood, males outnumber females by a considerable margin. The patients ages may range from 4 months to 55 years[104]; the majority of patients are younger than 5 years and nearly 90 percent of the tumors are discovered within the first decade.

There appears to be a slight predilection for the back and thigh. Less commonly, the inguinal region, anterior chest, forearm, and abdominal walls are involved.

Microscopically these tumors are composed of loosely arranged spindle cells and associated with a prominent myxoid stroma (Fig. 2-24A) or a heavily collagenized fibrous tissue. The tumors contain clefts, cystic or sinusoidal spaces (Fig. 2-24B), and lobules of fat that may appear atrophic (Fig. 2-25). These clefts and cystic or sinusoidal spaces often appear to be lined by plemorphic spindle cells and multinucleated giant cells having a "floretlike" arrangement of hyperchromatic nuclei immersed in an eosinophilic cytoplasm (Fig. 2-25). However, these lining cells stain negatively for factor VIII-related antigen.[103, 104] In the recurrent lesions, the giant cells may be scarce, and often there is a sprinkling of eosinophils. In the more cellular areas, the tumor may bear a superficial resemblance to myxoid dermatofibrosarcoma protuberans. Under the electron microscope, the fibroblastic nature of both the mononuclear and multinucleated cells is supported by the presence of numerous profiles of rough endoplasmic reticulum and a well developed Golgi apparatus.[103, 104, 106]

Differential Diagnosis. Because of the disturbing cellular pleomorphism, many of these cases have been confused with various types of malignant mesenchymal tumors.[102] Myxoid liposarcoma is readily distinguished by its superficial location, the lack of the characteristic capillary pattern, the absence of lipoblasts, and the young age of the patient. The floret giant cells may sometimes lead to the erroneous impression of the sclerosing phase of pleomorphic lipoma, which typically occurs in the shoulder or neck regions of male patients older than 45 years. The bland appearance of the giant cells, the patient's age, and the absence of a distinct vascular network will permit separation from a myxoid malignant fibrous histiocytoma.

Prognosis. Despite the cellular pleomorphism, these lesions pursue a benign clinical course. In the reported series, about 50 percent of the tumors recurred locally. These recur-

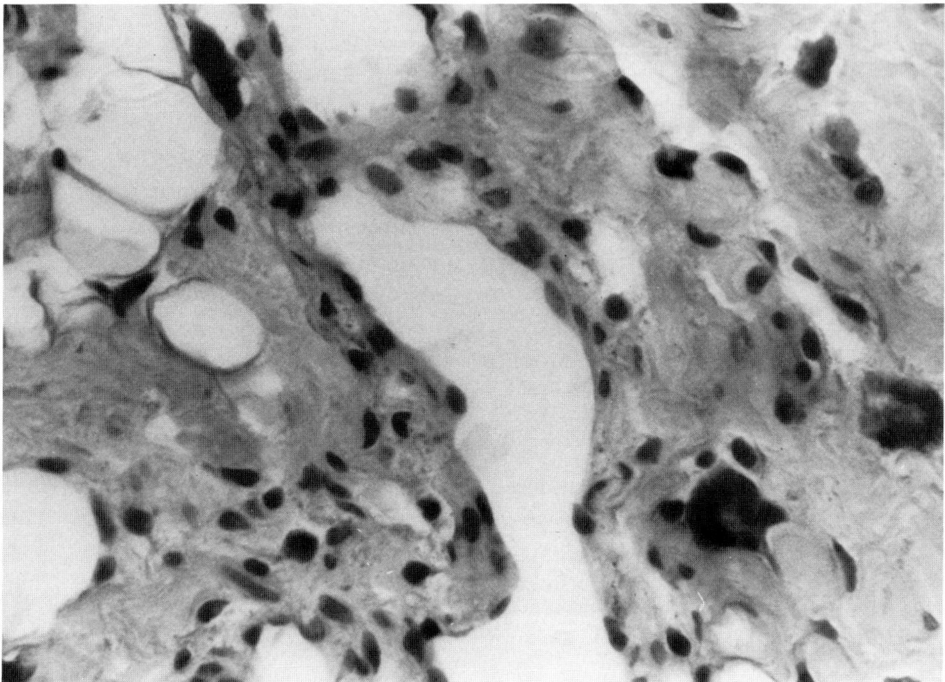

Fig. 2-25. Giant cell fibroblastoma demonstrating floretlike giant cells associated with an entrapped lobule of adipose tissue, a feature reminiscent of pleomorphic lipoma. (H&E, × 500.)

rences, however, appear related to involvement of the surgical margins since they were effectively treated by re-excision.[102, 103, 105]

FIBROSARCOMA

Before elctron microscopy and immunohistochemistry became routine tools in diagnostic pathology, fibrosarcoma was certainly overdiagnosed. Nonetheless, the differential diagnosis of the various "spindle cell tumors" still remains a difficult and challenging task. The major difficulty in diagnosing fibrosarcoma is the identification of the spindle cells as fibroblasts and the recognition of the tumor as sarcoma. Therefore, fibrosarcoma is conveniently defined as a malignant tumor of fibroblasts showing no evidence of other line of differentiation.[107] Because of their markedly different clinical behavior, fibrosarcomas in adults and those occurring in infancy and childhood are discussed separately.

Adult-type Fibrosarcoma

For many years, fibrosarcoma (adult-type) was considered the most commonly occurring somatic soft tissue sarcoma, however, thanks to the recent advances in the diagnosis and classification of "spindle cell tumors," fibrosarcomas currently comprise less than 12 percent of all sarcomas.[108]

Fibrosarcoma may occur anywhere in the body, but its most frequent location is the fascia between the muscles of the extremities, particularly the thigh. The trunk, subcutaneous tissue, periosteum, and the retroperitoneum are often involved, whereas fibrosarcoma in the head and neck region is uncommon. Fibrosarcoma is mostly encountered between the ages of 30 and 50, with a median age at diagnosis of 39.4[109] to 47.7 years.[108] Although most studies indicate a slightly higher incidence in women,[109] some have reported a predilection for the male sex.[108, 110]

Fibrosarcomas that arise in scar tissues (cica-

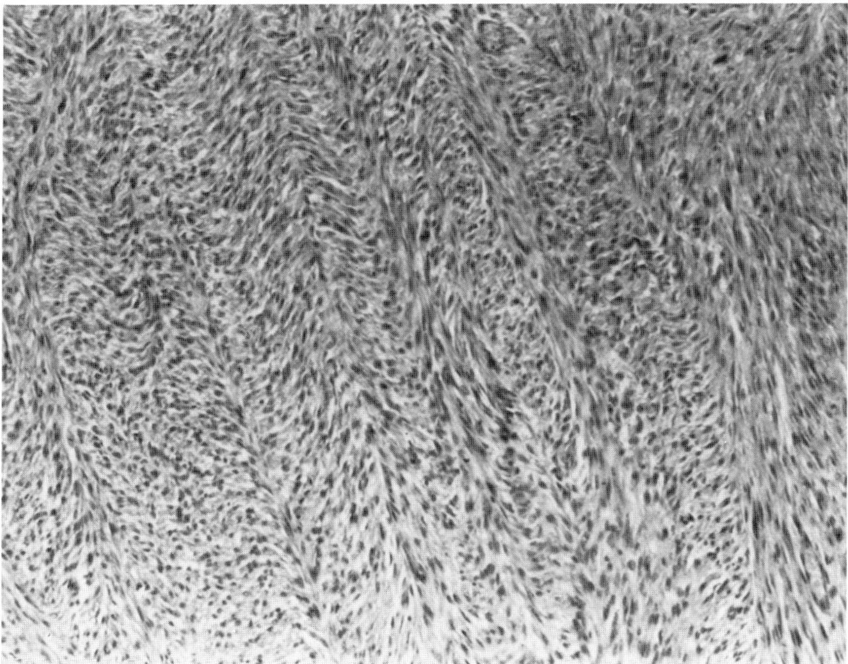

Fig. 2-26. Adult-type fibrosarcoma displaying great uniformity of neoplastic fibroblasts and the characteristic "herringbone" pattern. (H&E, × 125.)

tricial fibrosarcoma)[111] or develop at the sites of thermal[109, 112] and radiation injuries[113, 114] have been documented. Unlike the "spontaneous" fibrosarcomas, these tumors are usually found in the subcutis.

Depending on the cellular maturity and the amount of collagen produced by the tumor cells, the histologic picture may vary considerably. Fibrosarcomas typically consist of interlacing fascicles of fusiform or spindle-shaped cells wrapped by reticulin fibers, often forming a characteristic "herringbone" pattern (Fig. 2-26). In some cases, the neoplastic cells are separated by thick, wirelike collagen fibers. In others, the cells have a more rounded appearance, but are associated with dense hyalinized collagen. Foci of osseous or cartilaginous metaplasia may be observed. In poorly differentiated variants, the neoplastic cells are small, more ovoid or rounded, and less well-oriented. They produce only scant reticulin fibers and the fascicular pattern is often absent.

Although cells may show a moderate pleo-morphism (Fig. 2-27), multinucleated and/or mononucleated tumor giant cells are not a characteristic feature of this neoplasm. Mitotic activity varies, but mitotic figures are usually numerous in poorly differentiated variants. Areas of necrosis and hemorrhage are common in large tumors.

Differential Diagnosis. As already stated,[115] fibrosarcoma is not readily distinguished from other spindle cell tumors, such as malignant fibrous mesothelioma, monophasic fibrous type of synovial sarcoma, malignant schwannoma, leiomyosarcoma, and malignant fibrous histiocytoma, without immunohistochemical or ultrastructural studies. Similarly, fibrosarcoma in the head and neck region may be problematic since it mimics the cellular form of fibromatosis, desmoplastic or neurotropic malignant melanoma, or spindle cell carcinoma.

Benign processes that are likely to be mistaken for fibrosarcomas include nodular fasciitis, fibrous histiocytoma, and musculoaponeurotic fibromatosis. The differential diagnosis of

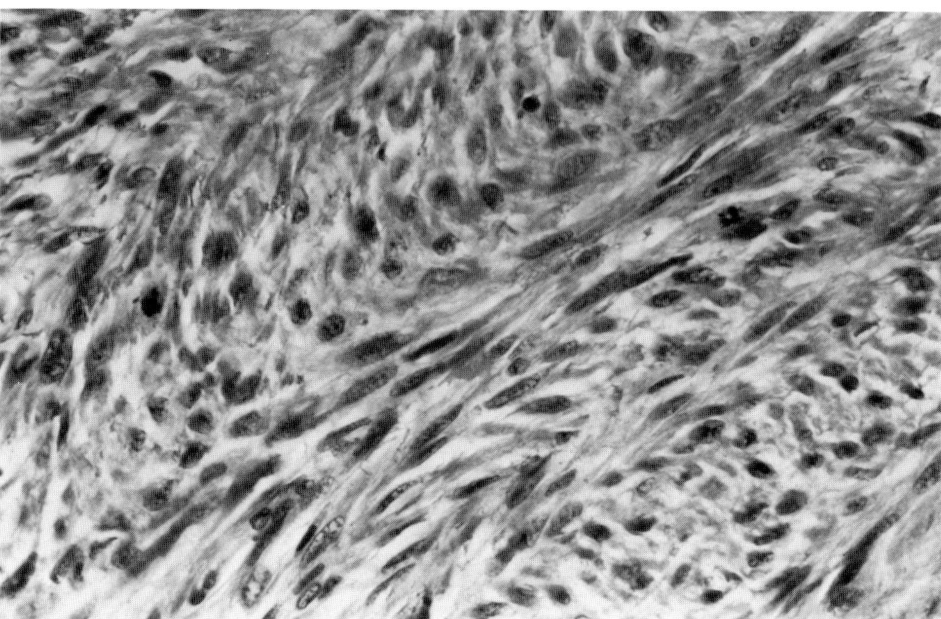

Fig. 2-27. Fibrosarcoma showing a more variable cellular pattern and frequent mitotic figures. (H&E, × 500.)

most of these tumors is discussed elsewhere in this chapter.

Prognosis. The reported survival and recurrence rates vary considerably. The 5-year survival rate ranges from 60 percent[108] to 70 percent,[110] while the 10-year rate is 57 percent[108] to 60 percent.[116] The reported recurrence rates span from 28 percent[73] to 48[116]–57 percent.[108]

If recurrence increases the risk of metastasis, the degree of differentiation is the most significant factor in determining the final outcome of patients. Distant tumor spread occurs exclusively by way of the blood stream, hence, the lung is the principal metastatic site, followed by vertebrae and skull. Lymph node metastasis is rare (up to 11 percent).[117]

Radical local excision together with en block regional node dissection[117] or a wide margin of normal tissue is generally considered to be the treatment of choice. When adequate margins cannot be obtained, amputation or excision followed by radiotherapy is necessary. In high-grade fibrosarcomas, adjunctive, systemic chemotherapy is indicated for frequent occurrence of subclinical or microscopic metastases.[118]

Congenital and Infantile Fibrosarcoma

Fibrosarcoma in newborns and infants, designated as congenital,[119] infantile, or juvenile fibrosarcoma,[120] displays histologic features similar to those occurring in adults, however, its clinical course is more favorable. Unlike the adult type of fibrosarcoma, neither the degree of cellularity and number of mitotic figures nor the extent of necrosis correlates well with the clinical behavior. Despite rapid growth and a high cellularity, most infantile fibrosarcomas are cured by wide local excision.[90]

The tumor usually presents as a nontender painless mass that may grow rapidly. In the majority of cases, the mass is discovered during the first year of life. According to the series of Chung and Enzinger,[90] the tumor was present at birth in about 38 percent of the cases, and 50 percent of the tumors were found during the first 3 months of life. The patients' ages ranged from newborn to 4 years, and males predominated slightly (1.5 : 1).

Unlike adult fibrosarcomas, which are most common in the thigh,[108] infantile fibrosarcomas

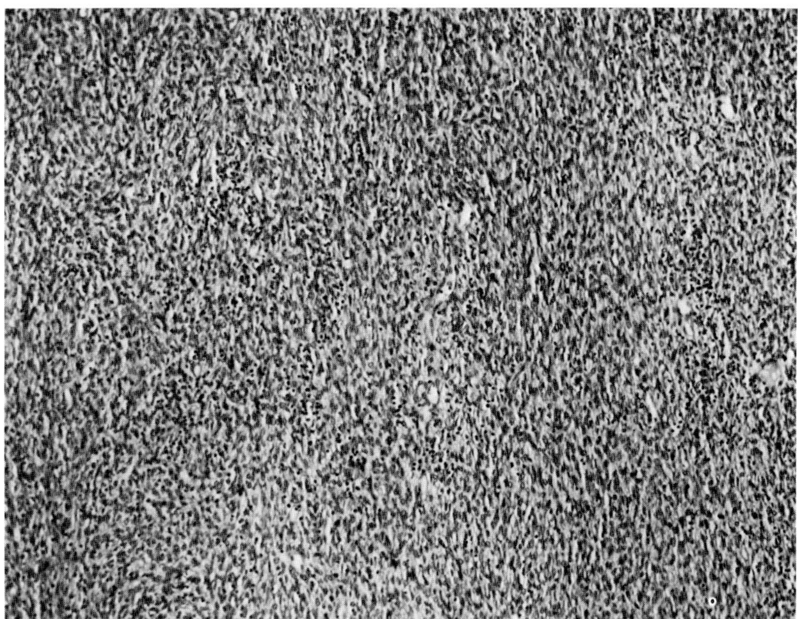

Fig. 2-28. Infantile fibrosarcoma of the right flank in a 4-week-old girl exhibiting poorly differentiated tumor cells and a sprinkling of lymphocytes. (H&E, × 125.)

affect chiefly the distal portions of the extremities, especially the ankle, foot, and lower leg, followed by the regions of the hand, wrist, and forearm.

Tumor size varies considerably from a few centimeters in diameter to extremely large tumors that may virtually replace the entire distal portion of the involved extremity. Radiologically a soft tissue mass may be associated with cortical thickening, bending deformities, and, rarely, destruction of underlying bone.

Microscopically the tumors consist of small round or spindle-shaped cells exhibiting variable amounts of collagen production. Tumors with a minimal amount of collagen are composed of small, round, immature-appearing cells (Figs. 2-28 and 2-29). Tumors with a greater amount of collagen, on the other hand, bear a close resemblance to adult-type fibrosarcoma (Fig. 2-30) and consist of uniform spindle-shaped cells with ill-defined cytoplasm and little nuclear pleomorphism.

Multinucleated giant cells are extremely rare. Mitotic figures are common, but their number varies from tumor to tumor and from area to area of the same neoplasm. Scattered mononuclear inflammatory cells, particularly lymphocytes, are a frequent and at times prominent feature that may help to distinguish the infantile from the adult-type fibrosarcoma. Not uncommonly, there are prominent cleftlike or cavernous vascular spaces accompanied by foci of endothelial proliferation and hemorrhage, which may mimic an angiosarcoma. Sometimes, the neoplastic cells are arranged about gaping endothelium-lined vascular spaces (Fig. 2-31) in a hemangiopericytomalike fashion.[90, 121]

Ultrastructurally fibroblasts in varying stages of differentiation were described,[122, 123] although the presence of a histiocytic component was also reported.[124]

Differential Diagnosis. The histomorphology of the infantile fibrosarcoma may be confused with that of other mesenchymal neoplasms, but its solid growth pattern, overall uniformity of the neoplastic cells with evidence of collagen production, and focal fascicular arrangement will permit a correct interpretation.

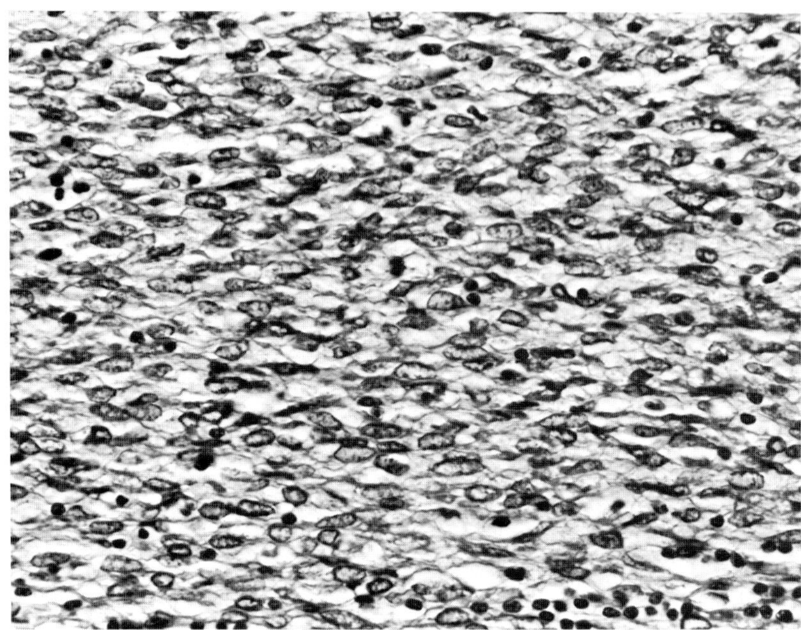

Fig. 2-29. High-power view of the tumor shown in Fig. 2-28. Note the immature-appearing fibroblasts associated with small round cells (lymphocytes). (H&E, × 500.)

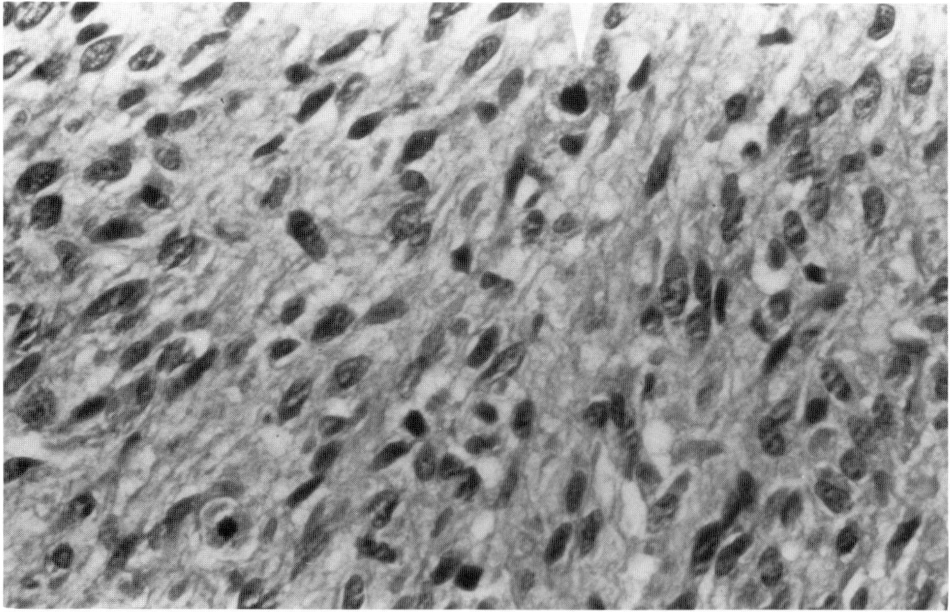

Fig. 2-30. Infantile fibrosarcoma revealing fascicular arrangement of more mature-appearing fibroblasts. Mitotic figures are readily found. (H&E, × 500.)

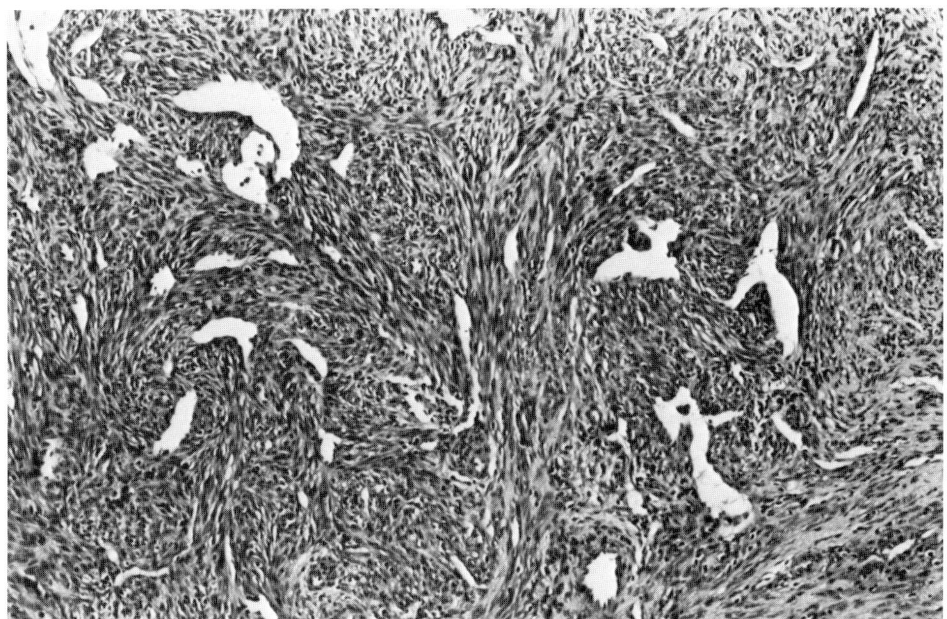

Fig. 2-31. Well-differentiated infantile fibrosarcoma with a hemangiopericytomalike pattern. (H&E, × 125.)

Likewise, the absence of rhabdomyoblasts and intracellular glycogen will help to distinguish it from embryonal rhabdomyosarcoma.

Infantile fibrosarcoma with a marked degree of vascularity may simulate an infantile hemangiopericytoma, but the latter is characterized by a distinct lobular arrangement and more regularly distributed dilated vascular spaces with a "staghorn" pattern. When a prominent inflammatory infiltrate is present, it may mimic inflammatory pseudotumor.[125] Unlike infantile fibrosarcoma, which occurs most commonly in the distal portions of extremities, inflammatory pseudotumors are mainly encountered in the abdomen, mediastinum, and visceral organs, and they may be associated with constitutional symptoms.

The cellular variant of infantile fibromatosis and fibrosarcoma may share a similar microscopic picture, and thus the differential diagnosis may be extremely difficult, although significant differences have been found between the two regarding the number of AgNORs.[126] Recent cytogenetic investigations did not reveal significant chromosomal aberrations in infantile fibrosarcoma[127, 128, 129] and the malignant properties of this tumor have been questioned.[129] Nevertheless, it appears preferable to include among infantile fibrosarcomas all fibroblastic tumors of infancy showing great cellularity and prominent mitotic activity.

Prognosis. Compared with adult-type fibrosarcoma, the clinical course of infantile fibrosarcoma is a more favorable one. Despite high local recurrence rates (43 percent), there is only about a 7.3 percent chance of developing metastatic spread.[130] The reported 5-year survival is 84 percent.[90]

The recurrent and nonrecurrent groups of tumors show no demonstrable differences concerning tumor site, age at onset, and size of tumor. Neither the degree of cellularity and number of mitotic figures nor the extent of hemorrhage or necrosis correlates well with the clinical behavior.

Despite rapid growth and high degree of cellularity, the majority of infantile fibrosarcomas are cured by wide local excision. Moreover, a

Table 2-2. Histologic Classification of Fibrohistiocytic Tumors[a]

Benign	Intermediate Malignancy	Malignant
Xanthoma	**Dermatofibrosarcoma protuberans**	**Atypical fibroxanthoma**
Juvenile xanthogranuloma	**Bednař tumor**	**Pleomorphic malignant fibrous histiocytoma (MFH)**
Reticulohistiocytoma		
Fibrous histiocytoma		**Myxoid MFH**
		Giant cell MFH
		Inflammatory MFH
		Angiomatoid MFH

[a] Boldface material denotes material discussed in text.

favorable response to preoperative chemotherapy and conservative surgery has recently been reported.[131]

FIBROHISTIOCYTIC TUMORS AND RELATED LESIONS

The term *fibrohistiocytic tumors* refers to a large group of lesions composed of a mixture of histiocytes and fibroblasts embedded in a variably collagenized stroma. This group encompasses both non-neoplastic lesions almost exclusively made up of a collection of foamy histiocytes, such as reactive xanthomatosis, and highly malignant tumors, such as malignant fibrous histiocytomas.

The histogenesis of these lesions is still under debate. Recent immunohistochemical and ultrastructural findings seem to confirm their origin from tissue histiocytes capable of behaving as "facultative fibroblasts," as originally proposed.[132, 133]

These tumors are commonly recognized as benign or malignant on the basis of their clinical course (Table 2-2). Dermatofibrosarcoma protuberans and its pigmented counterpart, the Bednař tumor, are listed separately under the heading, intermediate malignancy, although this term may be misleading, it generally refers to the locally infiltrative and destructive lesions characterized by a low metastatic potential.

In 1988 Enzinger and Zhang[134] reported 65 cases of a newly described entity, "plexiform fibrohistiocytic tumor" that bears some resemblance to both cutaneous fibrous histiocytoma and fibromatosis but differs from these lesions by its frequent occurrence in young individuals. Although the overall clinical outcome of these tumors was favorable, they recurred in one-third of the cases and in two of them metastasized to regional lymph nodes. Based on the histologic features, the authors were unable to predict the exact clinical behavior of the tumors.

Juvenile Xanthogranuloma (JXG)

The term *juvenile xanthogranuloma* was introduced in 1954 by Helwig and Hackney[135] to describe fibrohistiocytic lesions of infancy previously named "nevoxanthoendothelioma" by McDonagh in 1912.[136] This lesion shows a slight male predilection and may occur in all age groups; however, two frequency peaks are registered before the 4th year of life and in the 2nd and 3rd decade.[137, 138] The head and neck are the most commonly affected regions, followed by the trunk, and the upper and lower extremities. Visceral, palpebral, and intracranial involvement may also occur.[135, 139] Multiple lesions are found in about 20 percent of cases.[137, 138] JXG is never associated with lipid disorders.

Under the light microscope, JXG is a cellular lesion usually located in the dermis. The overlying epidermis and the cutaneous adnexa are generally spared. The tumor is composed of diffuse

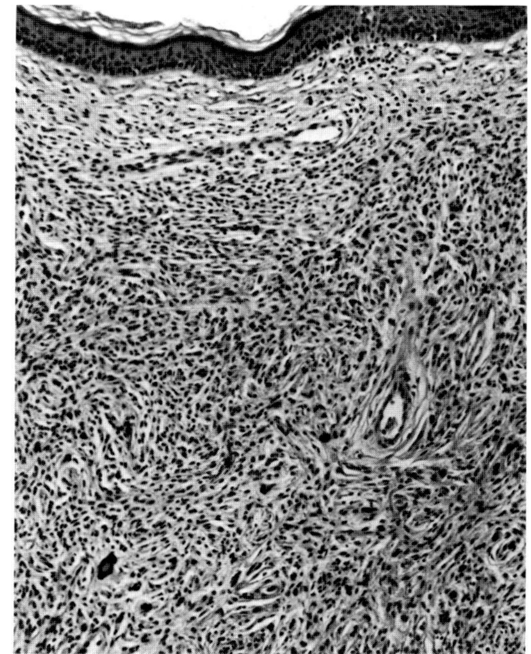

Fig. 2-32. Juvenile xanthogranuloma consisting of sheets of histiocytes accompanied by Touton giant cells. (H&E, × 125.)

sheets of polygonal histiocytic cells with an ill-defined, eosinophilic, and at times, finely vacuolated or foamy cytoplasm. A variable number of Touton giant cells, eosinophils, and other inflammatory cells are scattered throughout the tumor (Figs. 2-32 and 2-33). One to two mitotic figures per 10 high-power field may be observed.[138] Interstitial fibrosis may be seen at the periphery of the lesion.

The tumor cells show both the ultrastructural[140] and immunocytochemical (positivity to lysozyme, α_1-antichymotrypsin and α_1-antitrypsin[137]) characteristics of histiocytic cells. Recent evidences of reactivity to muscle-specific actin suggests a possible myofibroblastic line of differentiation for the tumor histiocytes.[12]

Differential Diagnosis. JXG that show a prevalence of xanthomatous cells may be confused for true xanthomas even though the latter are composed of a more uniform population of foamy histiocytes with a less prominent inflammatory background.

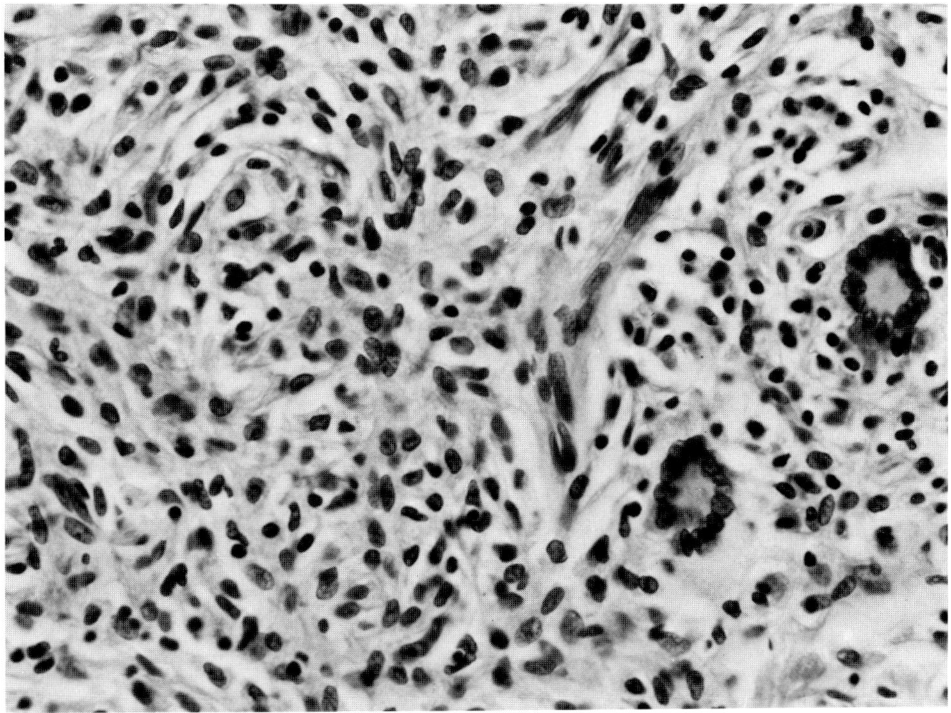

Fig. 2-33. Juvenile xanthogranuloma displaying various histiocytic cells admixed with mononuclear inflammatory cells and eosinophils. (H&E, × 500.)

When Touton-type giant cells are rare, the differential diagnosis will include the cutaneous forms of histiocytosis X. This diagnosis is favored by the involvement of the dermo–epidermal junction and the absence of typical Touton giant cells. However, in difficult cases, a confident diagnosis may be achieved by the unequivocal ultrastructural demonstration of Langerhans' granules in the tumor cells. Reactivity to S-100 protein is also considered a valuable tool in differentiating JFX from histiocytosis X. Mononuclear cells in JXG are in fact negative to S-100 protein.[137, 141] Although a scattered positivity to this antigen has been occasionally reported[138, 141] in JXG, it seems, however, mostly due to normal Langerhans' cells entrapped in the lesion.

Reticulohistiocytoma may also be considered in the differential diagnosis. Reticulohistiocytoma, a rare tumor of unknown etiology, occurs mainly in adults as a solitary nodule or as part of a systemic disease often associated with destructive arthritis.[142, 143] It is composed of atypical mono- or multinucleated histiocytic cells with large, eosinophilic "glassy" cytoplasms and neatly defined cellular borders. These atypical cells are absent in JXG.

Prognosis.   Simple surgical exicision is the treatment of choice, although in children multiple lesions are characterized by a high rate of spontaneous regression (83.3 percent).[137]

Fibrous Histiocytoma

Fibrous histiocytoma, the most common benign fibrous histiocytic proliferation, has been variously designated as *dermatofibroma*,[144] *histiocytoma cutis*,[11] *nodular subepidermal fibrosis*,[144] or *sclerosing hemangioma*[145] according to its different histologic features.

Fibrous histiocytoma is a painless solitary nodule slowly growing in the dermis or, more rarely, in deep soft tissues and visceral organs.[146] While it may occur anywhere on the body surface, the extremities are the most commonly involved region (Table 2-3). All age groups are affected, but it is more frequently diagnosed in the 3rd and 4th decades.[147]

The cutaneous lesions present as elevated

Table 2-3. Anatomic Sites of 342 Cases[a] of Fibrous Histiocytoma[b]

	N	%
Upper extremities	131	38.31
Upper girdle	26	7.60
Head and neck	28	8.18
Hands	14	4.09
Lower extremities	149	43.57
Lower girdle	16	4.67
Trunk	62	18.12

[a] Males: 175, Females: 167; M:F = 1.04; Mean age: 39 years.
[b] Observed at the Institute of Pathology, University of Padua, Padua, Italy.

nodules that at times appear black. In this case, the presence of the "dimple sign" may enable its distinction from malignant melanoma.[148]

Microscopically cutaneous fibrous histiocytoma is characterized by a poorly defined nodular proliferation of spindle cells, involving primarily the dermis and occasionally the subcutis. It consists of short fascicles of fibroblastic cells, which often display a vague storiform pattern (Fig. 2-34), accompanied by varying numbers of round histiocytic cells, siderophages, foam cells, and multinucleated foreign body or Touton-type giant cells. Native dermal collagen fibers are often entrapped within the tumor (Fig. 2-35).

Reticulin stains reveal a delicate network of reticulin fibers surrounding the individual cells. In long-standing lesions, the collagenous reaction frequently becomes exuberant and areas of desmoplasia and hyalinization may be prominent. The presence of vessels with thick, hyalinized walls and narrow lumen led to the use of the term "sclerosing hemangioma," presently abandoned. While cystic degeneration is rare, foci of extravasated red blood cells are common and may often give a brown pigmentation to the lesion.

The overlying epidermis often displays epithelial hyperplasia and hyperpigmentation. A zone of intact dermis ("free zone") is usually observed between the tumor and the overlying epidermis.[146]

Differences between superficial and deep fibrous histiocytomas are inconspicuous and in-

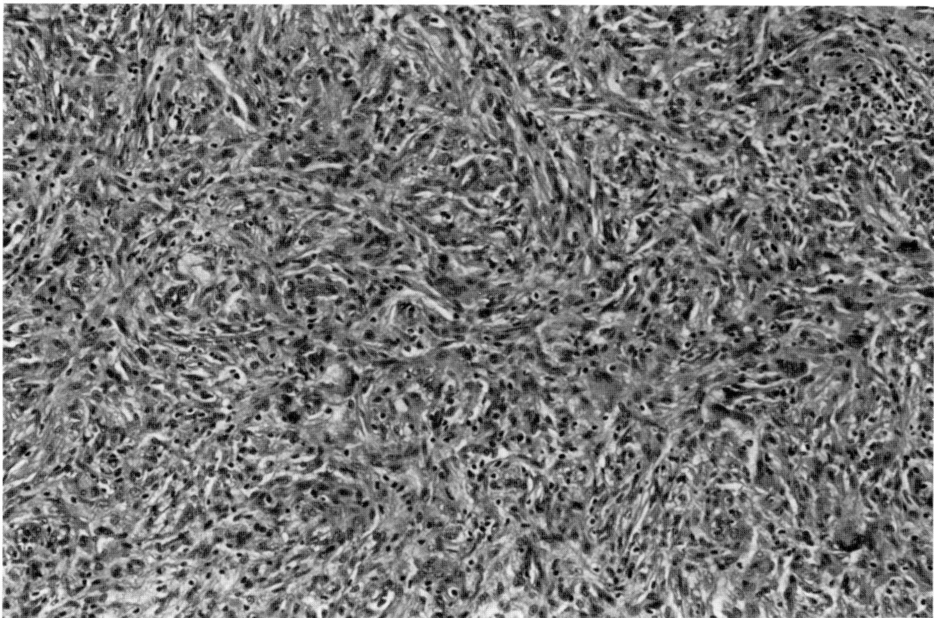

Fig. 2-34. Fibrous histiocytoma consisting of fibroblastic cells arranged in a vague storiform pattern accompanied by polygonal histiocytic cells, foam macrophages, multinucleated giant cells, and other chronic inflammatory cells. (H&E, × 125.)

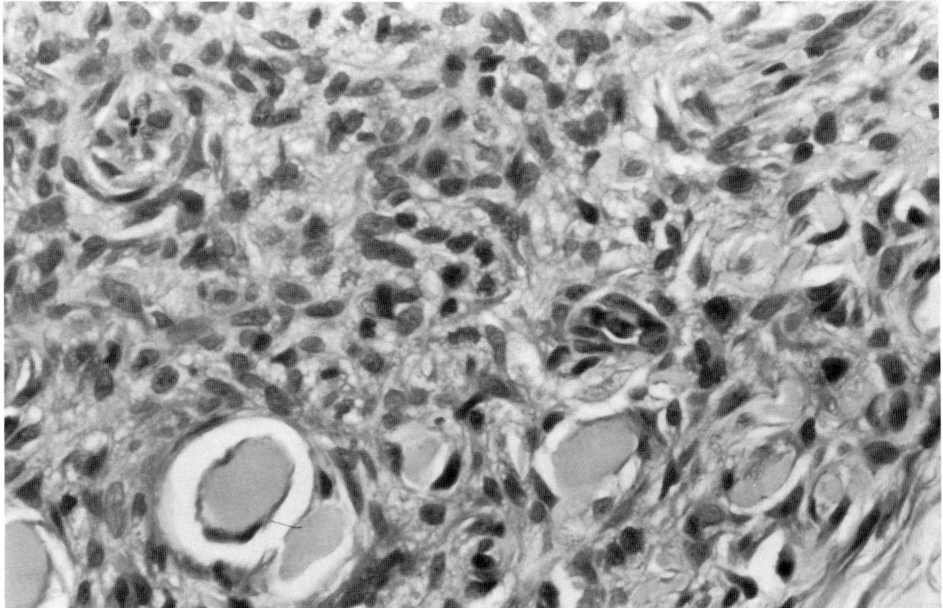

Fig. 2-35. Cutaneous fibrous histiocytoma showing ''entrapped'' dermal collagen fibers. (H&E, × 500.)

clude a more prominent fascicular or "storiform" pattern with more frequent myxoid and hyaline stromal changes in the latter.

Rarely there are prominent osteoclastlike giant cells mimicking a localized giant cell tumor of the tendon sheath. Occasionally the tumors display pleomorphic cells with hyperchromatic nuclei and eosinophilic cytoplasm; however, these are generally regarded as degenerative features.

Ultrastructural studies have shown a spectrum of cell types, namely cells resembling fibroblasts, myofibroblasts, and histiocytes. Intermediate tumor cells showing both fibroblastic and histiocytic differentiation have also been described.[149]

Differential Diagnosis. Fibrous histiocytomas are often confused with nodular fasciitis, particularly when a vague storiform pattern is observed. However, nodular fasciitis is typically composed of loosely arranged fascicles of feathery fibroblasts and myxoid areas containing extravasated erytrocytes and inflammatory cells. Curiously, siderophages are notably absent.

Fibrous histiocytomas occasionally may be mistaken for neurofibroma or leiomyoma. Neurofibroma, however, consists of bundles of comma-shaped spindle cells embedded in wavy, wiry collagen bundles that sometimes show foci of vague nuclear palisading. Although sclerotic forms of leiomyoma may superficially resemble fibrous histiocytoma, they are recognized by their fascicles or bundles of spindle cells with a plump eosinophilic cytoplasm and typical longitudinal myofibrils that are better demonstrated by phosphotungstic acid-hematoxylin (PTAH) or Masson trichrome stains. Hemangiopericytomalike areas may be found mainly at the periphery of deep fibrous histiocytoma. However, the differential diagnosis is usually forthcoming since true hemangiopericytoma is composed of uniform small cells with many "antler like" vessels and lacks a clear storiform pattern. Common blue nevus and desmoplastic melanoma may be mistaken for fibrous histiocytoma because of its location in the dermis, brown pigmentation, and dense connective tissue reaction.

Of course, fibrous histiocytoma must be distinguished from more aggressive forms of fibrohistiocytic neoplasms, such as the plexiform fibrohistiocytic tumor, dermatofibrosarcoma protuberans, and malignant fibrous histiocytoma. Unlike cutaneous fibrous histiocytoma, the plexiform fibrohistiocytic tumor is poorly demarcated and characterized histologically by a multinodular or plexiform proliferation of fibrohistiocytic cells associated with multinucleated giant cells and sometimes areas simulating a fibromatosis.

Dermatofibrosarcoma protuberans is characterized by a more uniform cellular proliferation and is composed of long fascicles of fibroblasts arranged in a distinct storiform pattern. Inflammatory cells, xanthoma cells, and multinucleated giant cells are generally absent. Moreover, unlike cutaneous fibrous histiocytoma, the overlying epidermis does not display hyperplastic changes. The distinction between fibrous histiocytomas and malignant fibrous histiocytoma is usually not difficult as the latter is a deeply situated tumor showing remarkable pleomorphism, areas of hemorrhage and necrosis, and prominent, often atypical, mitotic figures.

About 2 percent of fibrous histiocytomas may show considerable cellular atypia due to the presence of large foamy histiocytes with prominent nucleoli and bizarre multinucleated giant cells (atypical benign fibrous histiocytoma).[150–153] These features, nevertheless, occur only focally in an otherwise typical setting of fibrous histiocytoma and thus allow an easy distinction from superficial malignant fibrous histiocytomas (see also Atypical Fibroxanthoma).

Like other forms of malignant fibrous histiocytoma, angiomatoid MFH may be confused with fibrous histiocytoma due to its bland cytohistological appearance. Nevertheless it shows a greater degree of pleomorphism and mitotic activity and is composed of sheets of fibrohistiocytic cells separated by areas of hemorrhage and cystification and surrounded by nodular aggregates of lymphocytes and plasma cells.

Prognosis. Fibrous histiocytomas are benign tumors that are curable by local excision. The overall recurrence rate is approximately 5 percent.[154] The deeper the tumor, the greater the risk of recurrence, for these lesions tend to be larger and are less amenable to local excision.

FIBROHISTIOCYTIC TUMORS OF
INTERMEDIATE MALIGNANCY

Dematofibrosarcoma Protuberans

Dermatofibrosarcoma protuberans (DFSP) was described by Darier and Ferrand in 1924,[155] and was first called DFSP in 1925 by Hoffman.[156] However, DFSP may be a misleading term for this lesion because it is not a true sarcoma, nor is it exclusively localized in the dermis, and its histogenesis from fibroblasts or histiocytes is still under discussion. Nonetheless, as the term is unanimously recognized in the medical literature, it seems convenient to retain it.

DFSP may occur at any age, though it is most commonly found during early or mid-adult life. The mean age at diagnosis ranges from 27 to 40 years.[157, 158] Males are more commonly affected, with a predilection for the trunk and extremities,[158] but the scalp,[159] cosmetically sensitive areas of the head and neck,[160] upper aerodigestive tract,[161] and vulva[162] may also be involved.

DFSP usually presents as a firm slow-growing, long-standing plaque that eventually enters a phase of rapid multinodular growth. When fully developed, it manifests a typical "protuberant" appearance. In more than 50 percent of the patients, the overlying skin shows a red to blue discoloration.[157]

Grossly the lesion is deceptively circumscribed. Closer inspection reveals that it infiltrates the subcutaneous fat and occasionally the underlying muscle planes. Most lesions are firm, although some, especially if recurrent, may be soft and gelatinous.[163]

Histologically the tumor is characterized by a monotonous proliferation of uniform spindle cells arranged in a distinctive cartwheel or storiform pattern (Fig. 2-36). Little nuclear pleomorphism and a few inflammatory cells are ob-

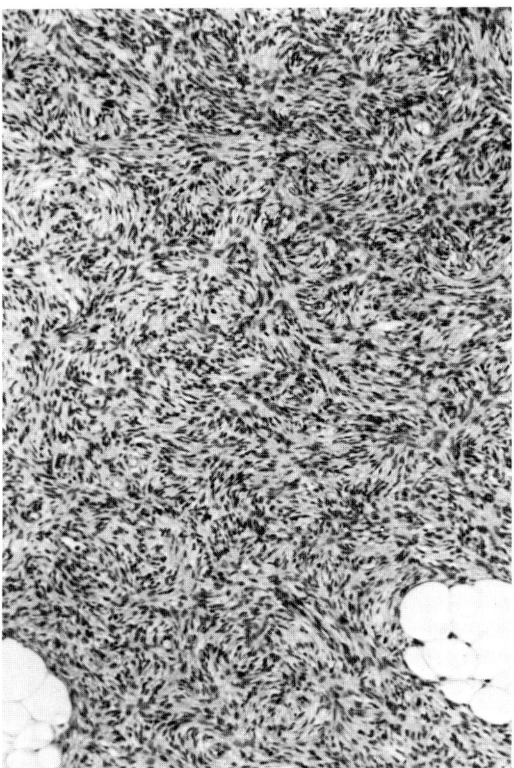

Fig. 2-36. Dermatofibrosarcoma protuberans showing bland-appearing slender spindle cells arranged in a characteristic storiform (curly) pattern. (H&E, × 125.)

served, while xanthoma cells and multinucleated giant cells are rare or absent. Mitotic figures (less than 5 per 10 high-power field)[158] are infrequent. A "grenz" zone of intact papillary dermis is found in the overwhelming majority of cases, while in only a few cases the tumor abuts on the epidermis. Neoplastic cells at the advancing margins appear more slender and spread along the subcutaneous fibrous septa infiltrating the fat lobules in a lacelike or honeycomb fashion. Myxoid areas are occasionally observed in the tumor. When the myxoid change is the predominant histological feature, the term *myxoid variant of DFSP* is applied.[163] In these cases, the storiform pattern is less apparent and the vascular pattern becomes more evident.

Occasionally hypercellular sharply demarcated areas displaying a fibrosarcomatous pat-

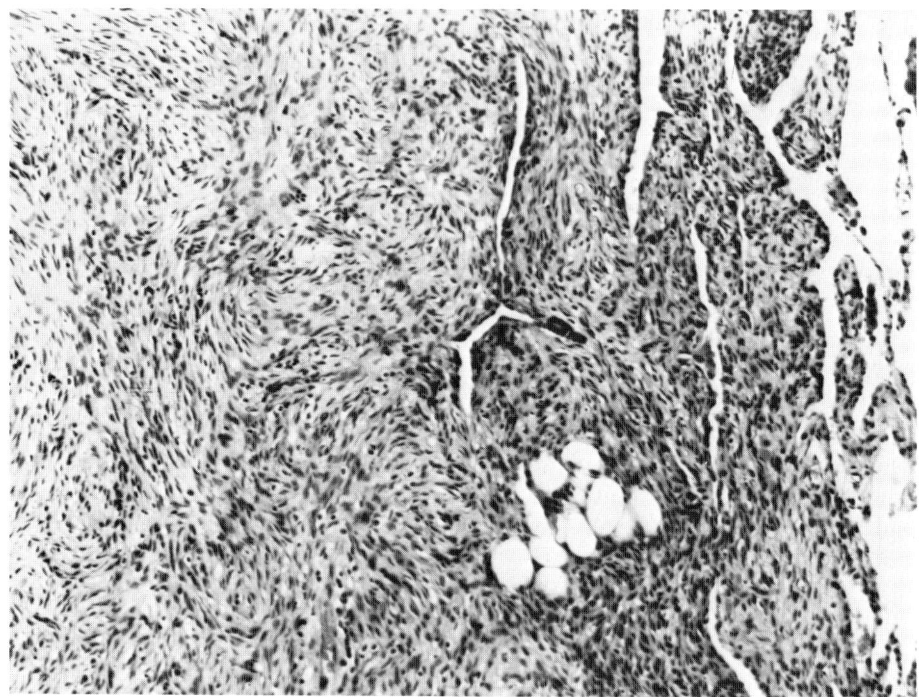

Fig. 2-37. Lung metastasis from a dermatofibrosarcoma protuberans. (H&E, × 125.)

tern may be observed in recurrent as well as in primary tumors.[164, 165] Areas resembling malignant fibrous histiocytoma are more rarely encountered, and mostly in recurrent lesions.[166, 167] Moreover, tumors showing transitional features of both DFSP and giant cell fibroblastoma[102, 168] have been reported.

The histogenesis of DFSP is still open to discussion. Neural,[169] histiocytic,[170–173] and fibroblastic[158, 174–176] origins have been variously proposed. Immunohistochemical studies, however, provided conflicting results regarding positivity to histiocytic markers, such as lysozyme, α_1-antitrypsin, α_1-antichymotrypsin,[158, 172, 176] and ferritin[172] and a fibroblastic origin of DFSP is currently favored.[176]

Prognosis. DFSP is characterized by a locally aggressive and destructive behavior, with occasional metastasis to regional lymph nodes[157, 177] and visceral organs,[178–182] usually to the lung (Fig. 2-37). The recurrence rate ranges from 20 percent[183] to about 50 percent of the cases,[157, 167] whereas metastatic rates of 14.3 percent[164] and 5.7 percent have been reported.[184] There is no conclusive evidence

that DFSP with fibrosarcomatous areas may be more aggressive than ordinary DFSP, although it is generally agreed that fibrosarcoma arising in a DFSP is far less aggressive than de novo fibrosarcoma.[164, 165]

Pigmented Dermatofibrosarcoma Protuberans (Bednař Tumor)

The Bednař tumor was first described in 1957 by Bednař, who considered it a storiform variant of neurofibroma.[185] It is now accepted as the pigmented counterpart of DFSP. This is a rare tumor, accounting for approximately 1 to 5 percent of all cases of DFSP.[186]

Histologically the lesion is indistinguishable from conventional DFSP. Scattered throughout the tumor are melanin-laden bipolar or multipolar dendritic cells that often are so heavily pigmented that cellular details may not be discernible (Fig. 2-38). Under the electron microscope, three types of cells can be recognized: fibroblast-like cells; cells resembling Schwann cells or perineural fibroblasts; and dentritic cells

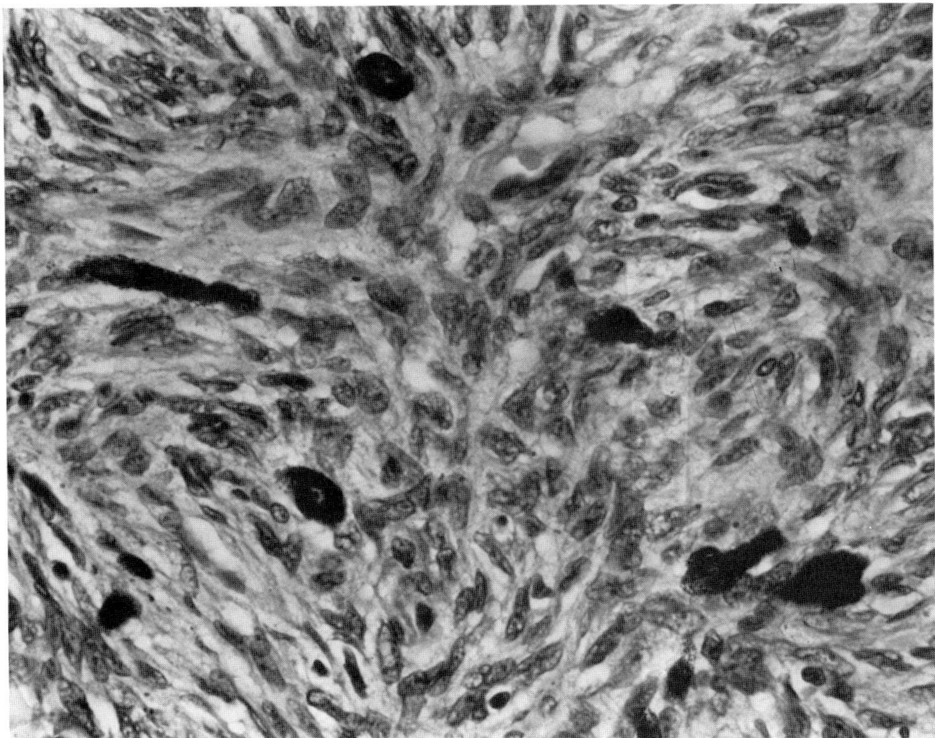

Fig. 2-38. High-power view of the tumor shown in Fig. 2-38. Note the melanin-laden dendritic cells with no discernible cellular detail. (H&E, × 500.)

containing melanosomes and premelanosomes.[186, 187]

Dupree et al.[186] considered pigmented cells a melanocytic differentiation of tumor cells, thus supporting the neural origin of DFSP. Fletcher et al.[187] suggested they might only represent entrapped epidermal and/or dermal melanocytes. Immunocytochemical studies did not clarify this point, for S-100 protein reactivity has been variously reported as negative[186] and positive.[187, 188] The origin of the pigmented cells is still uncertain.[189]

Differential Diagnosis. Although cellular forms of fibrous histiocytoma may resemble the Bednař tumor, they usually contain inflammatory and xanthoma cells, but not melanin-bearing dendritic cells. A tight storiform pattern may be encountered in neurofibromas, but these rarely contain pigmented cells and the spindle cells are always S-100 positive, unlike the invariably negative spindle cells in Bednař tumor. Because of the melanin-laden dendritic cells,

malignant melanoma and cellular blue nevus occasionally may enter the differential diagnosis. Unlike the Bednař tumor, however, they are composed of plump spindle or round cells that are heavily stained by anti S-100 protein antibodies.

Prognosis. The biologic behavior of the Bednař tumor is difficult to assess owing to the paucity of case reports. According to the series of Dupree et al.,[186] 11 percent of the cases recurred usually within 1 year of the initial excision, although distant metastases were not observed. Complete local excision and close follow-up appear to be the treatment of choice.

MALIGNANT FIBROUS HISTIOCYTOMA

Malignant fibrous histiocytoma (MFH) is a descriptive term used to designate tumors composed of fusiform fibroblastlike and round histiocytelike cells arranged in a storiform or cartwheel-like pattern. First reported by O'Brien and Stout in 1963,[190] MFH was recognized as a distinct entity in 1978 by Weiss and Enzinger.[191] Since then, MFH may be considered the most prevalent and frequently diagnosed malignant soft tissue tumor. According to reports, it accounts for 10 to 30 percent of all soft tissue sarcomas.[191–194]

The histogenesis of this tumor is a controversial issue. Ultrastructural studies have not been able to establish a definitive histogenesis because fibroblastlike and histiocytelike cells, as well as cells with both morphological characteristics, are commonly encountered; thus, a primitive mesenchymal cell was advanced as the putative cell of origin of this tumor.[195, 196] Similarly, immunocytochemical studies did not provide conclusive evidence of its histogenesis. The expression in both fibroblastlike and histiocytelike cells of histiocytic markers, such as cathepsin B, α_1-antitrypsin, and α_1-antichymotrypsin,[172, 194, 197–199] would partially support its origin from tissue fixed-histiocytes; however, lysozyme expression is frequently undetectable.[198, 200] Although some investigators[201, 202] reported a positive reaction to monoclonal antibodies recognizing determinants expressed by bone marrow-derived monocyte/macrophage cells, others have challenged an origin from the mononuclear phagocyte system[203, 204] and a primitive mesenchymal derivation is currently favored.[203–206] More recently, it was also suggested that MFH might not represent a distinct anatomic-clinical entity, but instead the final morphological picture of a dedifferentiation process involving other soft tissue sarcomas.[207]

Although pleomorphism is the essence of MFH, this tumor may display a broad spectrum of microscopic features depending on the relative percentage of its two major components; six different subtypes are commonly recognized (see Table 2-2). Indeed, MFH should not be considered a "wastebasket" where one may throw pleomorphic tumors for which a morphological diagnosis is not readily formulated. MFH-like areas, in fact, may be seen in many other malignant tumors, such as rhabdomyosarcoma, leiomyosarcoma, liposarcoma, and ma-

lignant schwannomas, as well as carcinomas and melanoma. Familiarity with these pitfalls should eliminate the overdiagnosis of MFH.

Although it is considered one of the most aggressive sarcomas, MFH shows a significantly variable prognosis in relation to several factors. Tumor size, depth, location, and histologic types, as well as the presence of inflammatory infiltrates, largely seem to govern the final patient outcome.[191, 208, 209] In general, the smaller, more superficial, and more distal the tumor, the better the prognosis.[208, 209]

Atypical Fibroxanthoma (Cutaneous Malignant Fibrous Histiocytoma)

Atypical Fibroxanthoma (AFX), first described by Helwig in 1963,[210] is a pleomorphic cutaneous tumor that typically arises on the sun-exposed skin of elderly individuals. The lesion is currently considered a fibrohistiocytic tumor of low-grade malignancy because of the occasional occurrence of metastasis.[211–213] Histologically this tumor is indistinguishable from the pleomorphic type of MFH and is best regarded as a cutaneous form of superficial MFH.

AFX usually presents as a solitary small, firm nodule on the sun-exposed skin of the head and neck of elderly persons. The median age is 69 years.[211] Although one-fourth of the cases are reported to occur in the trunk and extremities of younger people,[211] some of these cases may represent examples of atypical cutaneous fibrous histiocytoma.[153] Males are more frequently affected than females.[211, 214] Prolonged solar exposure and previous irradiation have been attributed a major role in the pathogenesis of AFX.[211]

Histologically AFX is typically confined to the dermis with no invasion of deeper structures. Cytologically this tumor is composed of spindle-shaped or large round and occasionally multinucleated cells, which often show marked pleomorphism and atypical mitotic figures. The neoplastic cells are arranged in vague fascicles, but an evident storiform pattern is rarely observed (Fig. 2-39). The overlying epidermis is

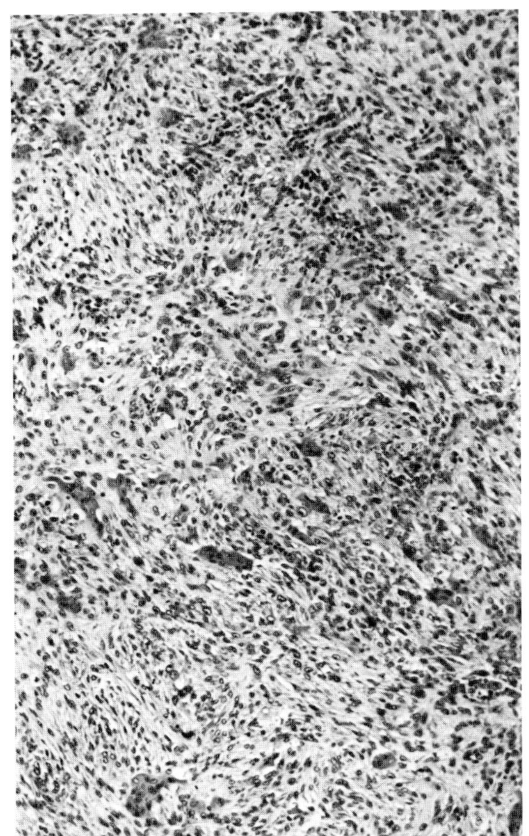

Fig. 2-39. Atypical fibroxanthoma from the right temple of a 73-year-old man. Note the malignant fibrous histiocytomalike area at the bottom. (H&E, × 125.)

atrophic and often ulcerated. The adjacent skin frequently displays solar elastosis, mild inflammation, and vascular ectasia (Fig. 2-40). Skin appendages are compressed and destroyed by tumor cells that may extend into the subcutaneous fat.

Like deeper MHF, AFX is composed of a mixture of cells with the ultrastructural characteristics of fibroblasts,[215] myofibroblasts,[216] and histiocytes.[217] Langerhans'-type histiocytes with diagnostic Birbeck granules have been also reported.[214, 217]

Differential Diagnosis. Cellular spindling and marked pleomorphism may be encountered in squamous cell carcinoma of the skin and malignant melanoma. In the large majority of cases, single cell keratinization, supported by positivity to keratin in the former and by the presence of junctional activity and S-100 protein in the latter, should permit a prompt distinction.

Occasionally pleomorphic multinucleated giant cells may be observed in superficial leiomyosarcomas. Unlike AFX, smooth muscle tumors are composed of spindle cells with blunt-ended nuclei organized in more orderly fascicles.

A greater challenge is the distinction from pleomorphic MFH. Tumors that extensively infiltrate the fascia and the underlying structures, and display necrosis or vascular invasion are more correctly classified as pleomorphic MFH because they show a higher risk of metastasis compared to typical cutaneous AFX.[211]

Prognosis. Although AFX may recur from 5 to 7 percent of the cases,[211, 218] the overall prognosis is excellent following conservative surgery. Metastases are infrequent; over 70 percent of so-called metastasizing AFX are associated with recurrence.[213] In view of the rarity of metastasis, complete locale excision is the treatment of choice. However, if AFX recurs as a large deeply located mass, it should be treated as a conventional MFH.

Malignant Fibrous Histiocytoma

Based primarily on conventional microscopy, deeper MFH are currently subdivided into five subtypes[219] (Table 2-2). Except for angiomatoid MFH, these subtypes share many features and are therefore discussed together.

MFH is characteristically a tumor of adult life with a peak incidence in the seventh decade.[191, 193, 207, 220] It is infrequent below the age of 40 years and exceptional in childhood.[221] About two-thirds of the cases occur in men. These tumors arise in the retroperitoneum or in the extremities, and are located close to the deep fascia or within skeletal muscle. In the extremities, they present as painless masses, whereas in the retroperitoneum they may give rise to constitutional symptoms, including anorexia, malaise, weight loss, and signs of increasing abdominal pressure. Hypoglycemia[191] and

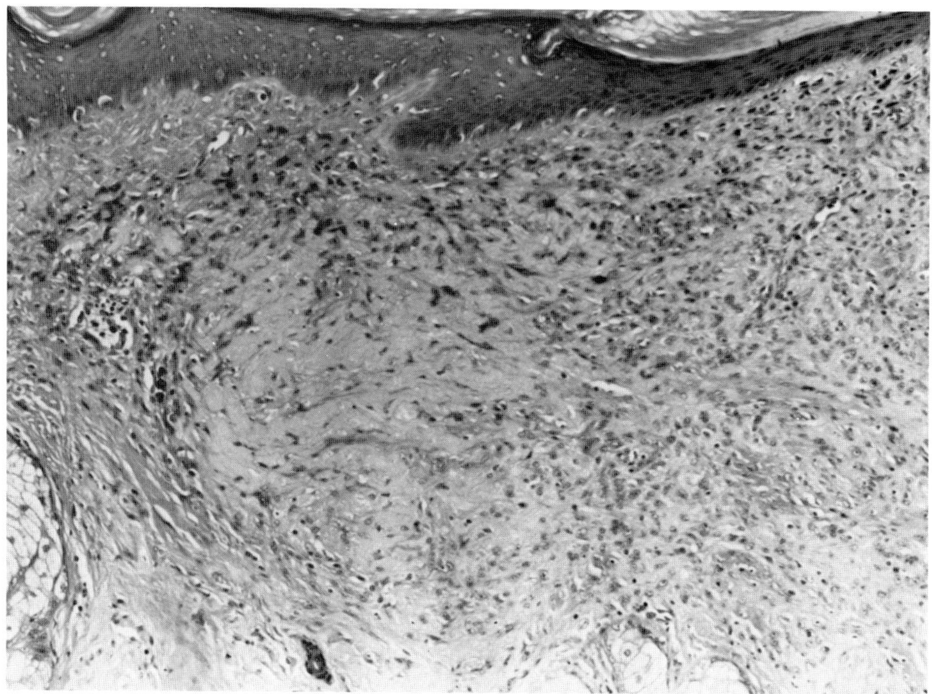

Fig. 2-40. Peripheral portion of an atypical fibroxanthoma showing solar elastosis. (H&E, × 125.)

leukemoid reaction[222, 223] are also described in association with MFH.

Most MFH are large, multilobulated masses with frequent areas of hemorrhage and necrosis. On the cut surface, they are whitish-gray, with the exception of the myxoid type, which is gelatinous or translucent, and the inflammatory type, which may have a yellow color due to the abundance of lipids.[146] These tumors occasionally present as hemorrhagic cystic masses simulating hematomas.

Pleomorphic MFH is the prototype of the group, and accounts for more than two-thirds of all cases.[191, 221] This tumor is composed of fascicles of plump, fusiform cells arranged in either a cartwheel or a storiform pattern. In most tumors, the storimform areas are associated with characteristic pleomorphic fields in which the neoplastic cells are round and histiocytoid with abundant eosinophilic cytoplasm. Scattered mono- or multinucleated giant cells, as well as striking often atypical mitotic figures are commonly found. Lymphocytes, plasma cells, and

some lipid-laden histiocytes are also seen (Fig. 2-41). Necrosis is the rule rather than the exception. Myxoid areas, due to the accumulation of acid mucopolysaccharides, often alternate with areas of sclerosis and hyalinization.

In about 20 percent of the cases, the myxoid areas make up more than 50 percent of the tumor mass. These tumors are defined *myxoid MFH,* and apparently bear a more favorable prognosis.[220] In the past, this type of MFH was also referred to as *myxofibrosarcoma.*[224, 225] Microscopically this variant is composed of large hypocellular myxoid areas that blend into more cellular areas indistinguishable from pleomorphic MFH. In the myxoid areas, the storiform pattern is absent or less conspicuous, while the vasculature is more prominent (Fig. 2-42). The cells in the myxoid areas may have a deceptively bland appearance, simulating normal or reactive fibroblasts. Occasional vacuolated cells resembling lipoblasts may also be present, but unlike true lipoblasts, these vacuoles contain acid mucin and no neutral fat.[220, 226]

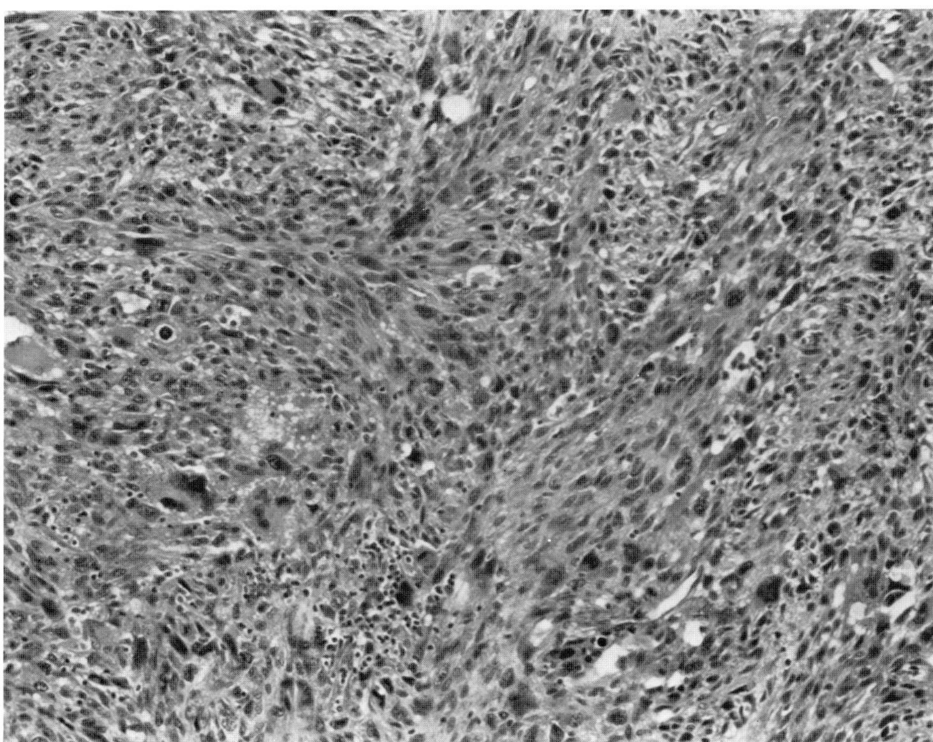

Fig. 2-41. Pleomorphic malignant fibrous histiocytoma showing short fascicles of plump fibroblastlike cells intimately associated with more rounded histiocytes and multinucleated giant cells. (H&E, × 125.)

A distinct multinodular growth pattern and the presence of a large number of osteoclastlike giant cells in an otherwise conventional pleomorphic MFH defines *giant cell type MFH,* also known as *giant cell tumor of the soft parts.*[227] At low magnification, this tumor strongly resembles giant cell tumor of bone, although the benign-looking multinucleated osteoclastlike cells appear interspersed with bizarre highly pleomorphic giant cells occasionally containing phagocytic vacuoles. Metaplastic osteoid or mature bone may be encountered at the tumor periphery.[227] At the ultrastructural level, the presence of chondroblastlike and osteoblastlike cells,[228] in addition to the cell types commonly observed in the pleomorphic type of MFH,[229] may raise the question of a close histogenetic link between giant cell MFH and extraskeletal osteosarcoma. Nevertheless, we prefer to classify giant cell tumors with only focal osteochondroid differentiation as giant cell MFH.[230]

The term *inflammatory MFH* is currently used to designate retroperitoneal tumors that in the past have been variously named as retroperitoneal xanthogranuloma, xanthosarcoma, or inflammatory fibrous histiocytoma.[149, 222, 231] Unlike other forms of MFH, this lesion is typically located in the retroperitoneal space and its diagnostic hallmark is the presence of xanthoma cells and polymorphonuclear leukocytes. This lesion, in fact, consists of sheets of histiocytic cells with acute and chronic inflammatory cells (Figs. 2-43 and 2-44)in a background of hyaline material with scant collagen. The majority of the histiocytic cells are laden with lipid material and appear xanthomatous. Most of the xanthoma cells appear bland, often with pyknotic nuclei, but some display nuclear atypia and mitotic activity. Scattered multinucleated giant cells are commonly observed throughout the tumor. The highly vascularized areas of the tumor occasionally bear a superficial resemblance to granulation

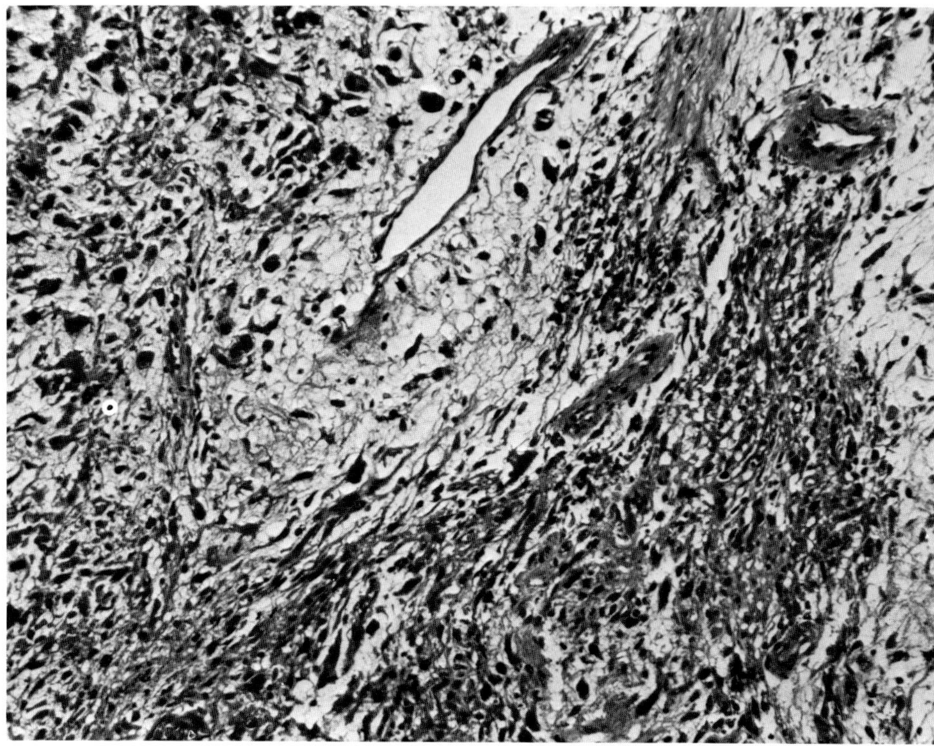

Fig. 2-42. Myxoid malignant fibrous histiocytoma. Note the myxoid zones that abut cellular areas. (H&E, × 125.)

tissue (Fig. 2-44). Nevertheless, transition to more spindled areas with a fascicular or a storiform pattern is generally observed.

Differential Diagnosis. Pleomorphic sarcomas, in particular liposarcoma and rhabdomyosarcoma, are the principal differential diagnoses of pleomorphic MFH. The pleomorphic variant of liposarcoma, however, lacks a distinct whorled or storiform pattern, whereas typical lipoblasts are commonly found. The differentiation from pleomorphic rhabdomyosarcoma may also cause some difficulty. However, the diagnosis of this very rare tumor and, in the absence of distinct cytoplasmic cross-striations, relies on ultrastructural and/or immunocytochemical findings (see also Ch. 4). Moreover, dedifferentiated sarcomas (i.e., liposarcoma, chondrosarcoma, malignant nerve sheath tumors, and leiomyosarcoma) show areas that are virtually indistinguishable from MFH. Nonetheless, adequate tumor sampling and the observation of more specific areas of differentiation should lead to a correct diagnosis.

Anaplastic carcinomas and metastatic malignant melanoma[232] at times may be misinterpreted as MFH. The diagnosis of MFH in an unusual clinical setting (e.g., when a tumor involves primarily visceral organs or major lymph node groups) should always be questioned. Stains for mucin and glycogen in conjunction with cytokeratin positivity are generally helpful in recognizing anaplastic carcinomas. Likewise, the presence of scattered nevoid areas, and a strong and diffuse positivity to S-100 protein will support the diagnosis of malignant melanoma.

The distinction from a benign fibrous histiocytoma or dermatofibrosarcoma protuberans is not a problem due to the absence of pleomorphism and necrosis. Plexiform fibrohistiocytic tumor is characterized by its occurrence in younger patients, the smaller size and superficial location

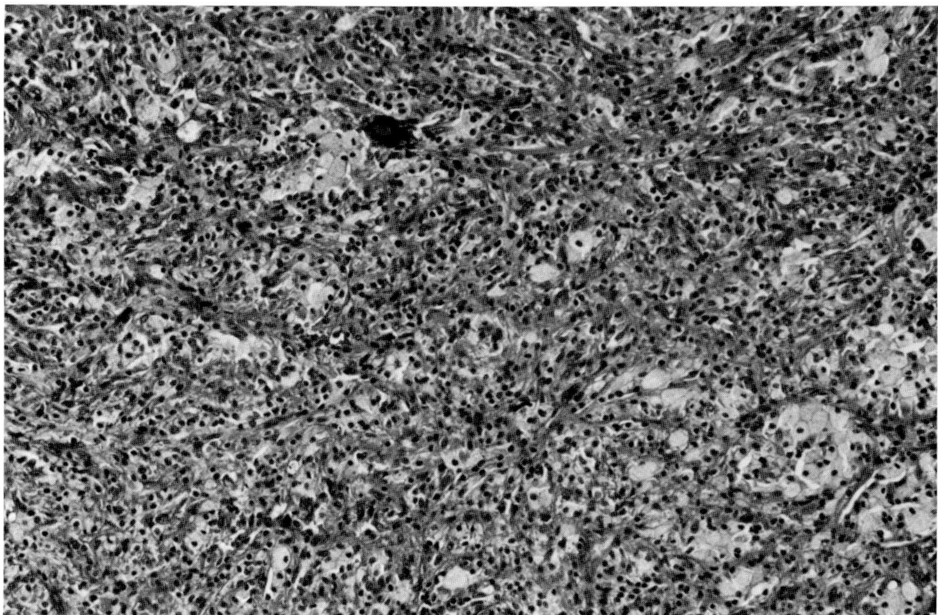

Fig. 2-43. Inflammatory malignant fibrous histiocytoma revealing sheets of inflammatory cells, foam macrophages, plump spindle cells resembling fibroblasts, and occasional multinucleated giant cells. (H&E, × 125.)

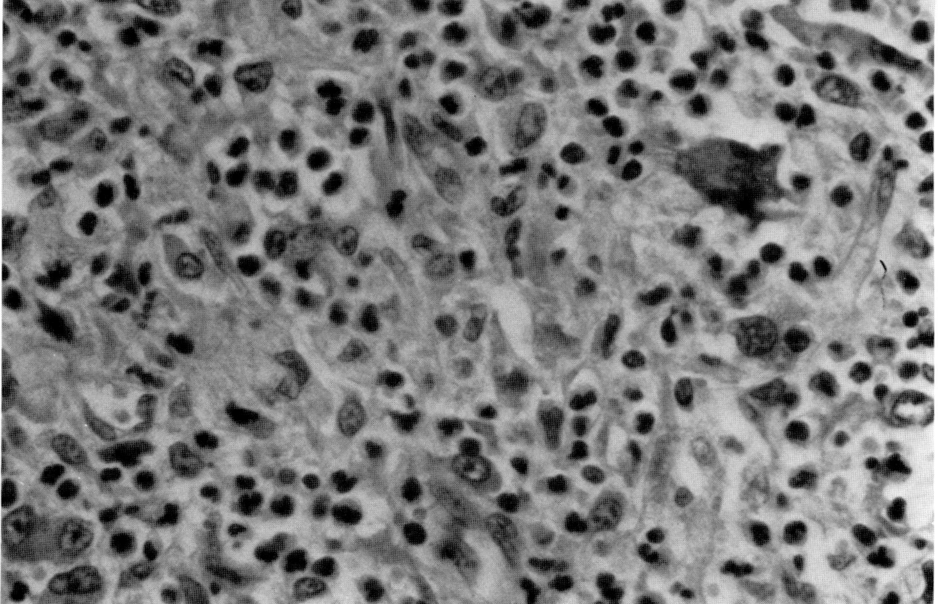

Fig. 2-44. High-power view displaying a mixture of acute and chronic inflammatory cells, intermingled with neoplastic histiocytes set in a background reminiscent of granulation tissue. (H&E, × 500.)

of the lesion, and the presence of fibromatosis-like areas.

Benign myxoid lesions, such as myxoma and nodular fasciitis, may enter the differential diagnosis with myxoid MFH. Bland cytological features and the absence of a prominent vascular network readily distinguish myxomas from MFH, while the absence of atypical mitotic figures and highly pleomorphic cells differentiate nodular fasciitis. The distinction from myxoid liposarcoma is more difficult. The presence of unequivocal lipoblasts (see also Ch. 3), pools of amorphous eosinophilic material, and a delicate plexiform vasculature favor the diagnosis of myxoid liposarcoma over MFH.

Giant cell MFH must be differentiated from giant cell tumor of bone with soft tissue extension. Unlike the bone tumor, giant cell MFH displays a distinct multinodular growth pattern and does not produce significant bone defects. Inflammatory MFH is distinguished from reactive xanthomatous processes by findings of the cellular atypia and mitotic activity.

Prognosis. With the exception of the myxoid and inflammatory types, local recurrences or metastases will develop in one-half of the patients and the overall 5-year survival rate ranges from 36[209] to 48 percent.[193] In the myxoid type, local recurrences develop in two-thirds of the cases, and metastases in about one fourth.[220] In the inflammatory type, metastases occur in about one-third of the patients[231]; recurrences are directly related to surgery, and rates range from 0 percent, after adequate wide excision, to 84 percent following incomplete excision.[209]

Metastasis usually occurs within two years of the initial diagnosis, and lung, liver, and bones are the most frequent metastatic sites. Lymph node metastases are reported in 4 to 17 percent of the cases.[207, 209] The degree of anaplasia and the number of mitotic figures do not correlate with the outcome,[221] while tumor depth, size, and anatomic site are highly significant factors. Less than 10 percent of tumors confined entirely within the subcutis with no fascial involvement undergo metastasis. When fascia is infiltrated, metastasis occurs in 27 per-

cent of cases, while 43 percent of cases with skeletal muscle involvement metastasize.[191] The 5-year survival rate ranges from 28 percent for MFH in the proximal portions of the body, to 75 percent for distal tumors. Retroperitoneal tumors show the lowest survival rate (14 percent).[207]

Prompt surgery, either radical local excision or amputation, is the treatment of choice for MFH. Systemic radio- or chemotherapy is also recommended as a palliative measure.[221]

Angiomatoid MFH is a rare variant of MFH and deserves special attention because of its peculiar anatomic-clinical characteristics. Since its first description by Enzinger in 1979,[233] about 200 cases have reported in the literature.[234–242] Unlike classic MFH, this tumor mainly affects children and young adults, with a median age of 14 years at diagnosis.[242] Congenital cases have also been reported.[240, 241] Ultrastructural and immunocytochemical studies favor a fibrohistiocytic[239, 241] rather than an endothelial origin,[234, 235, 237] and this tumor, in fact, invariably lacks factor VIII-associated antigen.

The lesions present as slow growing nodular or cystic masses in the lower dermis or subcutaneous tissues. The extremities are involved in more than 60 percent of the cases,[233, 241, 242] while head neck, and orbit and lymph nodes are rarely involved.[233, 234, 241, 243] A hemorrhagic tendency with no evidence of clotting defects or thrombocytopenia may be present, as well as general symptoms, such as anemia, fever with chills, and weight loss.[233]

The tumors are small, firm, and well circumscribed. The cut surface has a variegated appearance owing to the presence of brownish hemorrhagic areas and irregular blood-filled cystic spaces. Microscopically the tumors are composed of nodules of plump histiocytelike cells, interspersed with cystic areas of hemorrhage and a peripheral cuff of mononuclear inflammatory cells (Fig. 2-45). The neoplastic cells are uniform (Fig. 2-46) and giant cells are only occasionally encountered. A storiform pattern may be present, but it never is a prominent feature. Inflammatory cells consist of lympho-

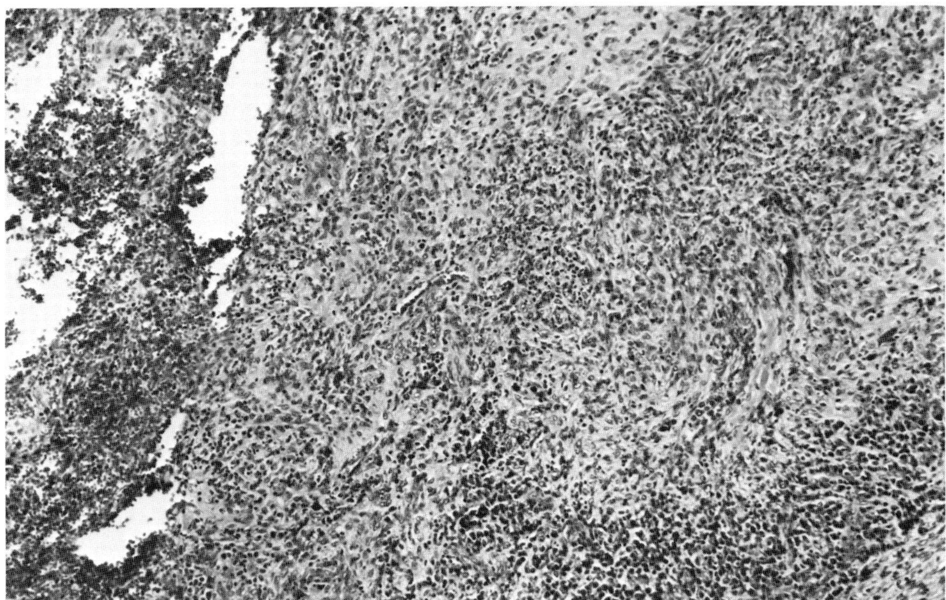

Fig. 2-45. Angiomatoid malignant fibrous histiocytoma consisting of a solid mass of histiocytoid cells with a vague storiform pattern, partially cuffed by a lymphoplasmacytic infiltrate and associated with a cystic space. (H&E, × 125.)

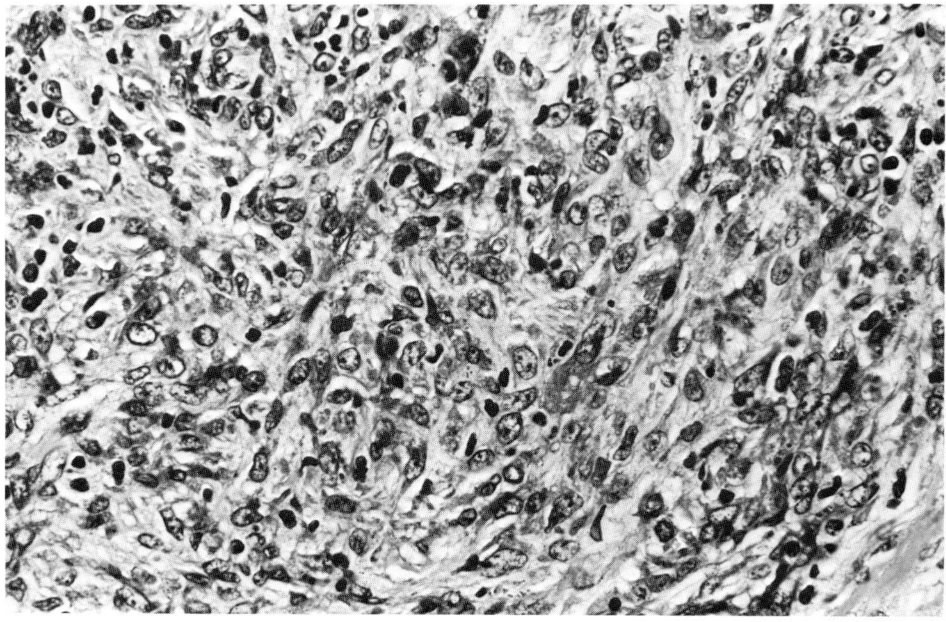

Fig. 2-46. High-power view of the solid area shown in Fig. 2-45. Note the uniform appearance of the histiocytoid cells. (H&E, × 500.)

cytes and plasma cells with prominent reactive centers. The tumor cells express vimentin, cathespin B, and α_1-antichymotrypsin, and are invariably negative to factor-VIII associated antigen.[241]

Differential Diagnosis. The large blood-filled cystic spaces may raise the suspicion of cystic hematoma, thrombosed vessel, or cavernous hemangioma. However, the multinodular aspect and the presence of large clusters of histiocytelike cells will clarify the diagnosis.

Prognosis. The clinical behavior is dramatically different from the other forms of MFH. Recurrence rates vary from about 60[233, 241] to 11 percent[242] of cases, and approximately 1 to 15 percent of the patients develop metastases.[233, 241, 242] This low metastatic potential seems partially explained by the tumor's diploid status,[241, 244] which strongly differs from the abnormal DNA content reported for classical MFH.[244] Conservative surgery with adequate margins, therefore, represents the treatment of choice.

REFERENCES

1. Majno G, Gabbiani G, Hirschel BJ et al: Contraction of granulation tissue in vitro: similarly to smooth muscle. Science 173:548, 1971
2. Skalli O, Schurch W, Seemayer T, et al: Myofibroblasts from diverse pathologic settings are heterogeneous in their content of actin isoforms and intermediate filament protein. Lab Invest 60:275, 1989
3. Darby I, Skalli O, Gabbiani G: Alpha-smooth muscle actin is transiently expressed by myofibroblasts during experimental wound healing. Lab Invest 63:21, 1990
4. Ghosh L, Ghosh BC, Das Gupta YK: Ultrastructural study of stroma in mammary carcinoma. Am J Surg 139:229, 1980
5. Balazs M, Kovacs A: The transitional mucosa adjacent to large bowel carcinoma—electron microscopy features and myofibroblast reaction. Histopathology 6:617, 1982
6. Seemayer TA, Schürch W, Lagacé R: Myofibroblasts in human pathology. Hum Pathol 12:491, 1981
7. Gabbiana G, Majno G: Dupuytrens' contraction: fibroblastic contraction? An ultrastructural study. Am J Pathol 66:131, 1972
8. Stiller D, Katenkamp D: Cellular features in desmoid fibromatosis and well-differentiated fibrosarcomas. An electron microscopic study. Virchows Arch [A] 369:155, 1975
9. Wirman JA: Nodular fasciitis, a lesion of myofibroblasts. An ultrastructural study. Cancer 38:2378, 1976
10. Craver JL, McDivitt RW: Proliferative fasciitis. Arch Pathol Lab Med 105:542, 1981
11. Katenkamp D, Stiller D: Cellular composition of so-called dermatofibroma (histiocytoma cutis). Virchows Arch [A] 367:3325, 1975
12. Bhawan J, Majno G: The myofibroblast: possible derivation from macrophages in xanthogranuloma. Am J Dermatopathol 11:255, 1989
13. Chung EB, Enzinger FM: Infantile myofibromatosis. Cancer 48:1807, 1981
14. Wargotz ES, Weiss SW, Norris HJ: Myofibroblastoma of the breast. Sixteen cases of a distinctive mesenchymal tumor. Am J Surg Pathol 11:493, 1987
15. Sappino AP, Schurch W, Gabbiani G: Differentiation repertoire of fibroblastic cells: expression of cytoskeleton proteins as marker of phenotypic modulations. Lab Invest 63:144, 1990
16. Ross R, Wight TN, Strandness E, Thiele B: Human atherosclerosis I. Cell constitution and characteristics of advanced lesions of the superficial femoral artery. Am J Pathol 114:79, 1984
17. Gown AM: The mysteries of the myofibroblast (partially) unmasked. Lab Invest 63:1, 1990
18. Dahl I, Angervall L: Pseudosarcomatous lesions of the soft tissues reported as sarcoma during a 6-year period (1958–1963). Acta Pathol Microbiol Scand [A] 85:917, 1977
19. Lattes R: Pseudosarcomatous lesions and "borderline" tumors of soft tissues. Historical review. Appl Pathol 6:154, 1988
20. Konwaler BE, Keasbey L, Kaplan L: Subcutaneous pseudosarcomatous fibromatosis (fasciitis). Am J Clin Pathol 25:241, 1955
21. Lauer DH, Enzinger FM: Cranial fasciitis of childhood. Cancer 45:401, 1980
22. Hutter RVP, Foote FW Jr, Francis KC et al: Parosteal fasciitis. A self-limited benign process that simulates a malignant neoplasm. Am J Surg 104:800, 1962
23. Chung EB: Pitfalls in diagnosing benign soft tissue tumors in infancy and childhood. Pathol Annu 20(2):323, 1985

24. Patchefsky AS, Enzinger FM: Intravascular fasciitis. A report of 17 cases. Am J Surg Pathol 5:29, 1981
25. Chung EB, Enzinger FM: Proliferative fasciitis. Cancer 36:1450, 1975
26. Enzinger FM, Dulcey F: Proliferative myositis. Report of 33 cases. Cancer 20:2213, 1967
27. Stiller D, Katenkamp D: The subcutaneous fascial analogue of myositis proliferans. Electron microscopic examination of two cases and comparison with myositis ossificans localisata. Virchows Arch [A] 368:361, 1975
28. Kitano M, Iwasaki H, Enjoji M: Proliferative fasciitis-a variant of nodular fasciitis. Acta Pathol Jpn 27:485, 1977
29. Chung EB, Enzinger FM: Fibroma of tendon sheath. Cancer 44:1945, 1979
30. Lundgren LG, Kindblom L-G: Fibroma of tendon sheath. A light and electron-microscopic study of 6 cases. Acta Pathol Microbiol Immunol Scand [A] 92:401, 1984
31. Sarma DP, Weilbaecher TG, Rodriguez FH Jr: Fibroma of tendon sheath. J Surg Oncol 32:230, 1986
32. Alguacil-Garcia, Unni KK, Goellner JR: Giant cell tumor of tendon sheath and pigmented villonodular synovitis. An ultrastructural study. Am J Clin Pathol 69:6, 1978
33. Azzopardi JG, Tanda F, Salm R: Tenosynovial fibroma. Diagn Histopathol 6:69, 1983
34. Cooper PH: Fibroma of tendon sheath. J Am Acad Dermatol 11:625, 1984
35. Järvi OH, Saxén E: Elastofibroma dorsi. Acta Pathol Microbiol Scand 51 (Suppl 144):83, 1961
36. Jarvi OH, Saxén AE, Hospu-Havu VK. et al: Elastofibroma-a degenerative pseudotumor. Cancer 23:42, 1969
37. Enzinger FM, Weiss SW: Soft Tissue Tumors. 2nd Ed. p. 123. CV Mosby Company, St. Louis, 1988
38. Mirra JM, Straub LR, Jarwi OH: Elastofibroma of the deltoid. A case report. Cancer 33:234, 1974
39. Weissman J, Smith DW: Fine structure of an elastofibroma. Cancer 22:671, 1968
40. Barr JR: Elastofibroma. Am J Clin Pathol 45:679, 1966
41. Nakamura Y, Okamoto K, Tanimura A et al: Elastase digestion and biochemical analysis of the elastin from an elastofibroma. Cancer 58:1070, 1986
42. Ramos CV, Gillespie W, Narconis RJ: Elastofibroma: a pseudotumor of myofibroblast. Arch Pathol Lab Med 102:438, 1978
43. Dixon AY, Lee SH: An ultrastructural study of elastofibromas. Hum Pathol 11:257, 1980
44. Harry RD, Kruger RL, McLaughlin CW: Elastofibroma dorsi: an unusual soft tissue tumor simulating sarcoma. Am J Surg 125:773, 1973
45. Stout AP: Juvenile fibromatosis. Cancer 7:953, 1954
46. Stout AP, Lattes R: Tumors of the soft tissues. In Atlas of Tumor Pathology. Second Series. Fascicle I. Armed Forced Institute of Pathology, Washington DC, 1967
47. Lattes R: Tumors of the soft tissues. In Atlas of Tumor Pathology. Second Series. Fascicle I/Revised. Armed Forces Institute of Pathology, Washington DC, 1981
48. Enzinger FM, Lattes R, Torloni R: 1969 Histological typing of soft tissue tumours. International Histological Classification of Tumours No. 3. World Health Organization, Geneva,
49. Allen PW: The fibromatoses: a clinicopathologic classification based on 140 cases. Part 1. Am J Surg Pathol 1:255, 1977
50. Häyry P, Reitamo JJ, Vihko R et al: The desmoid tumor. III. A biochemical and genetic analysis. Am J Clin Pathol 77:681, 1982
51. Häyry P, Reitamo JJ, Tötterman S et al: The desmoid tumor. II. Analysis of factors possibly contributing to the etiology and growth behavior. Am J Clin Pathol 77:674, 1982
52. Reitamo JJ, Häyry P, Nykyri E, Saxén E: The desmoid tumor. I. Incidence, sex-, age- and anatomical distribution in the finnish population. Am J Clin Pathol 77:665, 1982
53. Dahn I, Jonsson N, Lundh G: Desmoid tumors. A series of 33 cases. Acta Chir Scand 126:305, 1963
54. Burke AP, Sobin LH, Shekitka KM: Mesenteric fibromatosis. A follow-up study. Arch Pathol Lab Med 114:832, 1990
55. Rosen PP, Ernsberger D: Mammary fibromatosis. A benign spindle-cell tumor with significant risk for local recurrence. Cancer 63:1363, 1989
56. Wargotz ES, Norris HJ, Austin RM et al: Fibromatosis of the breast. A clinical and pathological study of 28 cases. Am J Surg Pathol 11(1):38, 1987
57. Rosenberg HS, Stenback WA, Spjut HJ: The fibromatoses of infancy and childhood. Perspect Pediatr Pathol 4:269, 1978

58. Brasfield RD, Das Gupta TK: Desmoid tumors of the anterior abdominal wall. Surgery 65:241, 1969

59. Yannopoulos K, Stout AP: Primary solid tumors of the mesentery. Cancer 16:914, 1963

60. Kim DH, Goldsmith HS, Quan SH et al: Intra-abdominal desmoid tumor. Cancer 27:1041, 1971

61. Burke AP, Sobin LH, Shekitka KM et al: Intra-abdominal fibromatosis. A pathologic analysis of 130 tumors with comparison of clinical subgroups. Am J Surg Pathol 14(4):335, 1990

62. Enzinger FM, Shiraki M: Musculo-aponeurotic fibromatosis of the shoulder girdle (extra-abdominal desmoid). Analysis of thirty cases followed up for ten or more years. Cancer 20:1131, 1967

63. Das Gupta TK, Brasfield RD, O'Hara J: Extra-abdominal desmoids: a clinicopathological study. Ann Surg 170:109, 1969

64. Barber HM, Galasko CSB, Woods CG: Multicentric extra-abdominal desmoid tumours. Report of two cases J Bone Joint Surg 55B:858, 1973

65. Rock MG, Pritchard DJ, Reiman HM et al: Extra-abdominal desmoid tumors. J Bone Joint Surg 66A:1369, 1984

66. Khorsand J, Karakousis CP: Desmoid tumors and their management. Am J Surg 149:215, 1985

67. Reye RDK: A consideration of certain subdermal "fibromatous tumours" of infancy. J Pathol Bacteriol 72:149, 1956

68. Enzinger FM: Fibrous hamartoma of infancy. Cancer 18:241, 1965

69. Mitchell ML, Di Sant'Agnese PA, Gerber JE: Fibrous hamartoma of infancy. Hum Pathol 13:586, 1982

70. Greco MA, Schinella RA, Vuletin JC: Fibrous hamartoma of infancy: an ultrastructural study. Hum Pathol 15:717, 1984

71. Shapiro L: Infantile digital fibromatosis and aponeurotic fibroma. Case reports of two rare pseudosarcomas and review of the literature. Arch Dermatol 93:37, 1969

72. Reye RKD: Recurring digital fibrous tumors of childhood. Arch Pathol 80:228, 1965

73. Enzinger FM: fibrous tumors of infancy. p 375. In Tumors of Bone and Soft Tissues. Year Book Medical Publishers, Chicago, 1965

74. Viale G, Doglioni C, Iuzzolino P et al: Infantile digital fibromatosis-like tumour (inclusion body fibromatosis) of adulthood: report of two cases with ultrastructural and immunocytochemical findings. Histopathology 12:415, 1988

75. Purdy LJ, Colby TV: Infantile digital fibromatosis occurring outside the digit. Am J Surg Pathol 8:787, 1984

76. Sarma DP, Hoffman EO: Infantile digital fibroma-like tumour in adult. Arch Dermatol 116:578, 1980

77. Beckett JH, Jacobs AH: Recurring digital fibrous tumors of childhood: a review. Pediatrics 59:401, 1977

78. Allen PW: The fibromatoses: a clincopathologic classification based on 140 cases, Part 2. Am J Surg Pathol 1:305, 1977

79. McKenzie AW, Innes FLF, Rack JM et al: Digital fibrous swellings in children. Br J Dermatol 83:446, 1970

80. Iwasaki H, Kikuchi M, Ohtlsuki I et al: Infantile digital Fibromatosis. Identification of actin Filaments in cytoplasmic inclusions by heavy meromyosin binding. Cancer 52:1653, 1983

81. Yun K: Infantile digital fibromatosis. Immunoistochemical and ultrastructural observation of cytoplasmic inclusions. Cancer 61:500, 1988

82. Jensen AR, Martin LW, Longino LA: Digital neurofibrosarcoma in infancy, J Pediatr 51:566, 1957

83. Allen PW: Recurring digital fibrous tumours of childhood. Pathology 4:215, 1972

84. Chung EB, Enzinger FM: Infantile myofibromatosis. Cancer 48:1807, 1981

85. Wiswell TE, Davis J, Cunningham BE et al: Infantile myofibromatosis: The most common fibrous tumor of infancy. J Pediatr Surg 23:314, 1988

86. Daimaru Y, Hashimoto H, Enjoji M: Myofibromatosis in adults (adult counterpart of infantile myofibromatosis). Am J Surg Pathol 13(10):859, 1989

87. Fletcher CDM, Achu P, Van Noorden S, Mckee PH: Infantile myofibromatosis: a light microscopic, histochemical and immunoistochemical study suggesting true smooth muscle differentiation. Histopathology 11:245, 1987

88. Morettin LB, Mueller E. Schreiber M: Generalized hamartomatosis (congenital generalized fibromatosis). Am J Roentgenol Rad Ther Nucl Med 114:722, 1972

89. Benjamin SP, Mercer RD, Hawk WA: Myofibroblastic contraction in spontaneous regression

of multiple congenital mesenchymal hamartomas. Cancer 40:2343, 1977

90. Chung EB, Enzinger FM: Infantile fibrosarcoma. Cancer 38:729, 1976

91. Remberger K, Krieg T, Kunze D et al: Fibromatosis hyalinica multiplex (juvenile hyalin fibromatosis): light microscopic, electron microscopic, immunohistochemical, and biochemical findings. Cancer 56:614, 1985

92. Ayala AG, Ro JY, Goepfert H et al: Desmoid fibromatosis: a clinicopathologic study of 25 children. Semin Diagn Pathol 3:138, 1986

93. Dehner LP, Askin FB: Tumors of fibrous tissue origin in childhood. A clinicopathologic study of cutaneous and soft tissue neoplasms in 66 children. Cancer 38:888, 1976

94. Fromowitz FB, Hurst LC, Nathan J et al: Infantile (desmoid type) fibromatosis with extensive ossification. Am J Surg Pathol 11:66, 1987

95. Butler JJ: Fibrous tissue tumors: Nodular fasciitis, dermatofibrosarcoma protuberans and fibrosarcoma, Grade I, desmoid type. p. 397. In Copeland MM, Martin R (eds): Tumors of Bone and Soft Tissue. Year Book Medical Publishers, Chicago, 1965

96. Keasbey LE: Juvenile aponeurotic fibroma (calcifying fibroma). A distinctive tumor arising in the palms and soles of young children. Cancer 6:338, 1953

97. Lichtenstein L, Goldman RL: the cartilage analogue of fibromatosis: A reinterpretation of the condition called "juvenile aponeurotic fibroma." Cancer 17:810, 1964

98. Goldman RL: The cartilage analogue of fibromatosis (aponeurotic fibroma). Further observation based on 7 new cases. Cancer 26:1325, 1970

99. Allen PW, Enzinger FM: Juvenile aponeurotic fibroma. Cancer 26:857, 1970

100. Keasbey LE, Fanselau HA: The aponeurotic fibroma. Clin Orthop 19:115, 1961

101. Chung EB, Enzinger FM: Chondroma of soft parts. Cancer 41:1414, 1978

102. Shmookler BM, Enzinger FM: Giant cell fibroblastoma: a peculiar childhood tumor (Abstract). Lab Invest 46:76A, 1982

103. Abdul-Karim FW, Evans HL, Silva EG: Giant cell fibroblastoma: a report of three cases. Am J Clin Pathol 83:165, 1965

104. Barr RJ, Young EM Jr, Liao S-Y: Giant cell fibroblastoma: an immunohistochemical study. J Cutan Pathol 13:301, 1986

105. Dymock RB, Allen PW, Stirling JM, et al: Giant cell fibroblastoma. A distinctive, recurrent tumor of childhood. Am J Surg Pathol 11:263, 1987

106. Chou P, Gonzales-Crussi F, Mangkornkanok M: Giant cell fibroblastoma. Cancer 63:756, 1989

107. Enzinger FM, Weiss SW (eds): Soft Tissue Tumors. 2nd Ed. p. 201. CV Mosby, St. Louis, 1988

108. Pritchard DJ, Soule EH, Taylor WF et al: Fibrosarcoma-a clinicopathologic and statistical study of 199 tumors of the soft tissues of the extremities and trunk. Cancer 33:888, 1974

109. Pack GT, Ariel IM: Fibrosarcoma of the soft somatic tissues. A clinical and pathologic study. Surgery 31:443, 1952

110. Castro EB, Hajdu SI, Fortner JG: Surgical therapy of fibrosarcoma of extremities. A reappraisal. Arch Surg 107:284, 1973

111. Stout AP: Fibrosarcoma. The malignant tumor of fibroblasts. Cancer 1:30, 1948

112. Fleming RM, Rezek PR: Sarcoma developing in an old burn scar. Am J Surg 54:457, 1941

113. Schwartz EE, Rothstein JD: Fibrosarcoma following radiation therapy. JAMA 203:296, 1968

114. Gane NFC, Lindup R, Strickland P et al: Radiation-induced fibrosarcoma. Br J Cancer 24:705, 1970

115. Enzinger FM, Weiss SW (eds): Soft Tissue Tumors. 2nd Ed. p. 210. CV Mosby, 1988

116. Mackenzie DH: Fibroma: a dangerous diagnosis. A review of 205 cases fibrosarcoma of soft tissues. Br J Surg 51:607, 1964

117. Bizer LS: Fibrosarcoma. Report of sixty-four cases. Am J Surg 121:586, 1971

118. Weiss SW: Proliferating fibroblastic lesions: from hyperplasia to neoplasia. Am J Surg Pathol 10(Suppl 1):14, 1986

119. Balsaver AM, Butler JJ, Martin RG: Congenital fibrosarcoma. Cancer 20:1607, 1967

120. Stout AP: Fibrosarcoma in infants and children. Cancer 15:1028, 1962

121. Iwasaki H, Enjoji M: Infantile and adult fibrosarcomas of the soft tissues. Acta Pathol Jpn 29:377, 1979

122. Gonzalez-Crussi F: Ultrastructure of congenital fibrosarcoma. Cancer 26:1289, 1970

123. Dahl I, Save-Soderbergh J, Angervall L: Fibrosarcoma in early infancy. Pathol Eur 8:193, 1973

124. Gonzales-Crussi F, Wielerhold MD, Sotelo-

Avila C: Congenital fibrosarcoma. Presence of a histiocytic component. Cancer 46:77, 1980

125. Dehner LP, Kaye V, Levitt C et al: Cellular inflammatory pseudotumor in young individuals: a lesion distinguishable from fibrous histiocytoma or myosarcoma? Lab Invest 44:14A, 1981

126. Egan MJ, Raafat F, Crocker J, Smith K: Nucleolar organiser regions in fibrous proliferations of childhood and infantile fibrosarcoma. J Clin Pathol 41:31, 1988

127. Speleman F, Cin PD, Depotter K et al: Cytogenetic investigation of a case of congenital fibrosarcoma. Cancer Genet Cytogenet 39:21, 1989

128. Mandahl N, Heim S, Ryhdolm A, Willen H, Mitelman F: Nonrandom numerical chromosome aberrations (+8, +11, +17, +20) in infantile fibrosarcoma. Cancer Genet Cytogenet 40;137, 1989

129. Wilson MB, Stanley W, Sens D, Garvin AJ: Infantile fibrosarcoma—a misnomer? Pediatr Pathol 10:901, 1990

130. Soule EH, Pritchard DJ: Fibrosarcoma in infants and children. A review of 110 cases. Cancer 40:1711, 1977

131. Ninane J, Gosseye S, Panteon E et al: Congenital fibrosarcoma. Preoperative chemotherapy and conservative surgery. Cancer 58:1400, 1986

132. Ozzello L, Stout AP, Murray MR: Cultural characteristics of malignant histiocytomas and fibrous xanthomas. Cancer 16:331, 1963

133. O'Brien JE, Stout AP: Malignant fibrous xanthomas. Cancer 17:1445, 1964

134. Enzinger FM, Zhang R: Plexiform fibrohistiocytic tumor presenting in children and young adults. An analysis of 65 cases. Am J Surg Pathol 12:818, 1988

135. Helwig EB, Hackney VC: Juvenile xanthogranuloma (nevoxantho-endothelioma). Am J Pathol 30:625, 1954

136. McDonagh JER: A contribution to our knowledge of the naevo-xantho-endotheliomata. Br J Dermatol 24:85, 1912

137. Sonoda T, Hashimoto H, Enjoji M: Juvenile xanthogranuloma. Clinicopathologic analysis and immunohistochemical study of 57 patients. Cancer 56:2280, 1985

138. Tahan SR, Pastel-Levy C, Bhan A, Mihm MC: Juvenile xanthogranuloma. Clinical and pathologic characterization. Arch Pathol Lab Med 113:1057, 1989

139. Webster SB, Reister HC, Harman LE Jr: Juvenile xanthogranuloma with extracutaneous lesions. A case report and review of the literature. Arch Dermatol 93:71, 1966

140. Gonzalez-Crussi F, Campbell RJ: Juvenile xanthogranuloma. Ultrastructural study. Arch Pathol 89:65, 1970

141. Janney CG, Hurt MA, Santa Cruz DJ: Deep juvenile xanthogranuloma. Subcutaneous and intramuscular forms. Am J Surg Pathol 15(2):150, 1991

142. Davies BT, Wood SR: The so-called reticulo-histiocytoma of the skin: a comparison of two distinct types. Br J Dermatol 67:205, 1955

143. Ehrlich GE, Young I, Nosheny SZ et al: Multicentric reticulohistiocytosis (lipoid dermatoarthritis). Am J Med 52:830, 1972

144. Rentiers PL, Montgomery H: Nodular subepidermal fibrous (dermatofibroma versus histiocytoma). Arch Dermatol Syph 59:568, 1949

145. Gross RE, Wolbach SB: Sclerosing hemangiomas: their relationship to dermatofibroma, histiocytoma, xanthoma and certain pigmented lesions of the skin. Am J Pathol 19:533, 1943

146. Gonzalez S, Duarte E: Benign fibrous histiocytoma of the skin. A morphologic study of 290 cases. Pathol Res Pract 174:379, 1982

147. Meister P, Konrad E, Krauss F: Fibrous histiocytoma: a histological and statistical analysis of 155 cases. Pathol Res Pract 162:361, 1978

148. Fitzpatrick TB, Gilchrest BA: Dimple sign to differentiating benign from malignant pigmented cutaneous lesions. N Engl J Med 296:1518, 1977

149. Fine G, Yang HY, Morales A et al: Ultrastructural study of histiocytomas (Abstract). Am Clin Pathol 67:214, 1977

150. Dahl I: Atypical fibroxanthoma of the skin. A clinicopathological study of 57 cases. Acta Pathol Microbiol Scand 84A:183, 1976

151. Leyva WH, Santa Cruz DJ: Atypical cutaneous fibrous histiocytoma. Am J Dermatopathol 8:467, 1986

152. Tamada S, Ackerman AB: Dermatofibroma with monster cells. Am J Dermatopathol 9:380, 1987

153. Beham A, Fletcher CDM: Atypical "pseudosarcomatous" variant of cutaneous benign fi-

brous histiocytoma: report of eight cases. Histopathology 17:165, 1990

154. Niemi KM: The benign fibrohistiocytic tumors of the skin. Acta Derm Venereol 50(Suppl 63):1, 1970

155. Darier J, Ferrand M: Dermatofibromas progressifs et recidivants ou fibrosarcomas de la peau. Ann Dermatol Syph 5:545, 1924

156. Hoffman E: Uber das knollentreibende fibrosarkom der haut (dermatofibrosarkom protuberans). Dermat Ztschr 43:1, 1925

157. Taylor HB, Helwig EB: Dermatofibrosarcoma protuberans: a study of 115 cases. Cancer 15:717, 1962

158. Fletcher CDM, Evans BJ, Macartney JC, Smith N, Wilson Jones E, McKee PH: Dermatofibrosarcoma protuberans: a clinicopathological and immunohistochemical study with a review of the literature. Histopathology 9:921, 1985

159. Rockley PF, Robinson JK, Magid M, Goldblatt D: Dermatofibrosarcoma protuberans of the scalp: a series of cases. J Am Acad Dermatol 212:278, 1989

160. Schuller DE, Snyderman CH, Quivey JM: Dermatofibrosarcoma protuberans [clinical conference]. Head Neck 12(2):178, 1990

161. Frankenthaler R, Ayala AG, Hartwick RW, Goepfert H: Fibrosarcoma of the head and neck. Laryngoscope 100:799, 1990

162. Lambert WC, Aggress R, Figge DC et al: Dermatofibrosarcoma protuberans of the vulva. Gynecol Oncol 16:288, 1983

163. Frierson HF, Cooper PH: Myxoid variant of dermatofibrosarcoma protuberans. Am J Surg Pathol 7:445, 1983

164. Ding J, Hashimoto H, Enjoji M: Dermatofibrosarcoma protuberans with fibrosarcomatous areas. Cancer 64:721–729, 1989

165. Wrotnowski U, Cooper PH, Smookler BM: Fibrosarcomatous change in dermatofibrosarcoma protuberans. Am J Surg Pathol 12(4):287, 1988

166. Enzinger FM, Weiss SW (eds): Soft Tissue Tumors. 2nd Ed. p. 256. CV Mosby, St. Louis, 1988

167. O'Dowd J, Laidler P: Progression of dermatofibrosarcoma protuberans to malignant fibrous histiocytoma: report of a case with implications for tumor histogenesis. Hum Pathol 19:368, 1988

168. Beham A, Fletcher CDM: Dermatofibrosarcoma protuberans with areas resembling giant cell fibroblastoma: report of two cases. Histopathology 17:165, 1990

169. Hashimoto K, Brownstein MH, Jakobiec FA: Dermatofibrosarcoma protuberans: a tumor with perineural and endoneural cell features. Arch Dermatol 110:874, 1974

170. Ozzello L, Hamels J: The histiocytic nature of dermatofibrosarcoma protuberans: tissue culture and electron microscopic study. Am J Clin Pathol 65:136, 1976

171. Alguacil-Garcia A, Unni KK, Goellner JR: Histogenesis of dermatofibrosarcoma protuberans: an ultrastructural study. Am J Clin Pathol 69:427, 1978

172. Kindblom LG, Jacobsen GK, Jacobsen M: Immunohistochemical investigation of tumors of supposed fibroblastic-histiocytic origin. Human Pathol 13:834, 1982

173. Yoshida H, Matsui K, Hashimoto K: Dermatofibrosarcoma protuberans and its tissue culture study—ultrastructural, enzyme histochemical and immunological stydy. Acta Pathol Jpn 32:83, 1982

174. Gutierrez G, Ospina JE, de Baez NE et al: Dermatofibrosarcoma protuberans. Int J Dermatol 23:396, 1984

175. Escalona-Zapata J, Fernandez EA, Escuin FL: The fibroblastic nature of dermatofibrosarcoma protuberans. A tissue culture and ultrastructural study. Virchows Arch [A] 391:165, 1981

176. Lautier R, Wolff HH, Jones RE: An immunohistochemical study of dermatofibrosarcoma protuberans supports its fibroblastic character and contradicts neuroectodermal of histiocytic components. Am J Dermatopathol 12(1):25, 1990

177. Hirabashi S, Kajikawa A, Kanazawa K, Mimoto K: Dermatofibrosarcoma protuberans with regional lymph node metastasis: a case report. Head Neck 11(6):562, 1990

178. Bonnabeau RC, Stoughton WB, Armanious AW et al: Dermatofibrosarcoma protuberans: report of a case with pulmonary metastasis and multiple intrathoracic recurrences. Oncology 29:1, 1974

179. Brenner W, Schaefler K, Chhabra H et al: Dermatofibrosarcoma protuberans metastatic to a regional lymph node. Cancer 36:1987, 1975

180. Volpe R, Carbone A: Dermatofibrosarcoma protuberans metastatic to lymph nodes and

showing a dominant histiocytic component. Am J Dermatopathol 5:327, 1983

181. McPeak CJ, Cruz T, Nicastri AD: Dermatofibrosarcoma protuberans: an analysis of 86 cases—five with metastasis. Ann Surg 166:803, 1967

182. Kahn LB, Saxe N, Gordon W: Dermatofibrosarcoma protuberans with lymph node and pulmonary metastases. Arch Dermatol 114:599, 1978

183. Roses DF, Valensi Q, LaTrenta G et al: Surgical treatment of dermatofibrosarcoma protuberans. Surg Gynecol Obstet 162:449, 1986

184. Das Gupta TK: Tumors of Soft Tissues. p. 396. Appleton-Century-Crofts, Norwalk, 1983

185. Bednař B: Storiform neurofibromas of the skin, pigmented and nonpigmented. Cancer 10:368, 1957

186. Dupree WB, Langloss JM, Weiss SW: Pigmented dermatofibrosarcoma protuberans (Bednař tumor). A pathologic, ultrastructural, and immunohistochemical study. Am J Surg Pathol 9:630, 1985

187. Fletcher CDM, Theaker JM, Flanagnan A, Krausz T: Pigmented dermatofibrosarcoma protuberans (Bednař tumor): melanocytic colonization or neuroectodermal differentiation? A clinicopathological and immunohistochemical study. Histopathology 13:631, 1988

188. Nakamura T, Ogata H, Katsuyama T: Pigmented dermatofibrosarcoma protuberans. Am J Dermatopathol 9(1):18, 1987

189. Miyamoto Y, Morimatsu M, Nakashima T: Pigmented storiform neurofibroma. Acta Pathol Jpn 34:821, 1984

190. O'Brien JE, Stout AP: Malignant fibrous xanthomas. Cancer 17:1445, 1964

191. Weiss SW, Enzinger FM: Malignant fibrous histiocytoma. An analysis of 200 cases. Cancer 41:2250, 1978

192. Enterline HT: Histopathology of sarcomas. Semin Oncol 8(2):133, 1981

193. Enjoji M, Hashimoto H, Tsuneyoshi M et al: Malignant fibrous histiocytoma. A clinicopathologic study of 130 cases. Acta Pathol Jpn 30:727, 1980

194. Fisher C: The value of electronmicroscopy and immunohistochemistry in the diagnosis of soft tissue sarcomas: a study of 200 cases. Histopathology 16:441, 1990

195. Fu YS, Gabbiani G, Kaye GI et al: Malignant soft tissue tumors of probable histiocytic origin (malignant fibrous histiocytoma): general consideration and electron microscopic and tissue culture studies. Cancer 35:176, 1975

196. Taxy J, Battifora H: Malignant fibrous histiocytoma. A clinicopathologic and ultrastructural study. Cancer 40:254, 1977

197. du Boulay CEH: Demonstration of alpha-1-antitrypsin and alpha-1-antichymotrypsin in fibrous histiocytoma using immunoperoxidase technique. Am J Surg Pathol 6:559, 1982

198. Meister P, Hohne N, Conrad E, Eder M: Fibrous histiocytoma: an analysis of storiform pattern. Virchows Arch [A] 383:31, 1979

199. Elias JM: Immunohistopathology. A practical approach to diagnosis. p. 503. American Society of Clinical Pathologists, Chicago, 1990

200. Burgdof WHC, Duray P, Rosai J: Immunohistochemical identification of lysozyme in cutaneous lesions of alleged histiocytic nature. Am J Clin Pathol 75:162, 1981

201. Strauchen JA, Dimitriu-Bona A: Malignant fibrous histiocytoma. Expression of monocyte/macrophage differentiation antigens detected with monoclonal antibodies. Am J Pathol 124:303, 1986

202. Soini Y, Miettinen M: Immunohistochemistry of markers of histiomonocytic cells in malignant fibrous histiocytomas. A monoclonal antibody study. Pathol Res Pract 186:759, 1990

203. Wood GS, Beckstead JH, Turner RR et al: Malignant fibrous histiocytoma tumor cells resemble fibroblasts. Am J Surg Pathol 10:323, 1986

204. Genberg M, Mark J, Hakelius L et al: Origin and relationship between different cell types in malignant fibrous histiocytoma. Am J Pathol 135(6):1185, 1989

205. Rohol PJM, Kleijne J, van Basten CDH et al: A study to analyze the origin of tumor cells in malignant fibrous histiocytomas. A multiparametric characterization. Cancer 56:2809, 1985

206. Meister P: Malignant fibrous histiocytoma. History, histology, histogenesis. Pathol Res Pract 183:1, 1988

207. Brooks JJ: Designificance of double phenotypic patterns and markers in human sarcomas. A new model of mesenchymal differentiation. Am J Pathol 125:113, 1986

208. Kearney MM, Soule EH, Ivins JC: Malignant

fibrous histiocytoma. A retrospective study of 167 cases. Cancer 45:167, 1980

209. Bertoni F, Capanna R, Biagini R et al: Malignant fibrous histiocytoma of soft tissue. An analysis of 78 cases located and deeply seated in the extremities. Cancer 56:356, 1985

210. Helwig EB: Atypical fibroxanthoma. In tumor seminar. Tex Med 59:664, 1963

211. Fretzin DF, Helwig EB: Atypical fibroxanthoma of the skin. A clinicopathologic study of 140 cases. Cancer 31:1541, 1973

212. Jacobs DS, Edwards WD, Ye RC: Metastatic atypical fibroxanthoma of skin. Cancer 35:457, 1975

213. Helwig EB, May D: Atypical fibroxanthoma of the skin with metastasis. Cancer 57:368, 1986

214. Ricci A Jr, Cartun RW, Zakowski MF: Atypical fibroxanthoma. A study of 14 cases emphasizing the presence of Langerhans' histiocytes with implications for differential diagnosis by antibody panels. Am J Surg Pathol 12(8):591, 1988

215. Barr RJ, Wuerker RB, Graham JH: Ultrastructure of atypical fibroxanthoma. Cancer 40:736, 1977

216. Weedon D, Kerr JFR: Atypical fibroxanthoma of skin: an electron microscope study. Pathology 7:173, 1975

217. Alguacil-Garcia A, Unni KK, Goellner JR et al: Atypical fibroxanthoma of the skin. An ultrastructural study of two cases. Cancer 40:1471, 1977

218. Starink TM, Hausman R, Van Delden, Neering H: Atypical fibroxanthoma of the skin: presentation of 5 cases and review of the literature. Br J Dermatol 97:167, 1977

219. Enzinger FM: Malignant fibrous histiocytoma 20 years after Stout. Am J Surg Pathol 10(Suppl 1):43, 1986

220. Weiss SW, Enzinger FM: Myxoid variant of malignant fibrous histiocytoma. Cancer 39:1672, 1977

221. Weiss SW: Malignant fibrous histiocytoma. A reaffirmation. Am J Surg Pathol 6:773, 1982

222. Kyriakos M, Kempson RL: Inflammatory fibrous histiocytoma. All aggressive and lethal lesion. Cancer 37:1584, 1976

223. Vilanova JR, Burgos-Bretones J, Simon R et al: Leukaemoid reaction and eosinophilia in "inflammatory fibrous histiocytoma." Virchows Arch [A] 388:237, 1980

224. Leak LV, Caulfield JB, Burke JF et al: Electron microscopic studies on a human fibromyxosarcoma. Cancer Res 27:261, 1967

225. Angervall L, Kindblom L-G, Merck C: Myxofibrosarcoma. A study of 30 cases. Acta Pathol Microbiol Scand 85A:127, 1977

226. Tsuneyoshi M, Hashimoto H, Enjoji M: Myxoid malignant fibrous histiocytoma versus myxoid liposarcoma. A comparative ultrastructural study. Virchows Arch [A] 400:187, 1983

227. Guccion JG, Enzinger FM: Malignant giant cell tumor of soft parts. An analysis of 32 cases. Cancer 29:1518, 1972

228. van Haelst UJGM, de Haas Dorsser AH: Giant cell tumor of soft parts. An ultrastructural study. Virchows Arch [A] 371:199, 1976

229. Alguacil-Garcia A, Unni KK, Goellner JR: Malignant giant cell tumor of soft parts. An ultrastructural study of four cases. Cancer 40:244, 1977

230. Chung EB, Enzinger FM: Extraskeletal osteosarcoma. Cancer 60:1132, 1987

231. Kahn LB: Retroperitoneal xanthogranuloma and xanthosarcoma (malignant fibrous xanthoma). Cancer 31:411, 1973

232. Kindblom L-G: Malignant melanomas simulating soft tissue sarcoma. Proceedings of International Post-graduate Course on Soft Tissue Pathology. p. 32. Riva del Garde, Italy, April 18–21, 1990

233. Enzinger FM: Angiomatoid malignant fibrous histiocytoma: a distinct fibrohistiocytic tumor of children and young adults simulating a vascular neoplasm. Cancer 44:2147, 1979

234. Caballero LR, Rodriguez AC, Sopelana AB: Angiomatoid malignant fibrous histiocytoma of the orbit. Am J Ophthalmol 92:13, 1981

235. Sun CCJ, Toker C, Breitenecker R: An ultrastructural study of angiomatoid fibrous histiocytoma. Cancer 49:2103, 1982

236. Leu HJ, Makek M: Angiomatoid malignant fibrous histiocytoma. Arch Pathol Lab Med 110:466, 1986

237. Kay S: Angiomatoid malignant fibrous histiocytoma: report of two cases with ultrastructural observations of one case. Arch Pathol Lab Med 109:934, 1985

238. Kanter MH, Duane GO: Angiomatoid malignant fibrous histiocytoma: cytology of fine needle aspiration and its differential diagnosis. Arch Pathol Lab Med 109:564, 1985

239. Wegmann W, Heitz U: Angiomatoid malignant fibrous histiocytoma: evidence for the histiocytic origin of tumor cells. Virchows Arch [A] 406:59, 1985

240. Argenyi ZB, Van Rybroek JJ, Kemp JD, Soper RT: Congenital angiomatoid malignant fibrous histiocytoma: a light, immunopathologic, and electron-microscopic study. Am J Dermatopathol 10:59, 1988

241. Pettinato G, Manivel JC, De Rosa G et al: Angiomatoid malignant fibrous histiocytoma: cytologic, immunohistochemical, ultrastructural, and flow cytometric study of 20 cases. Mod Pathol 3:479, 1990

242. Costa MJ, Weiss SW: Angiomatoid malignant fibrous histiocytoma. A follow-up study of 108 cases with evaluation of possible histologic predictors of outcome. Am J Surg Pathol 14:1126, 1990

243. Seo SI, Frizzera G, Coates TD et al: Angiomatoid malignant fibrous histiocytoma with extensive lymphadenopathy simulating Castelman's disease. Pediatr Pathol 6:233, 1986

244. El-Naggar AK, Ro JY, Ayala AG et al: Angiomatoid malignant fibrous histiocytoma: a DNA flow cytometric analysis of 7 cases. Am J Clin Pathol 90:502, 1988

3

Tumors of Adipose Tissue

E. B. Chung, Andrea O. Cavazzana, Ambrogio S. Fassina

Tumors of adipose tissue represent the most common form of soft tissue neoplasm in adults, and most benign lipomatous lesions do not present any particular diagnostic problems. On the other hand, lipomatous soft tissue masses in children are uncommon.[1] Moreover, there exists a group of benign lipomatous tumors, including spindle cell and pleomorphic lipomas, lipoblastoma and lipoblastomatosis, and intramuscular lipoma, that may cause considerable diagnostic problems, and are occasionally mistaken for liposarcomas.

Atypical lipoma or well-differentiated lipomalike liposarcoma, round cell liposarcoma, and poorly differentiated or dedifferentiated liposarcoma are sometimes difficult to recognize and in some cases, have given rise to controversy. Nevertheless, a great variety of tumors of adipose tissue are well defined and easily classified (Table 3-1).

For a better understanding of lipomatous tumors, it is necessary to provide a short description of the principal cell types encountered in normal adipogenesis and a brief discussion of their significance in tumor diagnosis.

Embryologically, adipose tissue is known to develop between the 26th and 30th weeks of gestation from primitive mesenchymal cells, as evidenced by their ability to synthesize and store lipids.[2] Small lipid droplets are first seen to accumulate about either pole of the primitive spindle cell (prelipoblast). At the mid-stage of development, lipid droplets coalesce into larger droplets, which mold the centrally placed nucleus; at this stage, the cell has a "moruloid" appearance (*the multivacuolated lipoblast*). Occasionally a single medium-sized lipid droplet accumulates at one pole and pushes the nucleus toward the opposite pole (*the monovacuolated* or *signet ring lipoblast*). Finally, a large accumulation of lipid fills the cytoplasm and flattens the nucleus against the plasma membrane (*the adipocyte* or *mature fat cell*). This process of adipogenesis apparently no longer takes place once adulthood is reached.

Monovacuolated and/or multivacuolated lipoblasts are found in both benign and malignant tumors, therefore their presence per se does not necessarily connote malignancy, particularly in infancy and childhood. On the other hand, malignant lipoblasts, when present, are the hallmarks of liposarcoma regardless of the patient's age and the tumor location. Malignant lipoblasts are currently defined as lipoblasts with large pleomorphic and hyperchromatic nuclei, occasionally with prominent nucleoli. When the malignant lipoblasts are not present, the pathologist must be able to recognize unequivocal, multivacuolated lipoblasts among many "impostors," as their presence in tumors of adulthood is decisive for a diagnosis of liposarcoma.

The principal cellular phenotypes occurring in normal adipogenesis and related tumors are shown in Figure 3-1. Because of their greater specificity and the recent developments regarding their recognition, this chapter considers only those entities listed in bold print in Table 3-1.

Table 3-1. Histologic Classification of Adipose Tissue Tumors

Benign	Malignant
Lipoma	
Angiolipoma	
Spindle cell and pleomorphic lipoma	**Atypical lipoma**
Lipoblastoma and lipoblastomatosis	**Well-differentiated liposarcoma**
Angiomyolipoma	**Myxoid liposarcoma**
Myelolipoma	**Round cell liposarcoma**
Intramuscular lipoma	**Pleomorphic liposarcoma**
Diffuse lipomatosis	**Dedifferentiated liposarcoma**
Hibernoma	

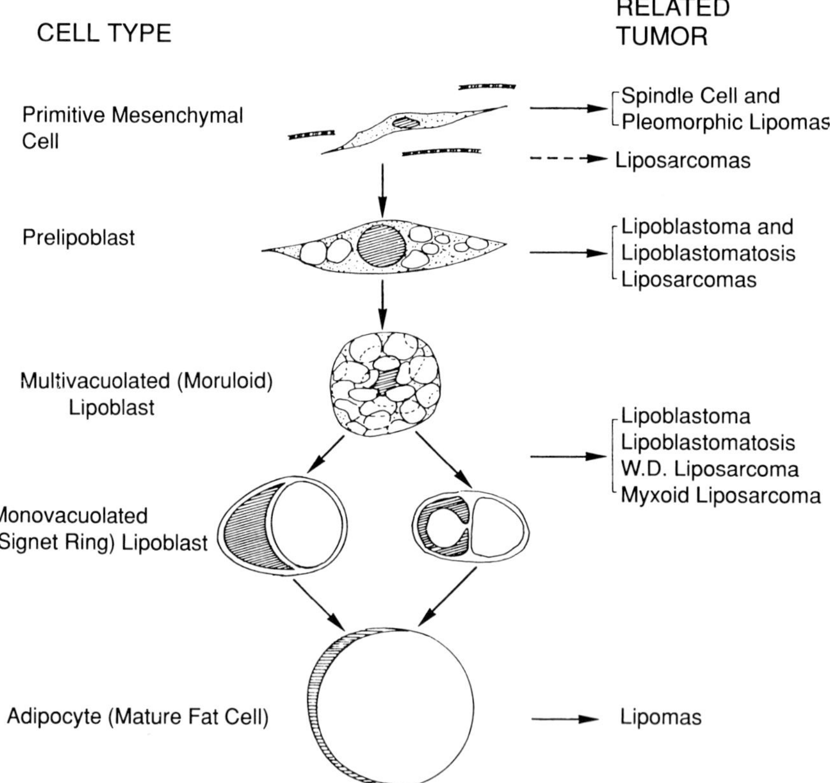

Fig. 3-1. Diagrammatic representation of the principal cell types occurring in normal adipogenesis and lipomatous tumors.

BENIGN TUMORS OF
ADIPOSE TISSUE

SPINDLE CELL AND PLEOMORPHIC LIPOMAS

A group of uncommon lipomas with typical clinical setting and gross appearance have been designated spindle cell and pleomorphic lipomas in view of their distinct microscopic features.[3, 4] Both types are believed to represent histogenetically related variants of the same tumor, in which the spindle cells correspond to the stellate mesenchymal cells of the primitive fat lobule.[5]

These tumors occur chiefly in male patients between 45 and 65 years of age and are most commonly found in the regions of the posterior neck and shoulder.[3, 4] Occasionally they are also found in women and young individuals, and at other anatomic sites.[6] They manifest as solitary, painless, slow-growing, firm nodules in the deep subcutaneous tissue that are often present for several years.

Grossly the tumor nodules resemble ordinary lipomas, except for gray-white gelatinous areas.

Microscopically spindle cell lipomas are characterized by a mixture of mature adipocytes and uniform spindle cells set in a mucoid matrix or intimately associated with mature collagen fibers (Figs. 3-2 and 3-3) and scattered mast cells. Occasionally the spindle cells predominate. The vascular pattern is generally inconspicuous.

As the name implies, pleomorphic lipomas display scattered bizarre giant cells, often with a "floret" appearance, and are usually embedded in dense collagenous tissue (Figs. 3-4 and 3-5). In some cases, transitional forms between spindle cell and pleomorphic lipomas are seen.

Differential Diagnosis

Spindle lipoma can be distinguished from liposarcoma with a predominant spindle cell pattern by uniformity of spindle cells and the absence of lipoblasts. Pleomorphic lipoma, on the other hand, closely resembles pleomorphic liposarcoma, as floretlike cells are common to both

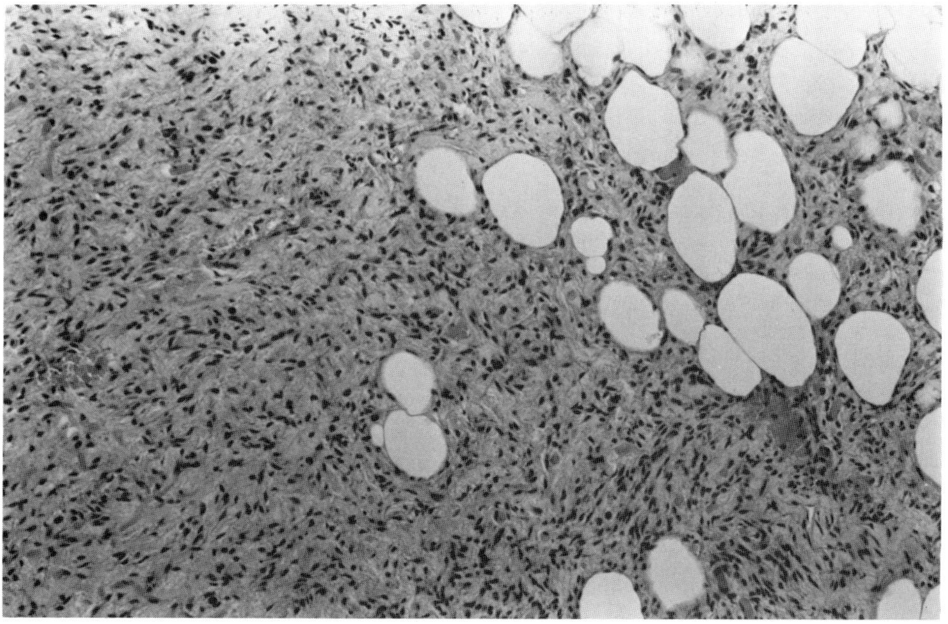

Fig. 3-2. Spindle cell lipoma showing a mixture of mature fat cells and uniform spindle cells that are associated with a myxoid matrix. (H&E, × 125.)

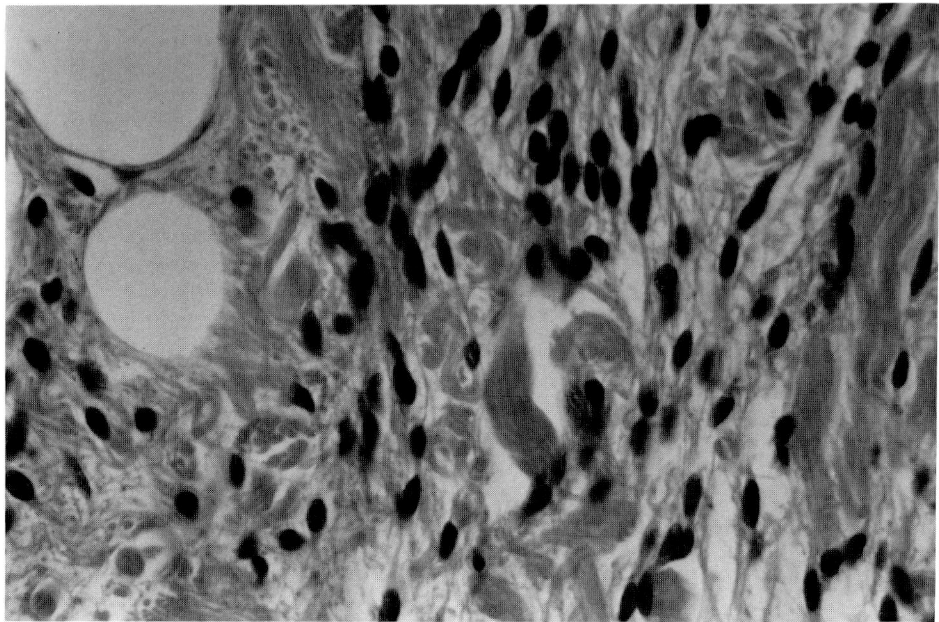

Fig. 3-3. Spindle cell lipoma in which small well-oriented spindle cells lacking nuclear pleomorphism are accompanied by bundles of mature collagen (H&E, × 500.)

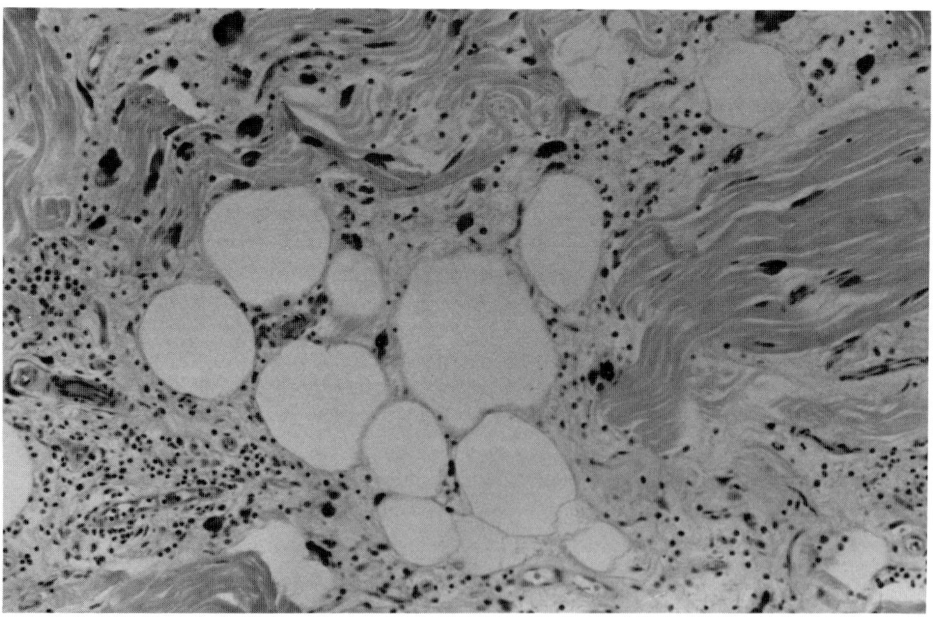

Fig. 3-4. Pleomorphic lipoma. Note the mixture of mature fat cells, multinucleated giant cells, and mononuclear inflammatory cells. (H&E, × 125.)

LIFE COLLEGE-LIBRARY
1269 Barclay Circle
Marietta, GA 30060

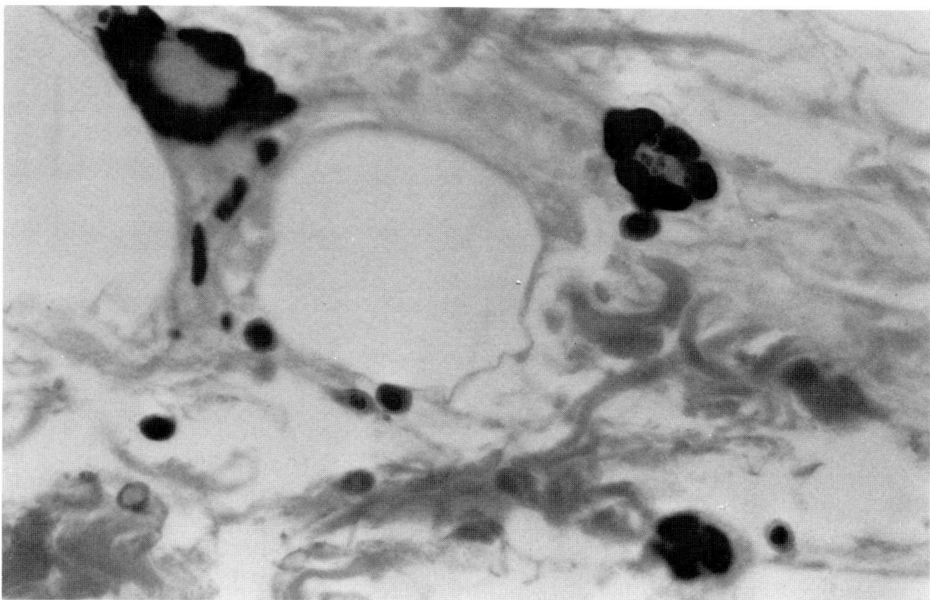

Fig. 3-5. Pleomorphic lipoma depicting characteristic floretlike giant cells. (H&E, × 500.)

tumors, but the former lacks unequivocal lipoblasts. A benign diagnosis is also supported by the superficial location and circumscription of the tumor, and its characteristic age distribution. Spindle cell lipoma of long duration may show a prominent vascular pattern that may be mistaken for a neoplasm of vascular origin.

Prognosis

The prognosis is excellent and local excision is adequate for cure in both spindle cell and pleomorphic lipomas.

LIPOBLASTOMA AND LIPOBLASTOMATOSIS

Although rare, benign tumors of developing fetal or embryonal adipose tissue occurring in infancy and early childhood often post considerable problems because their histologic picture closely resembles myxoid or well-differentiated liposarcoma.[7]

Lipoblastomatosis, a term first coined by Vellios et al.[8] in 1958, has been widely accepted as a distinct entity. It was further subdivided into two variants: lipoblastoma, which is circumscribed or encapsulated and superficial, and lipoblastomatosis, which is diffuse, infiltrative, poorly circumscribed, and deeply located.[9]

In the past, however, similar and related terms such as *lipoblastosis, lipoblastic tumor,* and *lipoblastoma* were used to describe tumors with an outright malignant appearance. The term *embryonal* or *fetal lipoma* was used as a synonym for benign lipoblastomatosis.

These benign lipogenic tumors are peculiar to children. They are most commonly found during the first three years of life and occasionally at birth. These tumors chiefly affect the extremities, (43 percent in the legs and 20 percent in the arms),[9] but they may also be found in the neck, trunk, and elsewhere. Most of the tumors are superficially located, whereas about 38 percent of cases were deep seated (lipoblastomatosis). They are generally asymptomatic and nontender. The time interval between initial discovery and removal of the mass may vary from a few days to 5 years, with a median of 6 months.

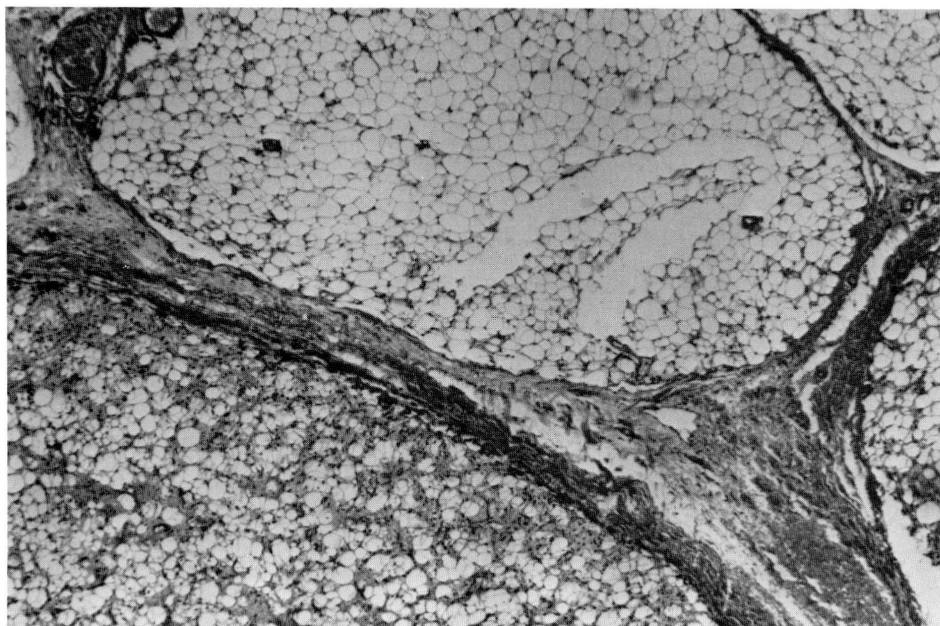

Fig. 3-6. Lipoblastoma revealing the typical multilobular pattern. Note the myxoid matrix and prominent vasculature within the lobules. (H&E, × 50.)

Radiologically, deep-situated lipoblastomatosis shows a focal periosteal reaction in close relationship to the overlying soft tissue mass.

Grossly the majority of the tumors are lobulated, globular and soft to rubbery. They usually measure 3 to 5 cm in diameter, but may range from 2 to 14 cm. The deep-seated tumors are generally encapsulated and often poorly circumscribed. The cut surfaces are pale yellow to white and frequently mottled, with solid or cystic gelatinous myxoid areas.

Microscopically both lipoblastoma and lipoblastomatosis are characterized by a lobular arrangement of immature fat cells, fibrous trabeculae of varying thickness, a prominent plexiform vascular pattern, and a myxoid stroma (Figs. 3-6 and 3-7). The lobular pattern, however, is less pronounced in the diffuse form. The constituent fat cells within the individual lobules show varying degrees of maturation or differentiation.

The mature adipocytes are often interspersed with various lipoblasts (Fig. 3-7), namely, multivacuolated, granular, monovacuolated, or signet ring types, and spindle or stellate-shaped cells (prelipoblasts). Mature fat cells are more common in the center of the individual lubules, and poorly differentiated cells are often embedded in a myxoid stroma rich in hyaluronidase-sensitive connective tissue mucin.

In some cases, hibernoma cells may be prominent. Mitotic figures are occasionally observed in mesenchymal or prelipoblastic-stage cells, but atypical forms are not observed. Foci of extramedullary erythropoiesis as well as cartilaginous metaplasia are occasionally found.

Differential Diagnosis

The major differential diagnosis involves myxoid or well-differentiated liposarcoma. Unlike liposarcoma, however, there are no lipoblasts with atypical or hyperchromatic pleomorphic nuclei (malignant lipoblasts) in either the circumscribed or diffuse form of lipoblastoma. Furthermore liposarcomas very rarely occur in children under 5 years of age.[10]

Diffuse lipoblastomatosis may be mistaken for an intramuscular lipoma, as both contain an admixture of residual striated muscle fibers.

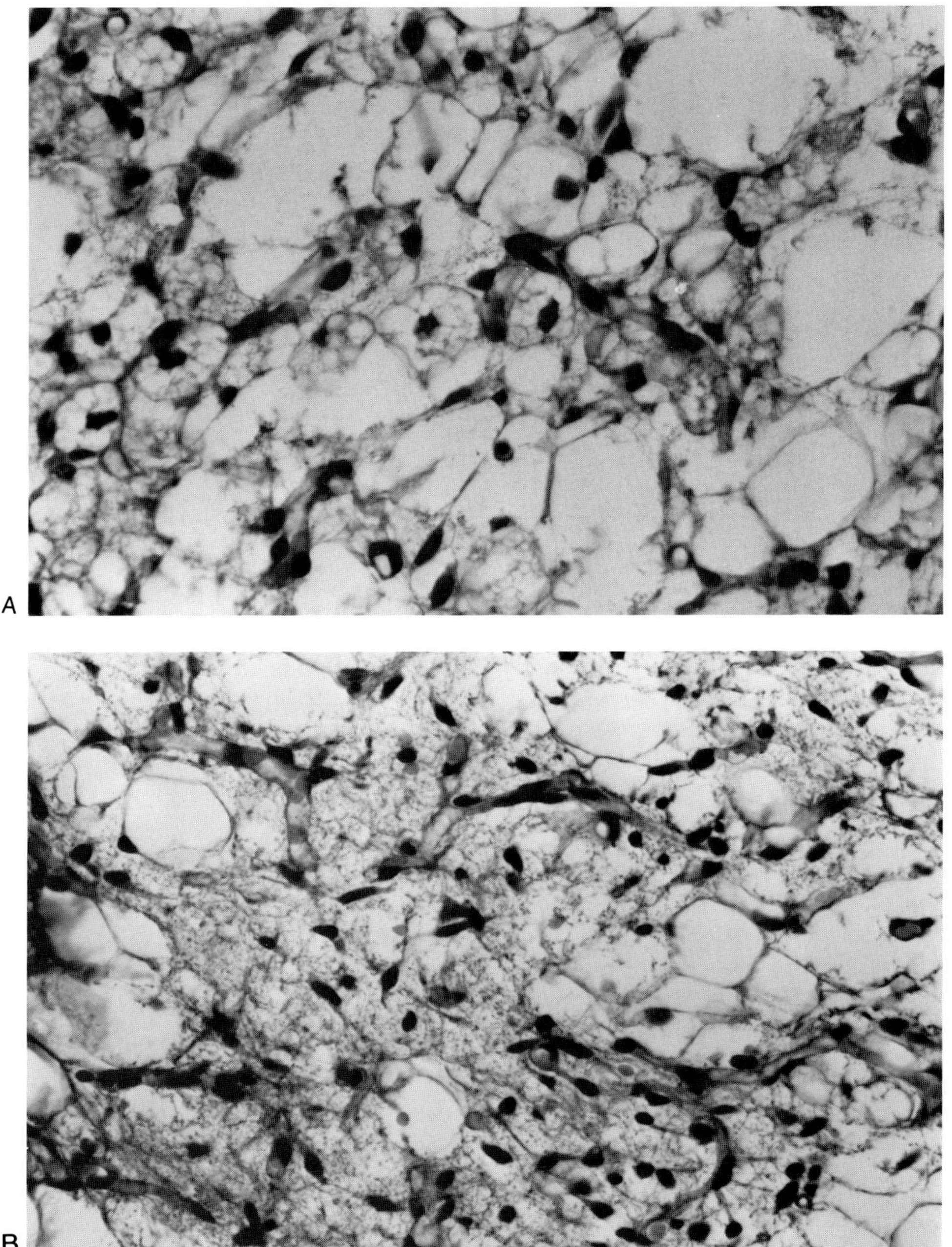

Fig. 3-7. Lipoblastoma. **(A)** Lipoblasts. Note the uniformity of cellular differentiation. **(B)** Plexiform capillaries traversing between immature fat cells. (H&E, × 500.)

Cases with broad fibrous tissue septa may be confused with infantile fibromatosis. Likewise, lipoblastomas may sometimes mimic myxomas or myxolipomas. The presence of unequivocal lipoblasts and a more or less pronounced plexiform capillary network—features that are not found in these latter tumors—should lead to the correct diagnosis.

Prognosis

The prognosis is excellent, although these tumors do recur occasionally. Recurrence, however, is usually attributable to incomplete removal of the tumor and is mostly encountered in the diffuse form (i.e., lipoblastomatosis).

INTRAMUSCULAR LIPOMA

Intramuscular lipomas are not uncommon. Their deep location, frequent large size, and infiltrative growth pattern often cause considerable concern, and they have been referred to as *infiltrating lipomas.*

Although all age groups are affected, these neoplasms are most commonly found in adults, with a median age of 44 years.[11] These tumors involve chiefly the large muscles of the extremities, especially the thigh, followed by the shoulder and chest wall. Unlike the more common subcutaneous lipomas, intramuscular lipomas are more frequent in males than females. Most tumors are slowgrowing and painless, although movement at times causes aching or pain.

The tumors vary considerably in size and are often large, some measuring 20 cm or more in diameter. On cross section, many are seen to involve irregularly both muscular and intermuscular tissue. Microscopically striated muscle is diffusely infiltrated by mature fat cells; associated muscular atrophy may be observed (Fig. 3-8). Lipoblasts or cells with atypical nuclei are not encountered (Fig. 3-9).

Differential Diagnosis

Because of its large size, deep location, and infiltrative pattern, this tumor may grossly mimic the features of a liposarcoma. Although

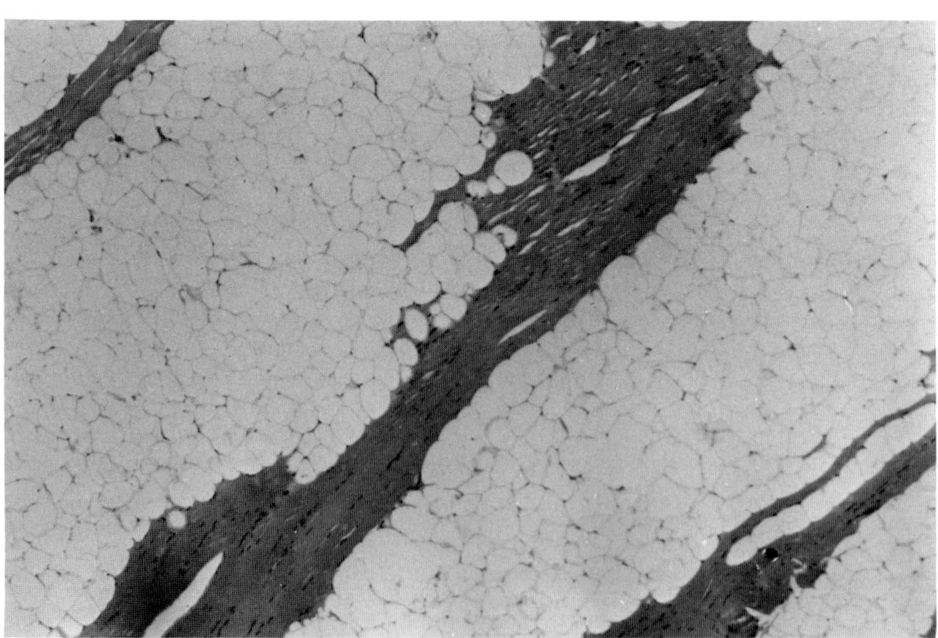

Fig. 3-8. Intramuscular lipoma. Note the striated muscle fibers in longitudinal section. (H&E, × 50.)

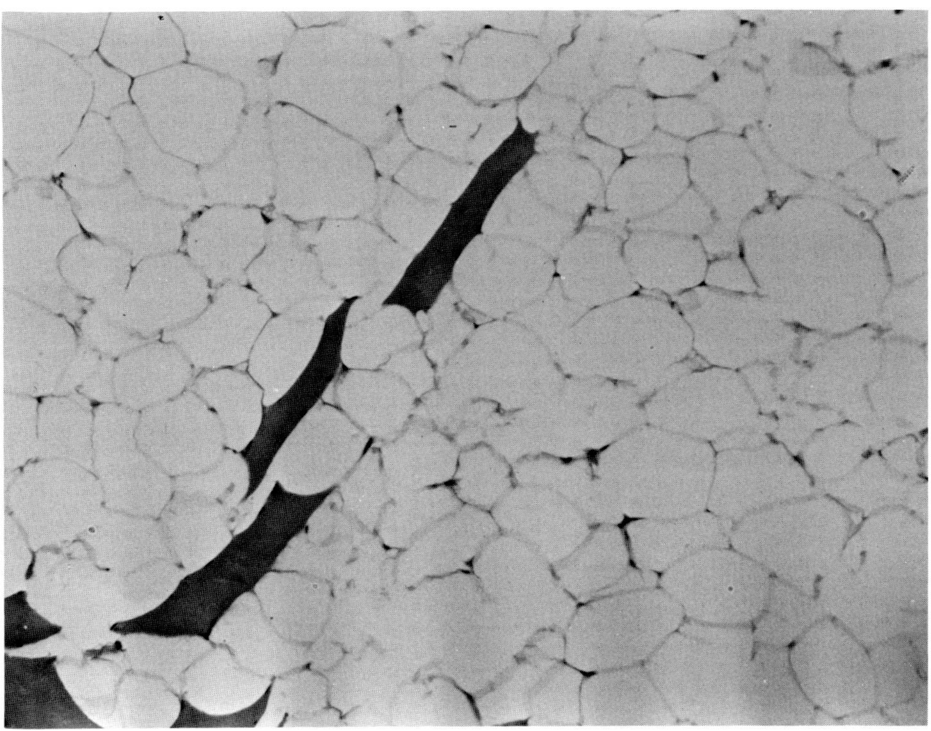

Fig. 3-9. Intramuscular lipoma showing complete lack of cellular atypism. (H&E, × 125.)

the absence of lipoblasts and cells with large hyperchromatic nuclei would support a benign diagnosis, careful tumor sampling is mandatory, as considerable portions of a well-differentiated liposarcoma may fail to demonstrate cells with atypical features.

When it occurs in children, this tumor may be mistaken for diffuse lipoblastomatosis. However, the absence of lipoblasts, a myxoid background, and a plexiform capillary pattern should help in making the correct diagnosis of intramuscular lipoma. The overgrowth of adipose tissue in an intramuscular hemangioma may mimic a richly vascularized intramuscular lipoma, and such lesions have been diagnosed as angiolipomas.

Prognosis

Recurrent rates following local excision have ranged from 3 percent[12] to 19 percent[13] to 62.5 percent.[14] Some patients have multiple recurrences, which are probably related to the adequacy of the excision and to the criteria used in distinguishing this lesion from well-differentiated liposarcoma.

MALIGNANT TUMORS OF ADIPOSE TISSUE (LIPOSARCOMAS)

Liposarcoma, in a strict sense, is a malignant infiltrative neoplasm characterized by the presence of lipoblasts in varying stages of differentiation. Thus, the presence of unequivocal lipoblasts is a prerequisite for formulating a diagnosis of liposarcoma, and their recognition is of utmost importance, especially in adults. On the other hand, vacuolated cells resembling lipoblasts are found in several lesions.[15] In fact, what one pathologist considers a lipoblast may be a histiocyte to another.[16]

Table 3-2. Relative frequency of 50 Cases of Liposarcoma According to Site[a]

	Well-differentiated	Myxoid	Round cell	Pleomorphic
Retroperitoneum	9	7	3	5
Extremities	3	14	7	2

[a] Observed at the Institute of Pathology, University of Padua, Padua, Italy.

Enzinger and Winslow,[17] in 1962, classified liposarcoma into four basic types: well-differentiated, myxoid, round cell, and pleomorphic. Subsequently, dedifferentiated liposarcoma was added.[18] Liposarcomas of the well differentiated type, particularly the lipomalike variant, are nearly always nonmetastasizing neoplasms. Thus, whether or not the term liposarcoma was justified for this group of tumors has been much discussed in the last few years, and the expression *atypical lipoma* was instead advanced[19] in analogy with the term *atypical fibroxanthoma* for superficially located cutaneous malignant fibrous histiocytoma.[20] Since their benign or malignant nature is still uncertain, we prefer to describe these tumors under the heading of malignant lipomatous tumors.

Liposarcoma is one of the most common soft tissue tumors in adults. Its peak incidence occurs during the 5th and 6th decades.[15, 16, 18, 21–25] It is extremely rare in children under 10 years of age,[10] and a slight male predominance has been reported.[24, 26] Liposarcoma occurs most frequently in the extremities, particularly the thigh, and in the retroperitoneum; the head and neck, paratesticular region, trunk, and mediastinum may also be involved. Liposarcomas of bone have rarely been described.[27–29] Multiple lesions are found in about 10 percent of the patients.[17, 24] Malignant transformation of a preexisting lipoma is an exceedingly rare event,[29–31] and its occurrence has been questioned.[17] Liposarcomas, particularly those located in the retroperitoneal area, may reach enormous sizes. Average weights of 8 kg for retroperitoneal and 1.5 kg for distal tumors have been reported.[17]

Grossly most liposarcomas are large, often well circumscribed and lobulated masses. The cut surface varies in appearance depending on the histologic type of the tumor. Some may have a myxoid or gelatinous aspect with foci of hemorrhage and necrosis, while others may show a yellow to orange or gray-white color due to the lipid content or the presence of fibrosis, respectively.

Liposarcoma classification is reported in Table 3-1, and the relative frequency of the different types according to site is shown in Table 3-2.

ATYPICAL LIPOMA

The term *atypical lipoma* was first used by Kindblom et al. in 1975[24] and was subsequently endorsed by Evans et al.[19] and Azumi et al.[32] These workers emphasized that a group of well-differentiated liposarcomas occurring in the subcutis or striated muscles, particularly those of somatic soft tissue, behave clinically as benign neoplasms. However, both spindle cell and pleomorphic lipoma were also included among the group of atypical lipomas.[33] Spindle cell and pleomorphic lipomas are benign, clinically and morphologically well-defined lipogenic tumors that have not been shown to undergo dedifferentiation.[3, 4, 34] It appears, therefore, that these tumors should be excluded from the category of atypical lipoma.

Atypical lipoma is histologically similar to well-differentiated liposarcoma of either the lipomalike or the sclerosing type (Fig. 3-10). It closely resembles ordinary lipoma. Unlike ordinary lipoma, however, atypical lipoma is characterized by the presence of atypical cells with hyperchromatic nuclei and equivocal lipoblasts that are more frequently observed in the fibrous septa of the tumor.

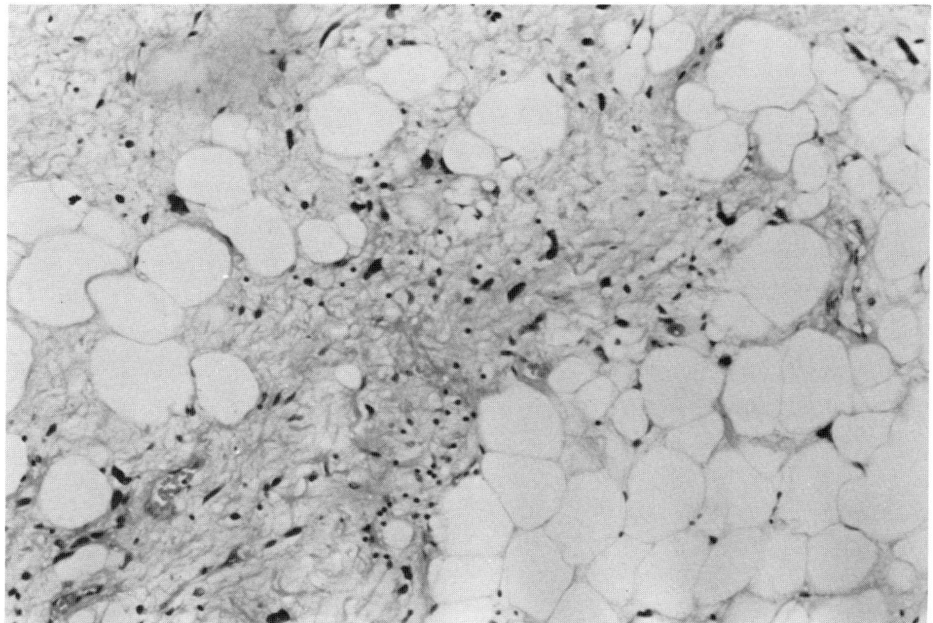

Fig. 3-10. Atypical lipoma simulating a well-differentiated sclerosing liposarcoma. (H&E, × 125.)

These tumors follow a benign clinical course and do not metastasize.[32, 35] However, four cases[35–37] showing features of dedifferentiated liposarcoma in recurrences have been reported. Therefore, if the term atypical lipoma has the advantage of sparing the patient mutilating surgery, the very remote possibility of a more aggessive behavior should always be considered, and a wide excision with long-term follow up is strongly recommended for these lesions.[37]

WELL-DIFFERENTIATED LIPOSARCOMA

This type comprises 20 to 30 percent of all liposarcomas[16, 18, 24] and is more frequently found found in the retroperitoneum. It includes three closely related subtypes, namely lipoma-like, sclerosing, and inflammatory.

The *lipomalike subtype* of well-differentiated liposarcoma is by far the most common. It closely mimics common lipoma, except for the presence of scattered hyperchromatic cells, isolated lipoblasts, and some variation in the size and shape of the lipocytes (Figs. 3-11 and 3-12). The malignant-appearing cells are often found in and about the fibrous septa or trabeculae. The *sclerosing type* is characterized by broad bands of fibrous tissue containing atypical or pleomorphic cells and occasional lipoblasts alternating with lobules of adipose tissue (Figs. 3-13 and 3-14). A prominent lymphoplasmacytic infiltrate within a background of lipogenic tumor with only scattered lipoblasts distinguishes the *inflammatory type* of well-differentiated liposarcoma (Fig. 3-15). Because of a paucity of typical lipoblasts, this liposarcoma variant is at times mistaken for an inflammatory lesion of adipose tissue.

MYXOID LIPOSARCOMA

Myxoid liposarcoma is by far the most common type of liposarcoma, accounting for 37 to 50 percent of all liposarcomas.[16–18, 24] It shows a clear predilection for the lower extremities[24]; in a series of 27 myxoid liposarcomas diagnosed at the Institute of Pathology of Padua University, 14 were localized in the lower extremities. The tumor is composed of round

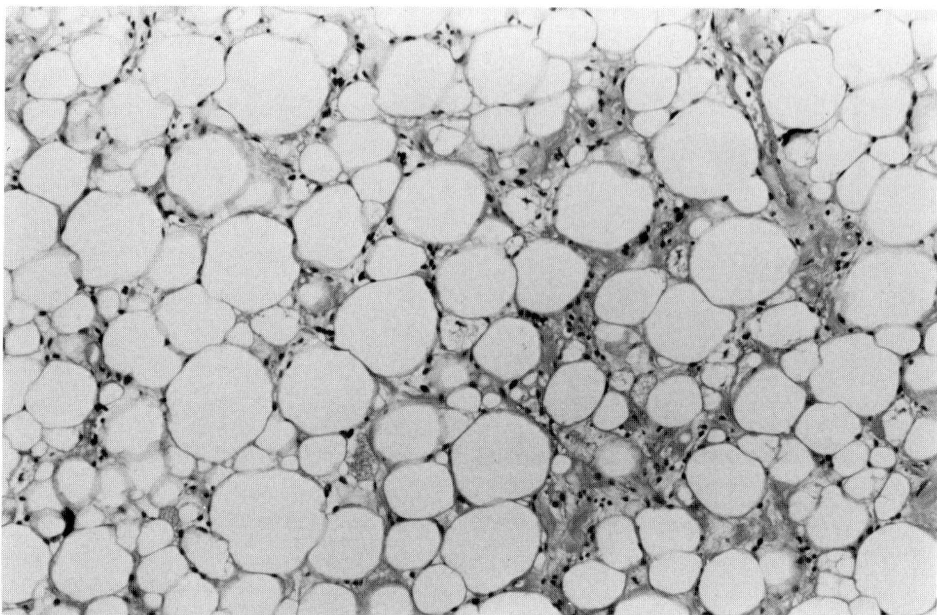

Fig. 3-11. Well-differentiated liposarcoma, lipomalike type, exhibiting scattered lipoblasts and atypical cells possessing hyperchromatic nuclei. (H&E, × 125.)

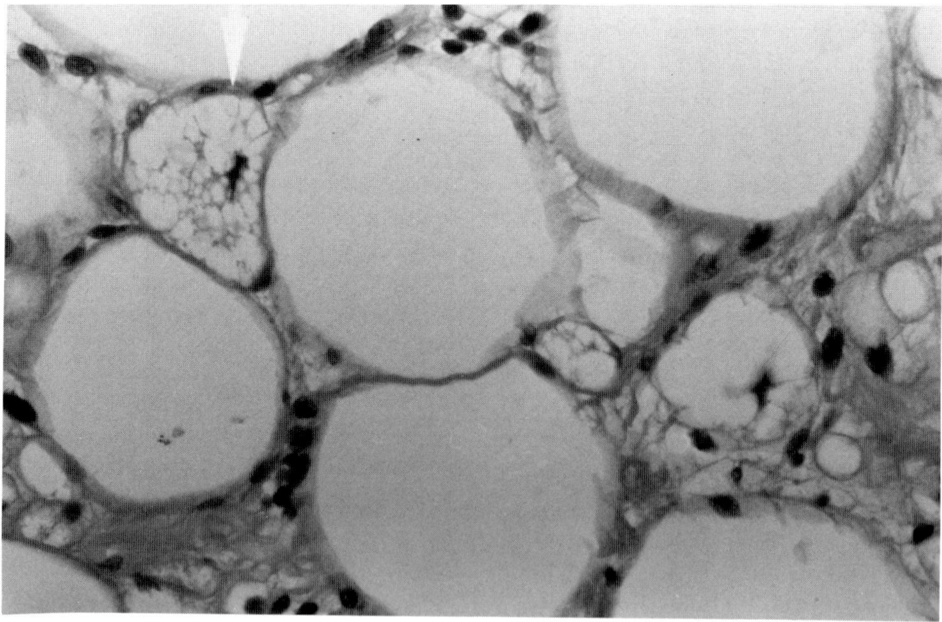

Fig. 3-12. High-power view of the same tumor shown in Fig. 3-11. Note the typical multivacuolated lipoblasts (one at arrow). (H&E, × 500.)

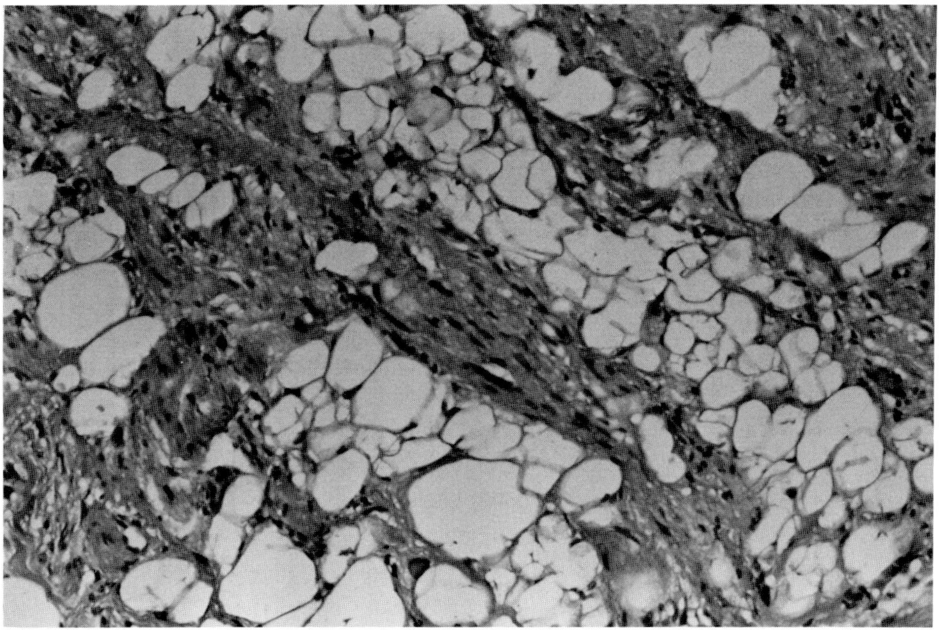

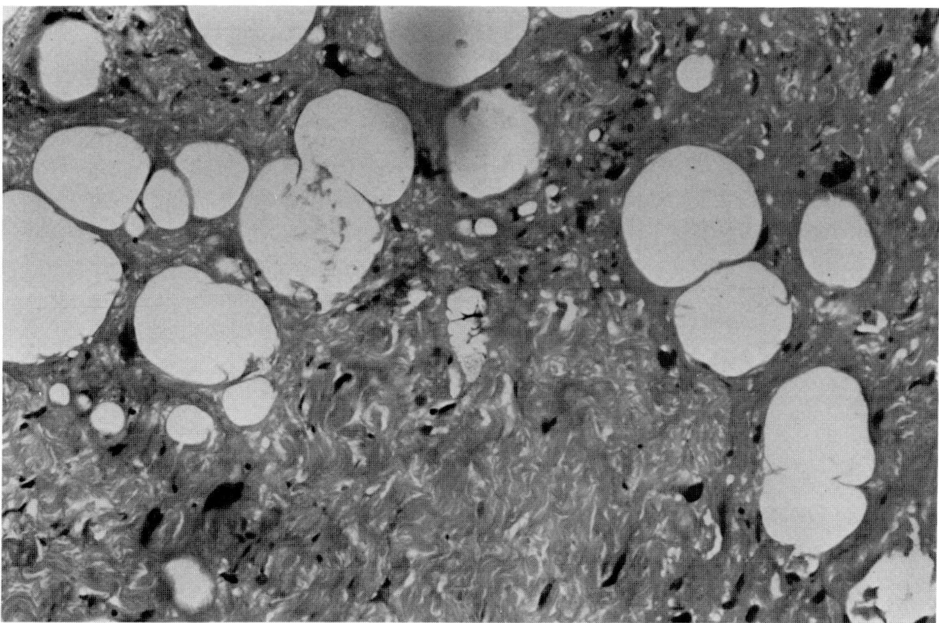

Fig. 3-13. Well-differentiated liposarcoma, sclerosing type. Note the variation in size and shape of the fat cells. Lobules of adipose tissue are separated by bands of fibrous tissue containing atypical cells. (H&E, × 125.)

Fig. 3-14. Different portion of the same tumor shown in Fig. 3-13. Note the dense collagenous fibrous stroma bearing lipoblasts and atypical pleomorphic cells. (H&E, × 125.)

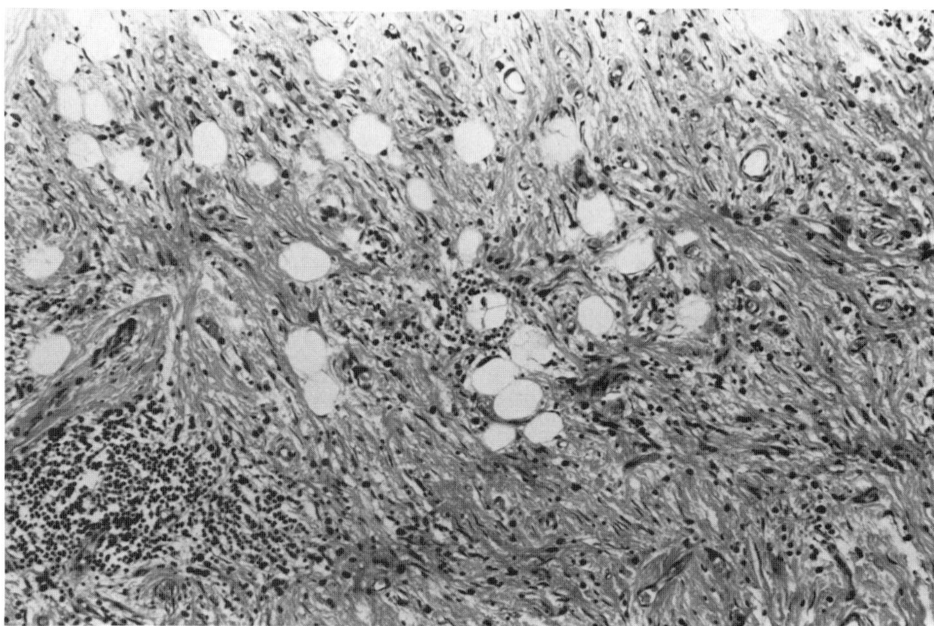

Fig. 3-15. Well-differentiated liposarcoma, inflammatory type, simulating an inflammatory process of adipose tissue. (H&E, × 125.)

to fusiform or stellate mesenchymal cells and lipoblasts in varying stages of differentiation set in a myxoid stroma rich in hyaluronidase-sensitive, acid mucopolysaccharides (Figs. 3-16 and 3-17). The tumor is often accompanied by a delicate plexiform capillary network (Fig. 3-16) and pools or lakes of this myxoid material are readily recognized (Fig. 3-18). The paucity of mitotic figures and lack of pleomorphism contrast with its rapid growth.

ROUND CELL LIPOSARCOMA

This variant comprises approximately 10 to 25 percent of all liposarcomas[16, 17, 24] and is considered a poorly differentiated form of myxoid liposarcoma.[18] The tumor is characterized by a proliferation of uniform round or oval cells having a clear or acidophilic granular cytoplasm and occasional evident nucleoli (Figs. 3-19 and 3-20). Transition to myxoid areas (Fig. 3-21), as well as to areas composed of short fascicles of spindle cells arranged in a storiform pattern, is frequently observed. Mitoses are more com-

mon, but the vascular pattern is less evident than in myxoid liposarcoma.

PLEOMORPHIC LIPOSARCOMA

Ten to 25 percent of the liposarcomas[16, 17] bear a close resemblance to pleomorphic MFH. These pleomorphic liposarcomas are, in fact, characterized by the presence of large mono- or multi-nucleated giant cells intermingled with many bizarre lipoblasts. Mitotic figures, often atypical, are a common finding (Figs. 3-22 and 3-23).

DEDIFFERENTIATED LIPOSARCOMA

The occurrence of pleomorphic MFH-like or fibrosarcomatous areas (Fig. 3-24) in a classic liposarcoma was described in 1944 by Stout.[21] In 1975 Kindblom[24] reported 24 cases of well-differentiated liposarcoma showing sharply demarcated pleomorphic areas. Later in 1979, Evans[19] first introduced the term dedifferentiated

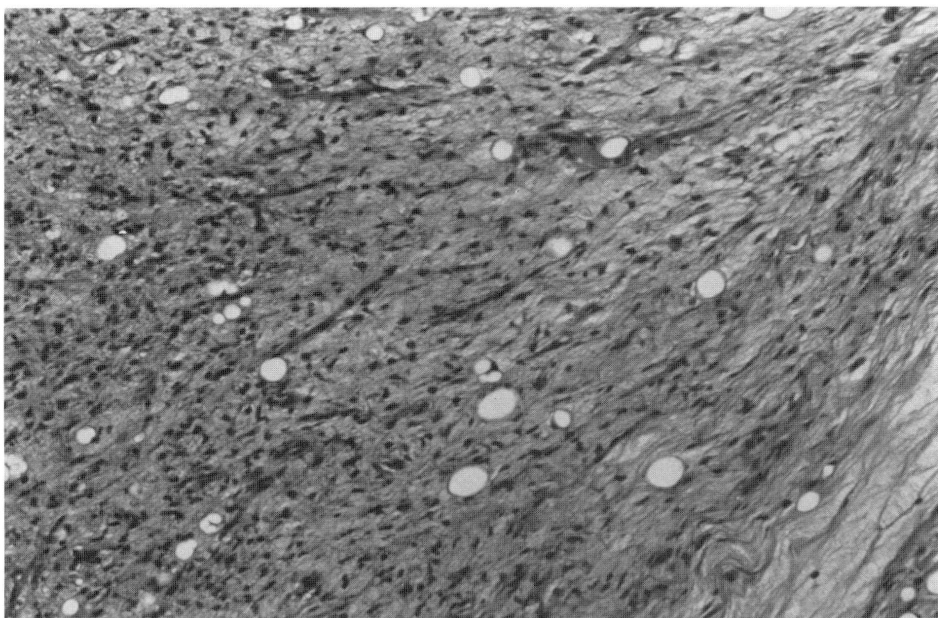

Fig. 3-16. Myxoid liposarcoma revealing scattered lipoblasts in different stages of maturation and a prominent plexiform capillary pattern set in an abundant myxoid stroma. (H&E, × 125.)

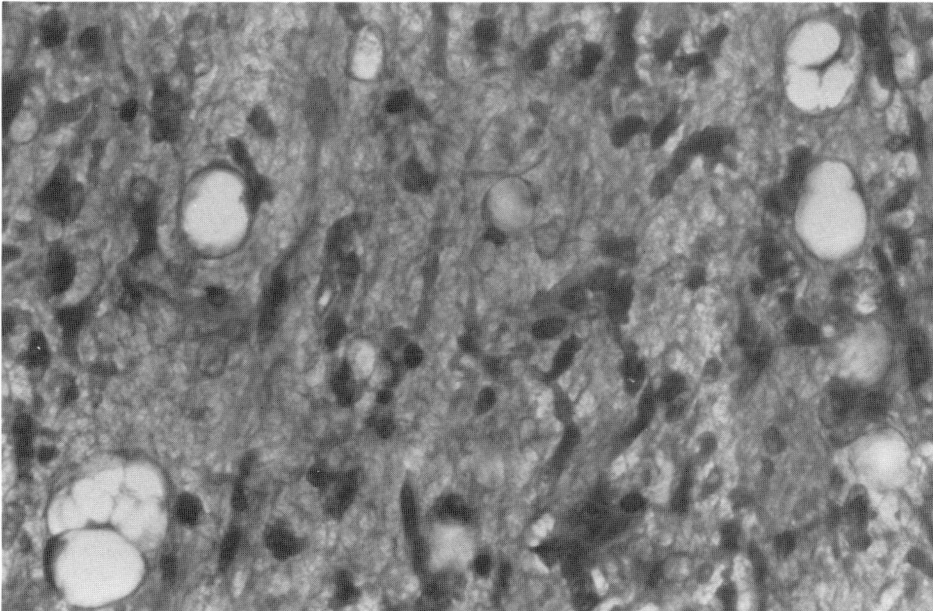

Fig. 3-17. High-power view of the same tumor shown in Fig. 3-16. Note the lipoblasts and spindling of tumor cells. (H&E, × 500.)

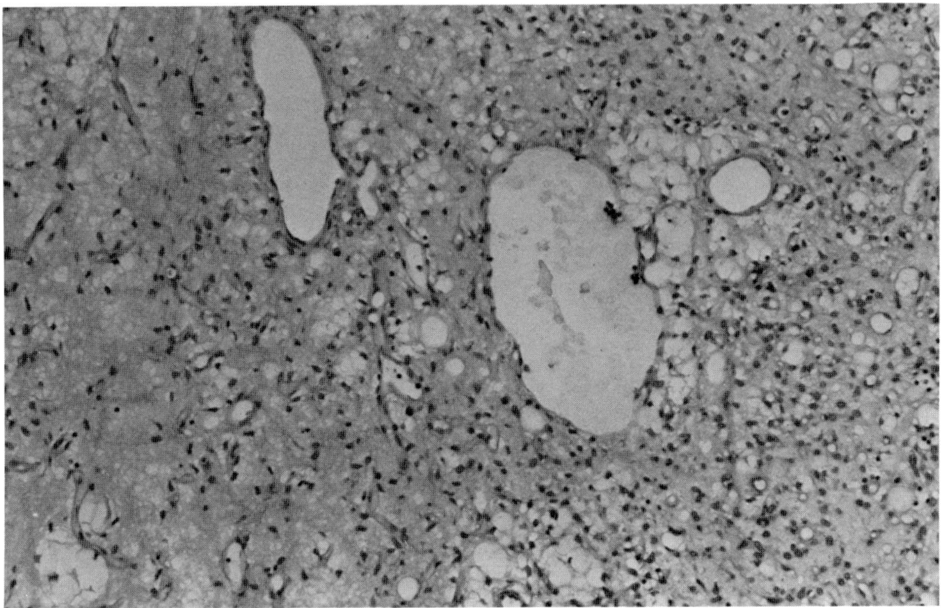

Fig. 3-18. Myxoid liposarcoma with pooling of myxoid material. (H&E, × 125.)

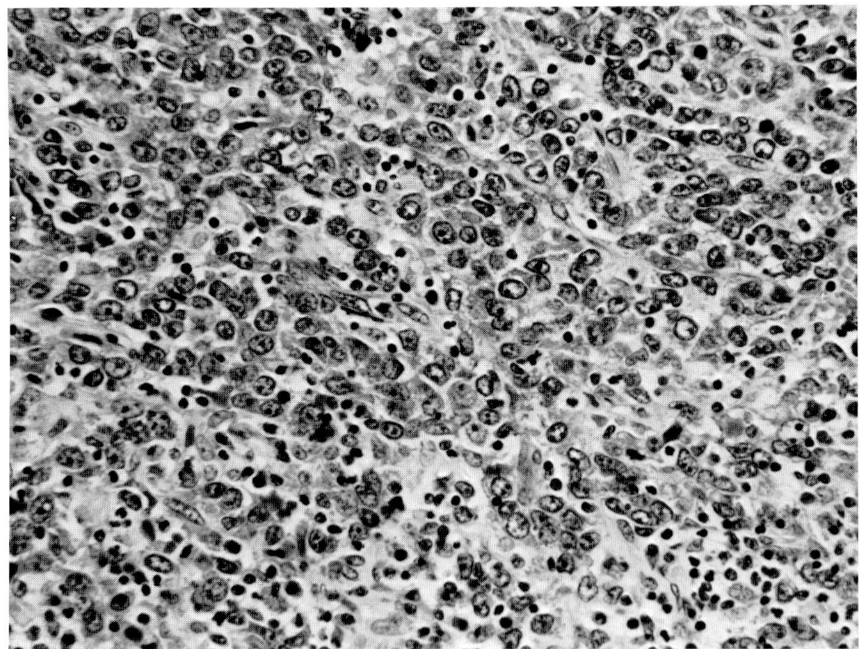

Fig. 3-19. Round cell liposarcoma. Diffuse proliferation of monomorphous round cells with prominent nucleoli, closely mimicking a large cell lymphoma. (H&E, × 250.)

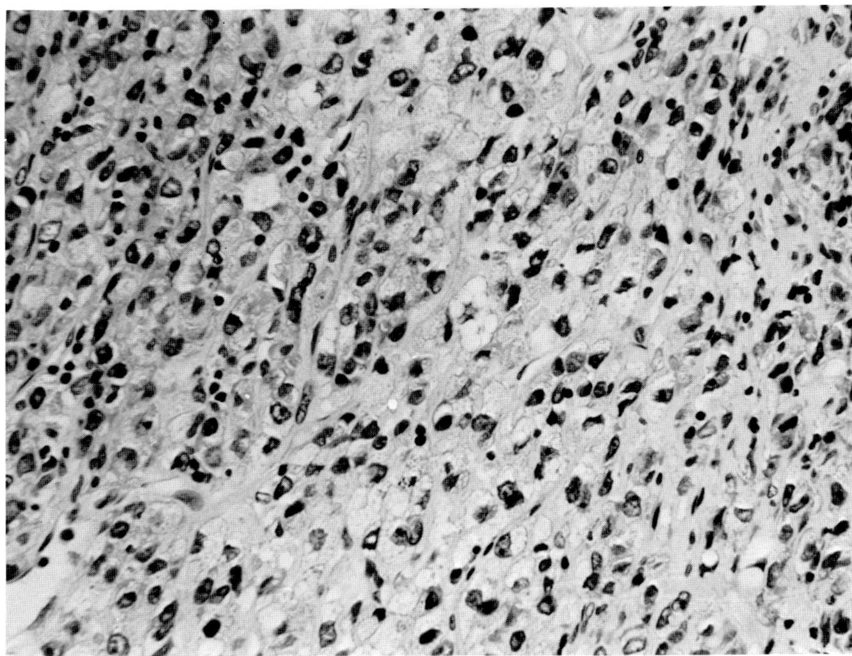

Fig. 3-20. Round cell liposarcoma (same tumor shown in Fig. 3-19). In the peripheral portion of the tumor, the neoplastic cells show granular cytoplasm and only occasional lipoblasts are appreciated. (H&E, × 250.)

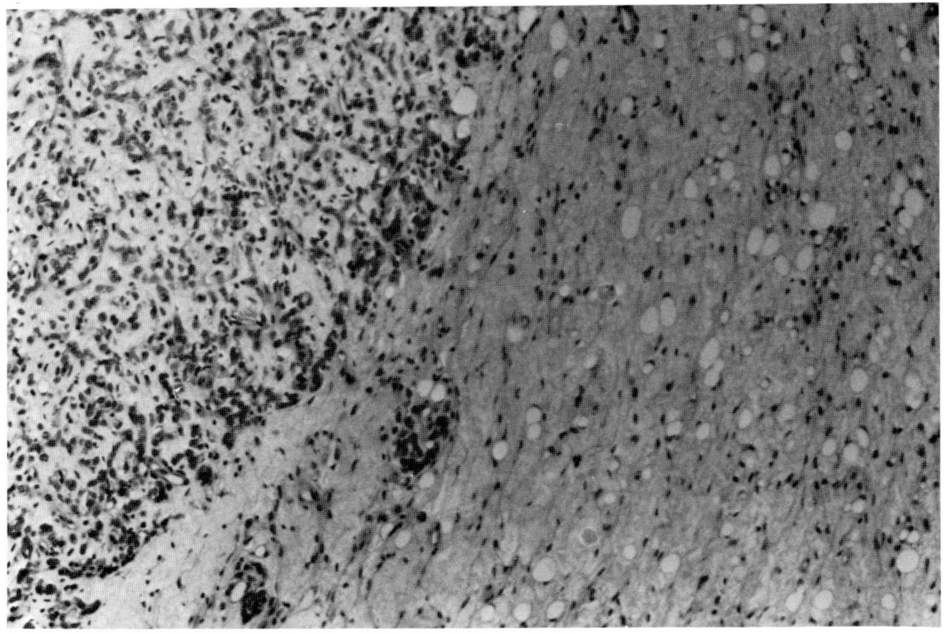

Fig. 3-21. Transition zone between myxoid and round cell liposarcoma. (H&E, × 125.)

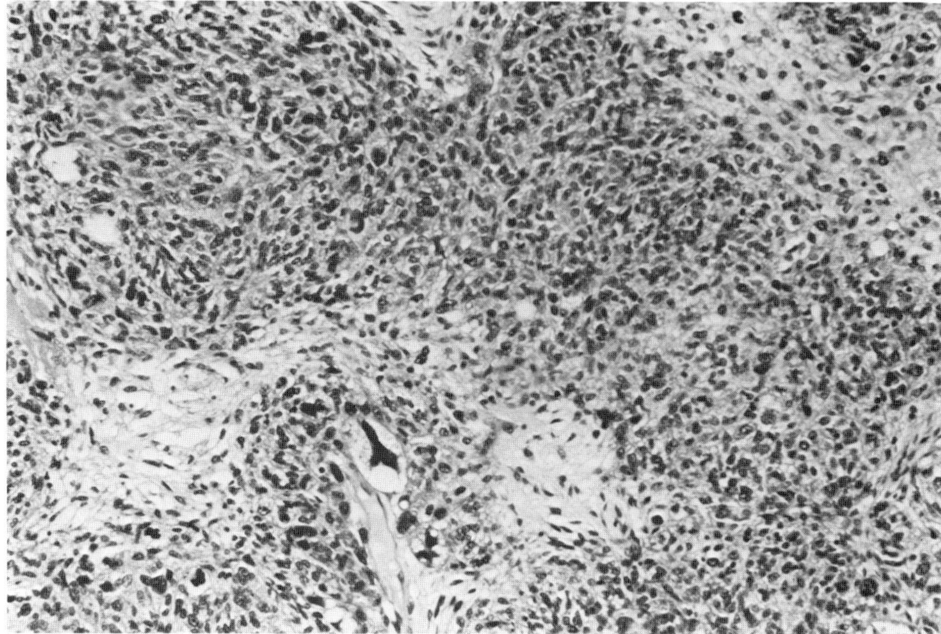

Fig. 3-22. Pleomorphic liposarcoma. Occasional lipoblasts are embedded in a background of pleomorphic neoplasm. (H&E, × 125.)

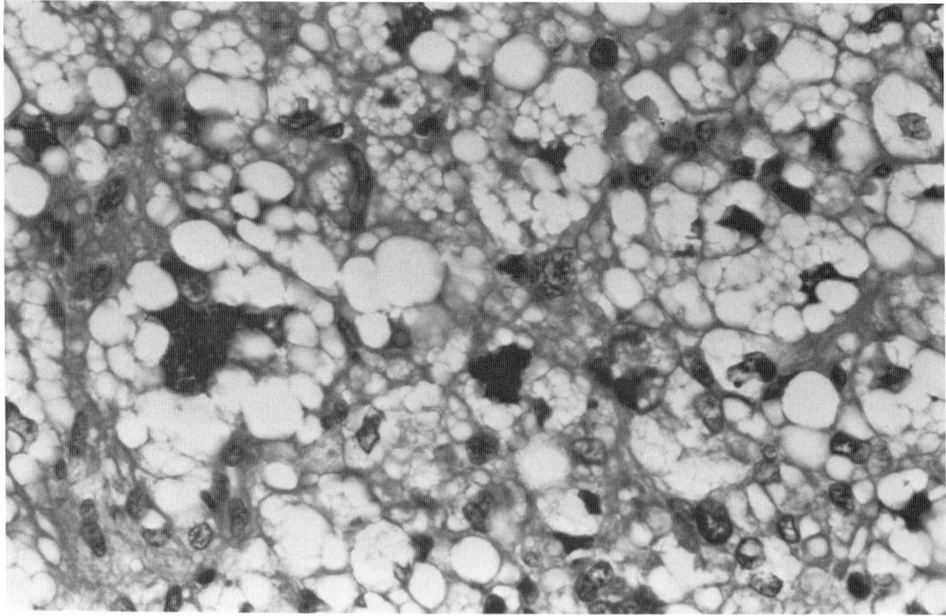

Fig. 3-23. Different portion of the same tumor shown in Fig. 3-22. Note the clustering of lipoblasts of various types, including bizarre forms. (H&E, × 500.)

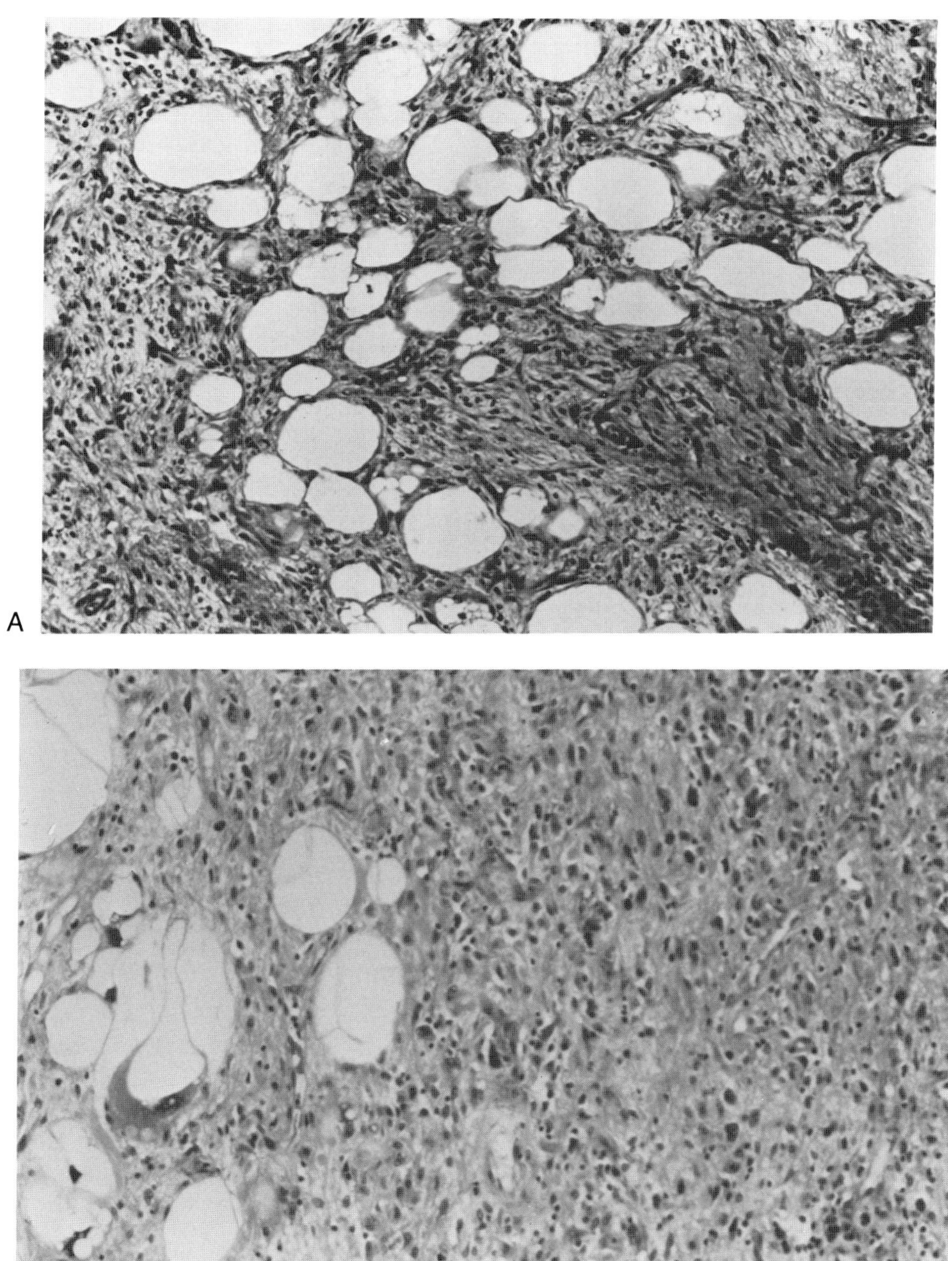

Fig. 3-24. Dedifferentiated liposarcoma. **(A)** Interdigitating junction of well-differentiated liposarcoma and malignant fibrous histiocytoma-like pattern. **(B)** Transition zone between a portion of well-differentiated liposarcoma and an undifferentiated sarcoma (H&E, × 125.)

Table 3-3. Principal Differential Diagnosis of Liposarcoma

Accessional Diagnosis	Age	Site	Revised Diagnosis
LPS	33	Thigh	MFH
LPS	70	Retroperitoneum	MFH
LPS myxoid	56	Thorax	MFH
LPS	62	Abdomen	MFH
LPS myxoid	68	Retroperitoneum	MFH
LPS myxoid	41	Trunk	MFH
LPS myxoid	21	Mesenterium	MNST
LPS	45	Retroperitoneum	MNST
LPS myxoid	82	Retroperitoneum	MNST
LPS myxoid	28	Neck	MNST
LPS	68	Mesenterium	Leiomyosarcoma
LPS myxoid	67	Abdomen	Leiomyosarcoma
LPS	40	Leg	Leiomyosarcoma
LPS	52	Knee	Myxoid chondrosarcoma
LPS	38	(unknown)	Myxoid chondrosarcoma
LPS myxoid	58	Retroperitoneum	Angiosarcoma
LPS round cell	17	Paravertebral	Rhabdomyosarcoma
LPS round cell	70	Stomach	Carcinoma
LPS	56	Shoulder	Intramuscular lipoma
LPS myxoid	67	Thigh	Intramuscular lipoma
LPS myxoid	28	Scapula	Pleomorphic lipoma

Abbreviations: LPS, liposarcoma not otherwise specified; MFH, malignant fibrous histiocytoma; MNST, malignant nerve sheath tumor.

liposarcoma to describe these tumors. The relative frequency of this entity ranges from 5 to 19 percent of the cases.[38, 24] The recognition and distinction of dedifferentiated liposarcoma from other histologic subtypes of liposarcoma seems justified by its more aggressive behavior. Metastasis are reported in half of the cases.

Differential Diagnosis

Before the recognition of MFH as a distinctive clinical and pathological entity, liposarcoma was the most frequently entertained diagnosis in soft tissue tumor pathology. In fact, in a series of 195 cases of previously diagnosed liposarcoma, the lipogenic nature was confirmed after histologic revision in only 95.[24] In a series of 90 liposarcoma diagnosed over a 15 year period from 1965 to 1980, at the Institute of Pathology of Padua University, we could confirm the original diagnosis in 66 cases. Table 3-3 shows the list of sarcomas that have been confused for a liposarcoma.

The most important problem facing a pathologist in the diagnosis of a liposarcoma is the recognition of unequivocal or acceptable lipoblasts in different stages of maturation, namely, multivacuolated, granular, monovacuolated signet-ring, spindle-shaped, and stellate lipoblasts. Characteristically, multivacuolated lipoblasts contain sharply defined lipid droplets that often indent the nuclei. Granular cells, resembling the cells of brown fat, are commonly found in round cell liposarcoma.

Vacuolated cells that may be confused with lipoblasts are frequently encountered in a variety of neoplasms as degenerative changes, as well as in mucin-producing or glycogen rich tumors such as poorly differentiated carcinomas or Ewing's sarcoma, or in MFH, and in the physaliferous cells of chordoma.

Well-differentiated liposarcoma in the retroperitoneal space should be distinguished from benign lesions containing mature adipose tissue such as angiomyolipoma,[39] and reactive lesions, such as xanthogranulomatous pyelonephritis. Bundles of smooth muscle fibers may be found in retroperitoneal liposarcoma[40] and may raise the suspicion of angiomyolipoma. The latter, however, is characterized by a more prominent vascular pattern due to the presence of thick walled vessels and the absence of atypical lipoblasts. The presence of a large collection of foamy macrophages, granulocytes, multinucleated foreign-body giant cells, and granulomatous foci around cholesterol crystals should allow the distinction of inflammatory processes from liposarcoma. Likewise, inflammatory reactions to silicon implants and fat necrosis may be separated from cutaneous forms of well-differentiated liposarcoma (atypical lipoma).

Many benign or malignant myxoid tumors enter the differential diagnosis with myxoid liposarcoma. Intramuscular myxoma may be overdiagnosed as liposarcoma due to its infiltrative growth pattern. Nevertheless, the paucity of vessels and absence of lipoblasts point more to myxoma than liposarcoma. Aggressive angiomyxoma of the female genital region can be differentiated by the absence of lipoblasts and the plexiform vascular pattern.

The higher mitotic activity and the prominent cellular pleomorphism of MFH contrast with the diagnosis of myxoid liposarcoma; furthermore, the cytoplasmic vacuoles do not contain lipids but stain for mucopolysaccharides. Since adipocytes and lipoblasts react positively to anti S-100 protein antibodies, this reaction has been recommended in separating liposarcoma from myxoid MFH.[41] Nodules of more orderly arranged rows of round, vacuolated cells embedded in a hyaluronidase-resistant myxoid background in the absence of a plexiform vascular pattern characterize myxoid chondrosarcoma. The presence of an elongated, eosinophilic cytoplasm in conjunction with positivity to muscle markers distinguish myxoid leiomyosarcoma from myxoid liposarcoma.

Large cell lymphoma, Ewing's sarcoma, and metastatic carcinoma should be considered in the differential diagnosis of round cell liposarcoma. The presence of areas showing clear lipogenic differentiation will generally clarify the diagnosis.

Prognosis

Liposarcomas are known to have high recurrence rates,[17, 24, 27, 35, 42] ranging from 46 percent[42] to 62 percent[24] (Tables 3-4 and 3-5). Retroperitoneal liposarcoma show higher recurrence rates than those located in the extremities,[24, 43] whereas round cell liposarcoma recur more frequently than myxoid and well-differentiated liposarcoma.[17, 24] Recurrences generally have the same histologic features of the primary tumor, although in 15 percent[24] to 37 percent[35] of the cases, they may show histologic aspects of dedifferentiation.

Table 3-4. Relative Frequency of Liposarcoma Recurrences According to Site[a]

Site	N	%	Median Time (months)
Retroperitoneum	7/11	63.6	18.8
Extremities	10/22	45.0	19.4
Others	3/7	42.8	16.3

[a] Observed at the Institute of Pathology, University of Padua, Padua, Italy.

Table 3-5. Relative Frequency of Liposarcoma Recurrences According to Histotypes[a]

Histologic Type	N	%	Median Time (months)
Well-differentiated	6/9	66.6	16.6
Myxoid	9/17	52.9	27
Round cell	2/6*	33.3	8
Pleomorphic	2/6*	33.3	13.3
Dedifferentiated	1/2	—	3

* These figures may be misleading since 5 patients with round cell liposarcoma and 4 patients with pleomorphic liposarcoma died of metastatic disease within 36 and 24 months after surgery respectively.

[a] Observed at the Institute of Pathology, University of Padua, Padua, Italy.

The 5-year survival rates range from 35 percent[24] to 41 percent[43] to 55 percent[24] to 71 percent[17] for retroperitoneal and distally located tumors respectively. The histological picture seems related to the final outcome. In one series[44] a 100 percent 5-year survival was reported for well-differentiated liposarcoma of the extremities, while 56 percent and 40 percent survival rates were found for pleomorphic and round cell liposarcoma. In another series,[24] 10-year survival rates of 73 percent and 60 percent have been reported for well-differentiated and myxoid liposarcoma respectively, whereas only 1 patient out of 13 (7 percent) with round cell liposarcoma survived.

Like many other sarcomas, radical excision of the tumor is the treatment of choice. In a series of 30 cases observed at Padua University, for whom clinical follow-up information was available, no differences in mortality were observed between patients treated by surgery alone and those receiving postsurgical radiotherapy. However, median survival times were 28.7 months and 42.5 months, respectively. Thus radiation therapy appears useful in controlling local disease[45] and in prolonging the disease-free interval.

REFERENCES

1. Kauffman SL, Stout AP: Lipoblastic tumors of children. Cancer 12:912, 1959
2. Simon G: Histogenesis. p. 101. In Renold AE, Cahill GF JR (eds): Handbook of Physiology. Sect. 5. Adipose Tissue. American Physiological Society, Washington, DC, 1965
3. Enzinger FM, Harvey DA: Spindle cell lipoma. Cancer 36:1852, 1975
4. Shmookler BM, Enzinger FM: Pleomorhic lipoma: a benign tumor simulating liposarcoma. A clinicopathologic analysis of 48 cases. Cancer 47:126, 1981
5. Bolen JW, Thorning D: Spindle cell lipoma: a clinical, light- and electron-microscopical study. Am J Surg Pathol 5:435, 1981
6. Sund S, Hordvik M, Maehle B et al: Large intramuscular spindle-cell lipoma. With review of the literature. APMIS 96:347, 1988
7. Bolen JW, Thorning D: Benign lipoblastoma and myxoid liposarcoma. A comparative light- and electron-microscopic study. Am J Surg Pathol 4:163, 1980
8. Vellios F, Baez JM, Shumacker HB: Lipoblastomatosis: a tumor of fetal fat different from hibernoma. Report of a case, with observation of the embryogenesis of human adipose tissue. Am J Pathol 34:1149, 1958
9. Chung EB, Enzinger FM: Benign lipoblastomatosis. An analysis of 35 cases. Cancer 32:482, 1973
10. Shmookler BM, Enzinger FM: Liposarcoma occurring in children: an analysis of 17 cases and review of the literature. Cancer 52:567, 1983
11. Enzinger FM: Benign lipomatous tumors simulating a sarcoma. p. 11. In Management of Primary Bone and Soft Tissue Tumors. Year Book Medical Publishers, Chicago, 1977
12. Kindblom L-G, Angervall L, Stener B et al: Intermuscular and intramuscular lipomas and hibernomas. A clinical, roentgenologic, histologic and prognostic study of 46 cases. Cancer 33:754, 1974
13. Fletcher CDM, Martin-Bates E: Intramuscular and intermusclar lipoma: neglected diagnoses. Histopathology 12:275, 1988
14. Dionne GP, Seemayer TA: Infiltrating lipomas and angiolipomas revisited. Cancer 33:732, 1974
15. Rossouw DJ, Cinti S, Dickersin GR: Liposar-

coma. An ultrastructural study of 15 cases. Am J Clin Pathol 85:649, 1986

16. Allen PW: Tumors and Proliferations of Adipose Tissue: A Clinicopathologic Approach. p. 131. Masson, New York, 1981

17. Enzinger FM, Winslow DJ: Liposarcoma. A study of 103 cases. Virchows Arch [A] 335:367, 1962

18. Evans HL: Liposarcoma. A study of 55 cases with a reassessment of its classification. Am J Surg Pathol 3:507, 1979

19. Evans HL, Soule EH, Winkelman RK: Atypical lipoma, atypical intramuscular lipoma, and well-differentiated retroperitoneal liposarcoma. A reappraisal of 30 cases formerly classified as well differentiated liposarcoma. Cancer 43:574, 1979

20. Enzinger FM: Atypical fibroxanthoma and malignant fibrous histiocytoma. Am J Dermatopathol 1:185, 1979

21. Stout AP: Liposarcoma. The malignant tumor of lipoblasts, Ann Surg 119:86, 1944

22. Enterline HT, Culberson JD, Rochlin DB et al: Liposarcoma. A clinical and pathological study of 53 cases. Cancer 13:932, 1960

23. Spittle MF, Newton KA, Mackenzie DH: Liposarcoma. A review of 60 cases. Br J Cancer 24:696, 1970

24. Kindblom L-G, Angervall L, Svendson P: Liposarcoma. A clinicopathological, radiographic and prognostic study. Acta Pathol Microbiol Scand [A] Suppl 253, 1975

25. Hajdu SI: Pathology of soft tissue tumors. p. 227. Lea & Febinger, Philadelphia, 1979

26. Reszel PA, Soule EH, Coventry MB: Liposarcoma of the extremities and limb girdles. A study of two hundred twenty-two cases. J Bone Joint Surg 48A:229, 1966

27. Stewart FW: Primary liposarcoma of bone. Am J Pathol 7:87, 1931

28. Kenan S, Klein M, Lewis MM: Juxtacortical liposarcoma. A case report and review of the literature. Clin Orthop 243:225, 1989

29. Milgram JW: Malignant transformation in bone lipomas. Skeletal Radiol 5:347, 1990

30. Sternberg SS: Liposarcoma arising within a subcutaneous lipoma. Cancer 5:975, 1952

31. Mariotti A, Bertaccini N: Studio sulla patogenesi del liposarcoma. Arch Ital Pat Clin 3:1456, 1959

32. Azumi N, Curtis J, Kempson RL et al: Atypical and malignant neoplasms showing lipomatous differentiation: a study of 111 cases. Am J Surg Pathol 11:161, 1987

33. Kindblom L-G, Angervall L, Fassina AS: Atypical lipoma. Acta Pathol Microbiol Scand Sect A 90:27, 1982

34. Azzopardi JC, Iocco J, Salm R: Pleomorphic lipoma: a tumor simulating liposarcoma. Histopathology 7:511, 1983

35. Evans HL: Liposarcomas and atypical lipomatous tumors: a study of 66 cases followed for a minimum of 10 years. Surg Pathol 1:41, 1988

36. Shimoda T, Yamashita H, Furusato M et al: Liposarcoma. A light and electron microscopic study with comments on their relation to malignant fibrous histiocytoma and angiosarcoma. Acta Pathol Jpn 30:779, 1980

37. Brooks JJ, Connor AM: Atypical lipoma of the extremities and peripheral soft tissues with dedifferentiation: implication for management. Surg Pathol 3:169, 1990

38. Enzinger FM, Weiss SW: Soft Tissue Tumors. 2nd Ed. p. 364. CV Mosby, St. Louis, 1988

39. Hruban RH, Bhagavan BS, Epstein JI: Massive retroperitoneal angiomyolipoma. A lesion that may be confused with well-differentiated liposarcoma. Am J Clin Pathol 6:805, 1989

40. Evans HL: Smooth muscle in atypical lipomatous tumors. A report of three cases. Am J Surg Pathol 8:714, 1990

41. Hashimoto H, Daimaru Y, Enjoji M: S-100 protein distribution in liposarcoma. An immunoperoxidase study with special reference to the distinction of liposarcoma from myxoid malignant fibrous histiocytoma. Virchows Arch [A] 405:1, 1984

42. Hashimoto H, Enjoji M: Liposarcoma. A clinicopathologic subtyping of 52 cases Acta Pathol Jpn 32:933, 1982

43. Kinne DW, Chu FCH, Huvos AG et al: Treatment of primary and recurrent retroperitoneal liposarcoma. Twenty-five years experience at Memorial Hospital. Cancer 31:53, 1973

44. Chang HR, Hajdu SI, Collin C, Brennan MF: The prognostic value of histologic subtypes in primary extremity liposarcoma. Cancer 64:1514, 1989

45. Shiu MH, Chu F, Castro EB et al: Results of surgical and radiation therapy in the treatment of liposarcoma arising in an extremity. Am Roentgenol 123:577, 1975

4

Tumors of Muscle Tissue

Vito Ninfo and Andrea O. Cavazzana

Striated and smooth muscles, the two main types of muscle tissue of the human body, differ considerably in structure. Smooth muscle tissue is widely distributed, and constitutes the major wall component of the gastrointestinal, respiratory, and genitourinary tracts, as well as blood vessels; in addition, ciliary muscle and the erector muscles of the skin, nipple, and scrotum are made up of smooth muscle fibers. Histologically, smooth muscle is composed of mononucleated spindle-shaped cells, arranged in small fascicles with the long axis parallel to the direction of contraction; the centrally placed nuclei have blunt edges and crenated surfaces. Ultrastructurally the eosinophilic cytoplasm is made up of closely packed, thin filaments with focal densities parallel to the long axis of the cell (Fig. 4-1). Glycogen as well as numerous pinocytotic vesicles are commonly present in the cytoplasm. A thin but distinct external lamina is generally observed around the cells.

Striated muscle, with few exceptions, represents the voluntary muscle component of the human body, contributing about 40 to 50 percent of its total weight.[1] The elementary unit is a long, syncytial cell, which is provided with hundreds of peripherally placed nuclei. The cytoplasm shows characteristic cross-striations owing to the proper alignment of the sarcomeres, which ultrastructurally are made up of thin (actin) and thick (myosin) filaments regularly organized by a rather granular, electron-dense line (Z band) perpendicular to the actin filaments (Fig. 4-2). Numerous mitochondria and clusters of glycogen granules are usually observed between myofibrils. The plasma membrane is coated by a basement membrane to which reticulin and collagen fibers are anchored.

TUMORS OF SMOOTH MUSCLE

Benign and malignant smooth muscle tumors show the same distribution and location as normal smooth muscle tissue. Thus, these neoplasms occur more frequently in the gastrointestinal, genitourinary, and respiratory tracts, are less common in the skin, and are fairly rare in deep soft tissues.

LEIOMYOMAS

Extravisceral leiomyomas are traditionally divided into two groups depending on their location (i.e., superficial or deep-seated). The former include so-called leiomyoma cutis and genital leiomyomas; leiomyoma cutis comprehends the vascular and pilar varieties.

Superficial Leiomyomas

Leiomyomas of the pilar erector muscle account for most (about 75 percent) of the superficial leiomyomas.[2,3] Adolescents or young adults are predominantly affected. These lesions present as painful, single or multiple cutaneous papules or nodules, measuring 1 to 2 cm in diameter, most commonly on the extensor surfaces of the extremities. The tumor is located in the middle dermis, and is separated from

91

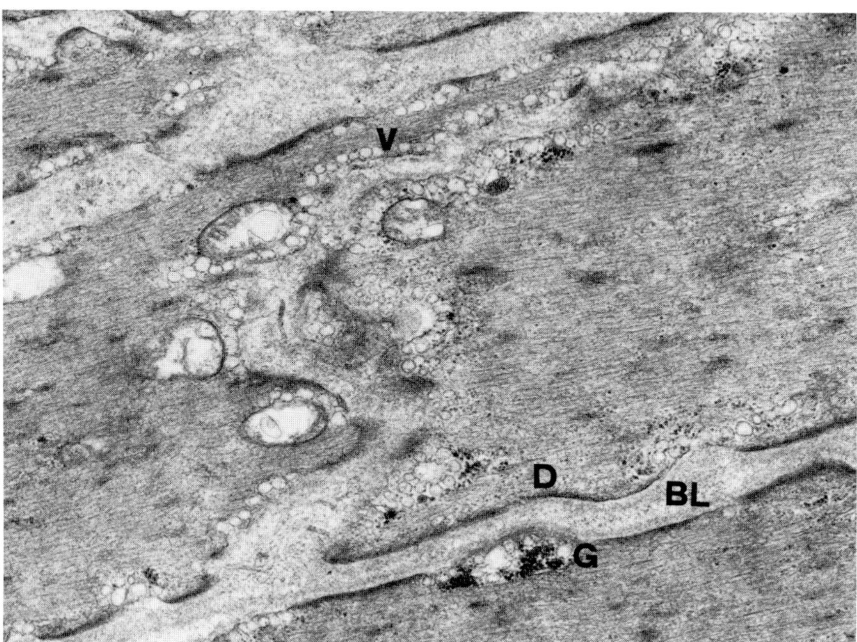

Fig. 4-1. Ultrastructurally the cytoplasm of smooth muscle cells is filled with thin filaments showing scattered focal densities parallel to their course. Subplasmalemmal densities (*D*), numerous micropinocytotic vesicles (*V*), small aggregates of glycogen (*G*), and a distinct basal lamina (*BL*) further characterize smooth muscle cells. (× 12,000.) (Courtesy of Dr. A. Parenti.)

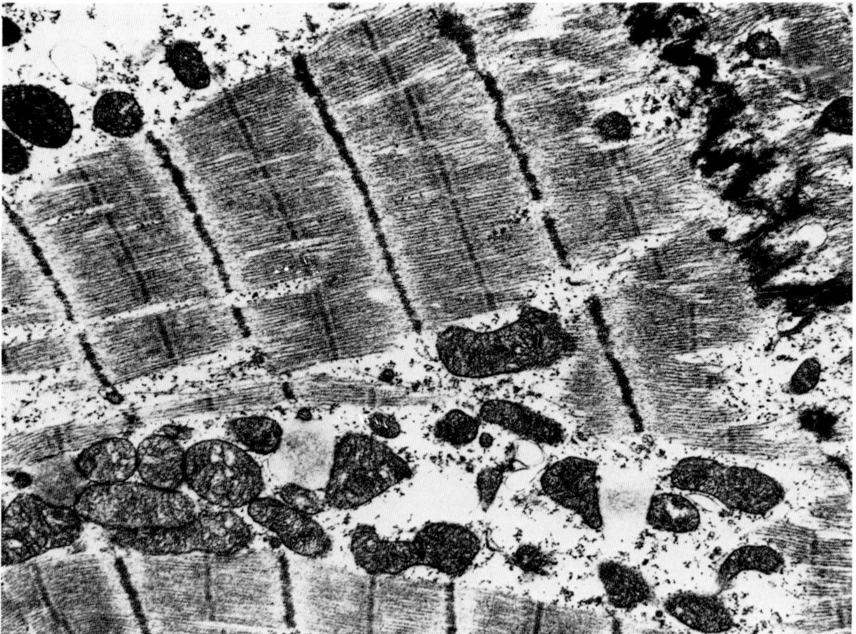

Fig. 4-2. In normal skeletal muscle, thick and thin filaments are regularly registered by a rather flocculent, transversally oriented Z band. (× 12,000.) (Courtesy of Prof M.L. Valente.)

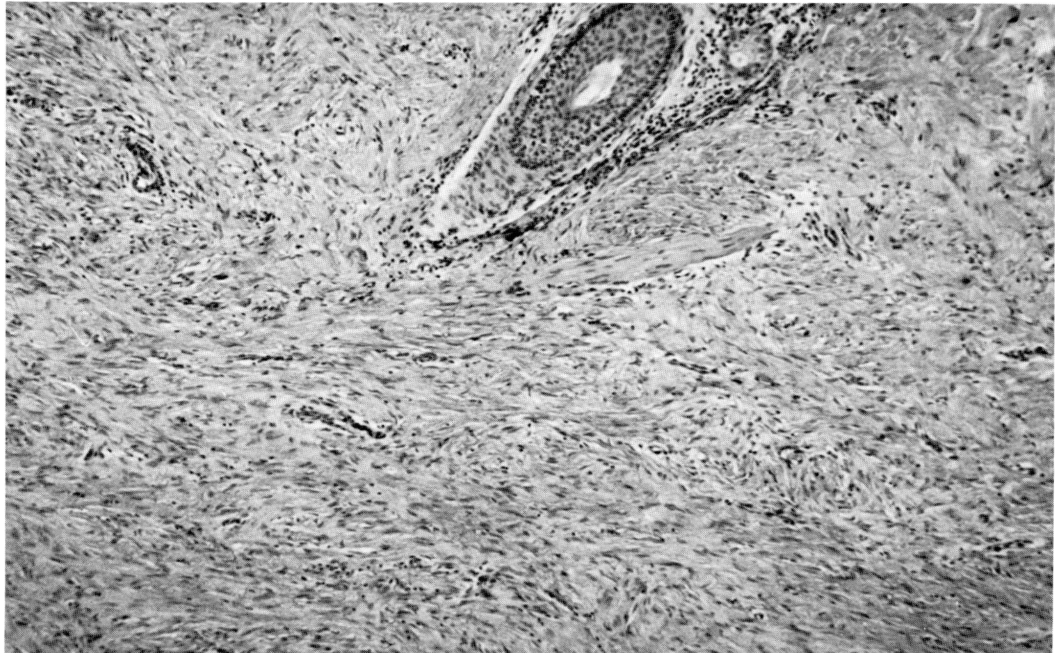

Fig. 4-3. Pilar leiomyoma. Bundles of smooth muscle fibers are associated with a hair follicle. (H&E, × 100.)

the overlying epidermis by a "grenz zone." On histologic examination, it is poorly demarcated, and made up of mature smooth muscle cells arranged in short interlacing bundles often surrounding hair follicles (Fig. 4-3). The differential diagnosis includes muscle nevi and cutaneous fibrohistiocytoma. Muscular hamartomas are often histologically indistinguishable, although they occur at earlier ages and are smaller. The absence of a distinct storiform pattern, foamy histiocytes, and inflammatory cells rules out cutaneous fibrohistiocytoma. Pilar leiomyoma is invariably benign, and no cases of malignant transformation have been reported.

Vascular leiomyomas are the second most common superficial type of leiomyoma, and constitute about 25 percent of the cases. Females are predominantly affected,[4] usually between the fourth and sixth decade of life.[4,5] Vascular leiomyomas are almost invariably located on the extremities, particularly the legs, in the deep dermis or subcutaneous tissue,[5] and present as small, solitary, painful nodules of about 1.5 to 2 cm in diameter. Histologically they consist of well-circumscribed nodules of proliferating smooth muscle cells arranged in a circumferential pattern around thickened vessels (Fig. 4-4). The venous or arterial nature of the affected vessels is often difficult to establish, although features suggesting an arteriovenous anastomotic origin are observed.[6] Foci of hyalinization, myxoid changes, and calcification are frequent. Like all other superficial leiomyomas, vascular leiomyomas may be mistaken for fibrous cutaneous tumors. Collagen and elastic stains are then useful to differentiate them from fibrous proliferations. In fact, leiomyomas are generally characterized by the presence of newly formed elastic fibers running parallel to the tumor fascicles, which are absent in fibrohistiocytic lesions of the skin.

Genital leiomyomas are much less common, and originate from the diffuse network of muscle fibers located in the deep dermis of the genital area. They present as solitary, small, painless masses. On histologic examination, they resemble pilar leiomyomas, but tend to be more cellular.[3]

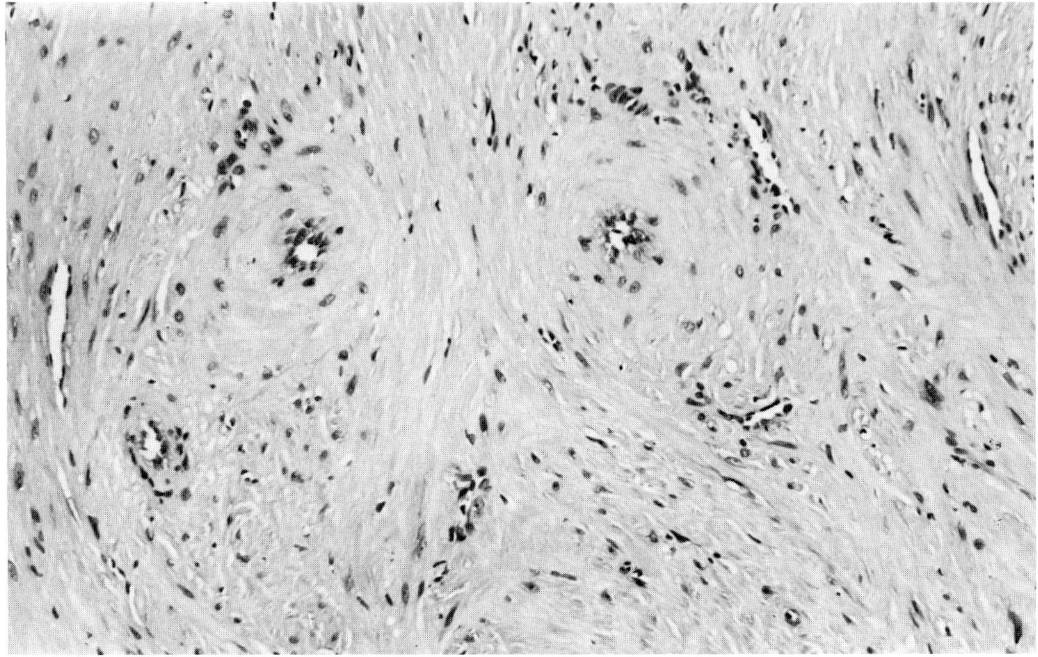

Fig. 4-4. Vascular leiomyoma. Numerous vessels encircled by spindle cells with plump nuclei arranged in circumferential fashion. (H&E, × 160.)

Leiomyomas of Deep Soft Tissues

Leiomyomas of deep soft tissues are rare, and only a few cases have been reported in the extremities or retroperitoneum.[7] These neoplasms occur at any age and both sexes are equally affected. They usually are larger than their cutaneous counterparts. Grossly leiomyomas of deep soft tissues are firm, well-circumscribed lesions. Microscopically they show features similar to those of cutaneous leiomyomas, although they appear more cellular. No mitotic activity is found, and pleomorphism is absent. Regressive changes, such as fibrosis, hyalinization, and calcification may be encountered in larger tumors.

LEIOMYOSARCOMAS

Leiomyosarcomas account for about 7 percent of all soft tissue sarcomas.[8, 9] These tumors usually occur in adults, with a clear female predomi-nance (M:F 1:3); they are rarely observed in children.[10] Most of these tumors are located in the uterus[11] and gastrointestinal tract.[12, 13] The most frequent extravisceral sites are the retroperitoneum,[14] the extremities,[9, 15 16] and the wall of large and medium-sized vessels (vascular leiomyosarcomas).[17–23]

Tumor size and shape vary considerably, depending on the site of origin. Deep-seated lesions, especially in the retroperitoneum, tend to be larger and frequently show degenerative and regressive changes, such as areas of necrosis, hemorrhage, and cyst formation. Superficial leiomyosarcomas are smaller (about 2 cm), and may be associated with epidermal changes, such as skin dimple, microscopic ulceration, and discoloration. Tumors arising from the vessel walls may exhibit either an intravascular polypoid appearance[21] or a predominant intramural pattern.[23] Microscopically leiomyosarcomas show a wide spectrum of cytohistologic features, ranging from well-differentiated, leiomyoma-like forms to poorly differentiated and pleo-

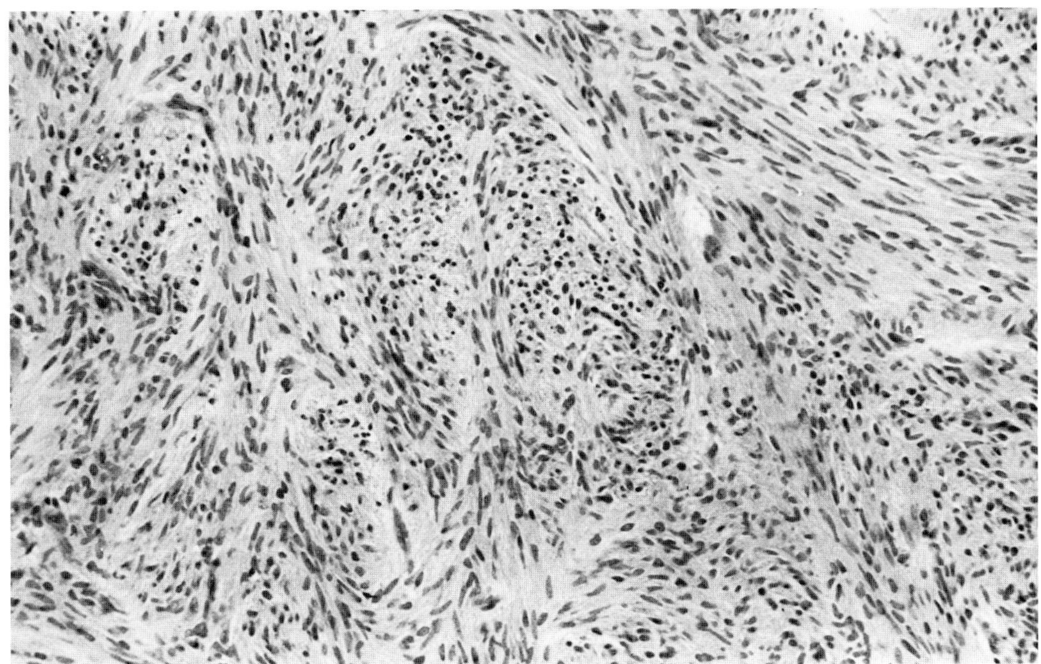

Fig. 4-5. Well-differentiated leiomyosarcoma with fascicles intersecting at right angles, producing circular silhouettes. (H&E, × 125.)

morphic leiomyosarcomas, which may mimic other soft tissue sarcomas.

The pattern of growth and the nuclear-cytoplasmic characteristics are the two most important diagnostic criteria.

Pattern of Growth

A fascicular pattern, with tumor bundles intersecting at right angles (Fig. 4-5), is the diagnostic architectural hallmark of a leiomyosarcoma. Both longitudinal and cross sections of circumferential silhouettes are observed side by side, producing a characteristic pattern of alternating fascicles or bundles (Figs. 4-5 and 4-6). This pattern is barely recognizable in moderately or poorly differentiated leiomyosarcomas owing to the less regular arrangement of the tumor fascicles (Fig. 4-7). A storiform pattern is also frequently observed, especially in recurrent tumors, which, at times, are exceedingly difficult or impossible to distinguish from malignant fi-

brous histiocytoma (MFH) (Fig. 4-8). Moreover, the tumor bundles may display either a regular nuclear alignment, which mimicks the palisades of a neurilemmoma (Fig. 4-9), or a perivascular arrangement in a hemangiopericytomalike pattern.

Cytology

Leiomyosarcoma cells are elongated, and typically possess blunt-ended, "cigar-shaped" nuclei (Fig. 4-6, inset). Perinuclear vacuoles, which may cause nuclear indentation, are frequent; the cytoplasm is fibrillar and intensely eosinophilic. Longitudinal myofibrils may be readily demonstrated in the well-differentiated forms by Masson's trichrome stain. Variable amounts of intracytoplasmic glycogen are usually present. Mononucleated or multinucleated MFH-like giant cells are seldom observed, especially in the pleomorphic variant of leiomyosarcoma (Fig. 4-8B).

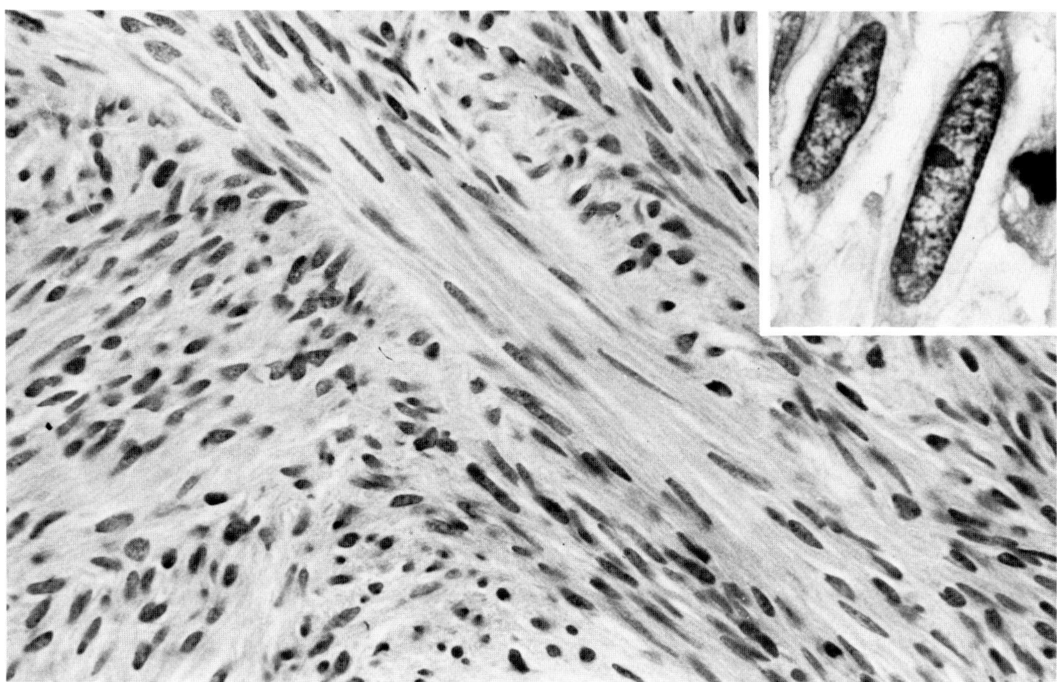

Fig. 4-6. At higher magnification well-differentiated leiomyosarcoma shows little cellular atypia. (H&E, × 250.) The spindle cells have bright eosinophilic cytoplasm and blunt-ended nuclei. (Inset × 1,000.)

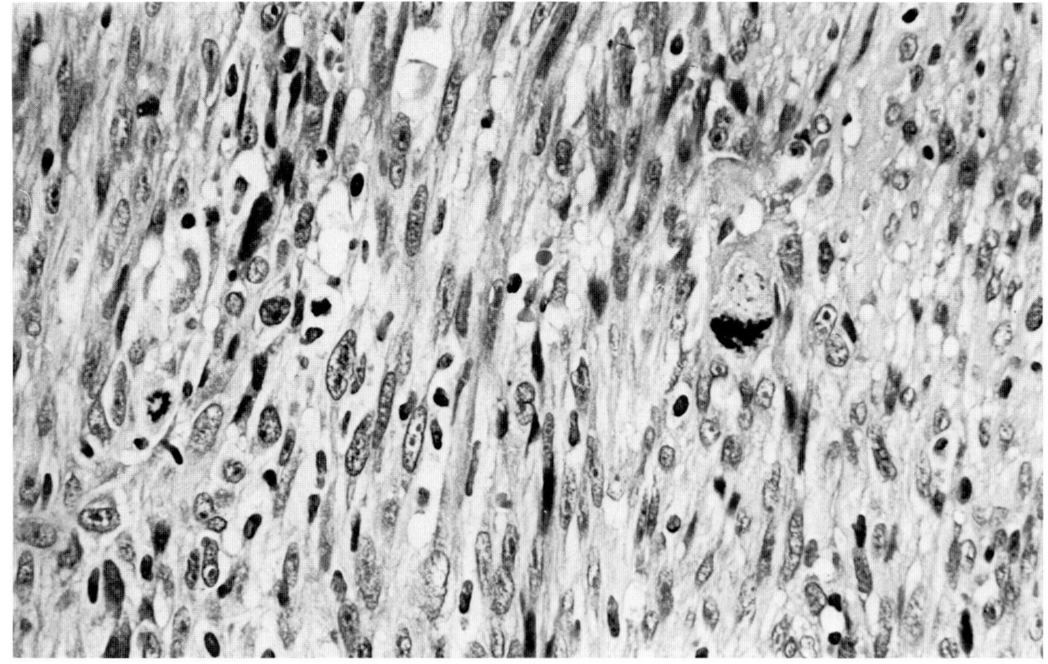

Fig. 4-7. In the poorly differentiated leiomyosarcoma, the typical alternating pattern is less evident (cf. Fig. 4-6) and mitoses, often atypical, are more numerous. (H&E, × 160.)

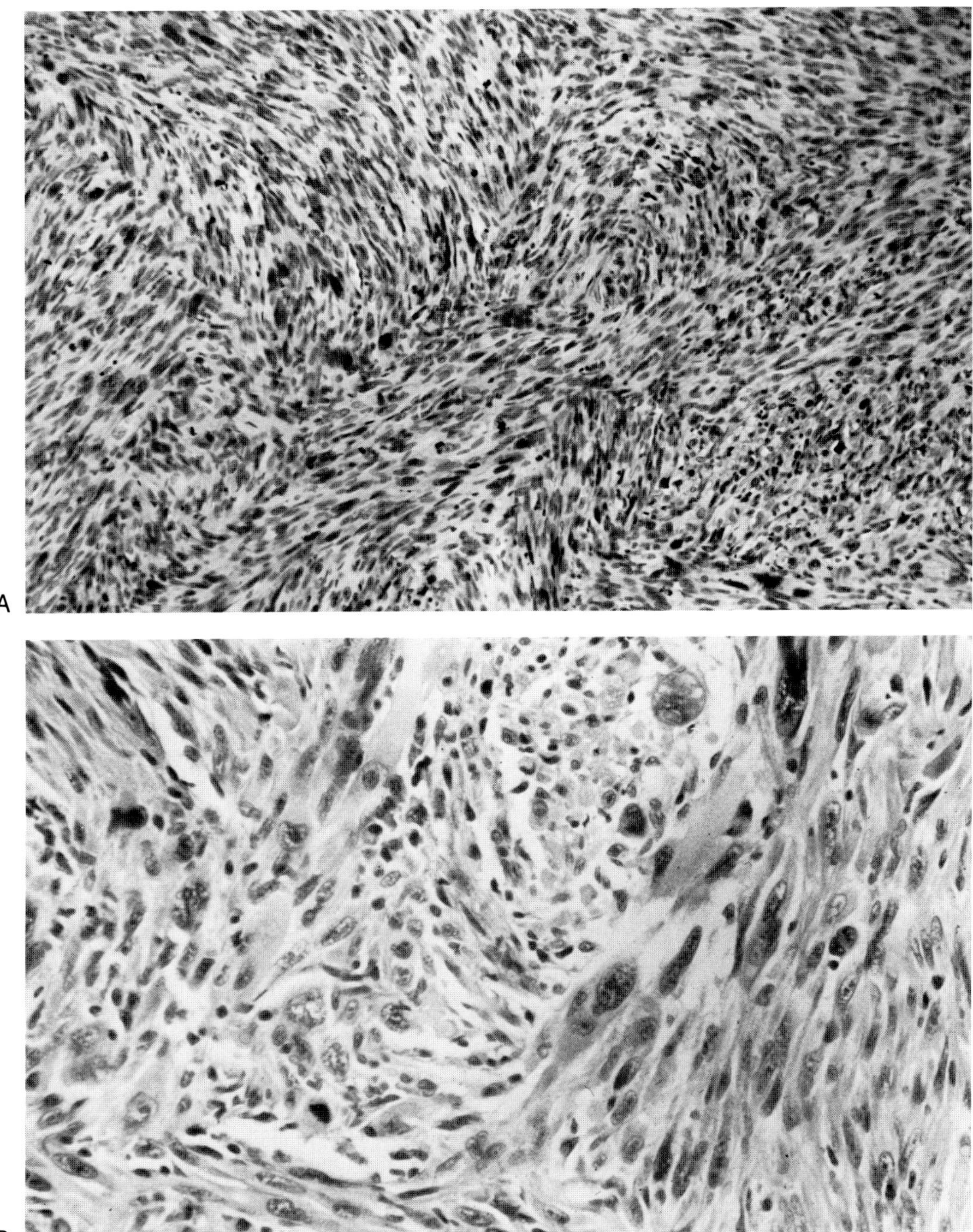

Fig. 4-8. A storiform pattern (**A**) and prominent cellular pleomorphism (**B**) reminiscent of an MFH are more frequently observed in recurrent leiomyosarcoma. (H&E, Fig. A × 100; Fig. B × 250.)

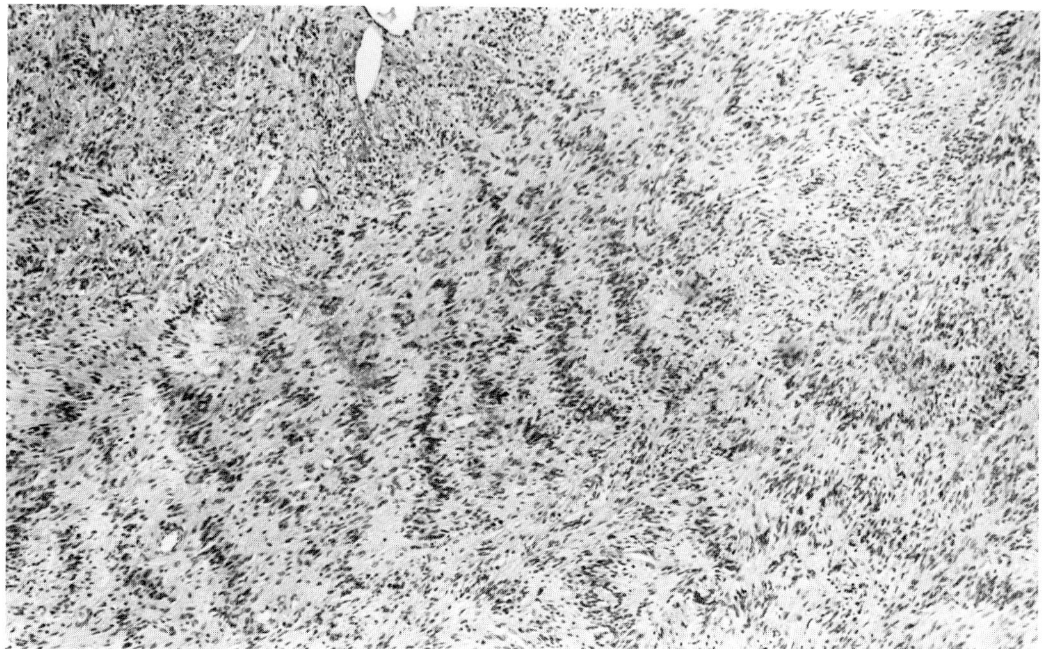

Fig. 4-9. Visceral leiomyosarcoma may show a rhythmic arrangement of nuclei (palisades) simulating a nerve sheath tumor. (H&E × 100.)

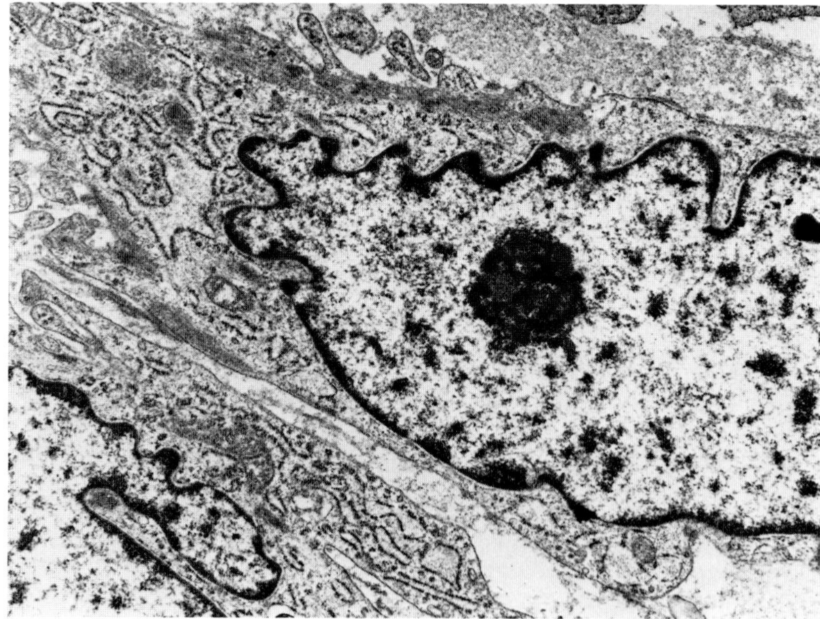

Fig. 4-10. A folded nucleus, few micropinocytotic vesicles, and arrays of thin filaments are the ultrastructural hallmarks of well-differentiated leiomyosarcoma. (× 8,000.)

Cellular differentiation, to a certain degree, corresponds with the ultrastructrual features. Well-differentiated leiomyosarcomas are characterized by numerous thin intracytoplasmic filaments, focal densities, subplasmalemmal pinocytotic vesicles, and a distinct, thin external lamina (Fig. 4-10).[24] In poorly differentiated forms, these features are less evident; thin filaments, focal densities, and pinocytotic vesicles are rare, and the external lamina is often incomplete or absent.[25]

Immunohistochemically leiomyosarcomas show a broad reactivity to many muscle markers, such as vimentin, actin, desmin, and smooth muscle myosin, as well as to basal lamina components, including laminin and type IV collagen.[26–30] Reactivity to keratin monoclonal antibodies, however, was recently demonstrated in both normal and neoplastic smooth muscle cells.[31, 32]

Differential Diagnosis

Although the above cytoarchitectural features are rather typical for leiomyosarcoma, other spindle cell sarcomas may occasionally pose difficult diagnostic problems. Fibrosarcoma and malignant nerve sheath tumors (MNST) may also display a fasciculated pattern. In these cases, trichrome and periodic acid-Schiff (PAS) stains are of utmost importance in the differential diagnosis; fibrosarcoma and MNST are PAS negative and fail to demonstrate any fibrillar cytoplasmic component. The presence of pleomorphic giant cells raises the possibility of a MFH. Cytoplasmic, diastase-sensitive PAS positivity in addition to positivity for muscle markers differentiate leiomyosarcoma from MFH.

Monophasic fibrous synovial sarcoma occasionally enters the differential diagnosis; a nodular growth pattern, a prominent mast cell infiltrate, small foci of clear cells, and keratin positivity will favor a diagnosis of synovial sarcoma rather than leiomyosarcoma. Table 4-1 summarizes the principal differential diagnostic features between leiomyosarcoma and other spindle cell sarcomas.

Reactive fibroblastic lesions, particularly in the genitourinary region, may closely resemble leiomyosarcoma.[33,34] These pseudotumors may be differentiated from leiomyosarcoma by a previous surgical history and the microscopic finding of a loose myxoid and inflammatory background.

Table 4-1. Differential Diagnosis of Leiomyosarcoma

	LS	FS	MNST	SS	MFH
Pattern	Fascicular	Herringbone	Whorls	Nodular	Storiform
Nuclear shape	Cigar	Sharp-pointed	Comma	Spindle	Anaplastic
Giant cells	+	−	+	−	+ +
Fibrillary cytoplasm (Masson)	+	−	−	−	−
PAS+/diastase+	+	−	−	−	−
Elastic fibers	+*	−	−	−	−
S-100	−	−	+/−	−	+/−
Keratin	+/−	−	−	+	−
Desmin	+	−	−	−	−

LS, leiomyosarcoma; FS, fibrosarcoma; MNST, malignant nerve sheath tumor; SS, synovial sarcoma; MFH, malignant fibrous histiocytoma.
* In the case of vascular leiomyosarcoma.

Prognosis

Although it is well recognized that leiomyosarcoma is a highly malignant tumor, the diagnostic criteria for malignancy in smooth muscle tumors are still unascertained. The number of mitoses required for such a diagnosis varies greatly depending on the anatomic site, and ranges from 10 to 2 mitoses per 10 high-power fields (hpf) for uterine and cutaneous tumors, respectively. As a general rule, the larger and deeper the tumor, the less favorable the final prognosis. Tumors larger than 6 cm in diameter in the gastrointestinal tract or 7.5 cm in the retroperitoneum should be considered malignant regardless of their mitotic activity or cytological appearance.[14, 35] Dermal tumors rarely metastasize (0 to 10 percent),[15] but subcutaneous and retroperitoneal tumors metastasize in 40 and 60 percent of the cases, respectively. The overall 5-year survival rate is about 60 percent, ranging from 29 percent for retroperitoneal tumors[14] to 100 percent for dermal lesions.[9]

EPITHELIOID SMOOTH MUSCLE TUMORS

Epitheloid smooth muscle tumors, unusual variants of smooth muscle tumors, are composed of round, epithelial-like cells, often arranged in a nodular rather than a fasciculated pattern. These tumors are more commonly found in the gastrointestinal tract and only exceptionally in soft tissues.[36, 37] Benign and malignant forms share many histologic features. In fact, both are characterized by nodules of round or short spindle cells, with clear or slightly eosinophilic cytoplasm. The nuclei are centrally located, although cytoplasmic vacuoles may occasionally displace them to the periphery to give a signet ring cell appearance (Fig. 4-11). However, this feature is not observed on frozen sections or ultrastructurally,[38] and should be considered an artifact attributable to formalin fixation.[39] Within the tumor nodules, cells are arranged in sheaths or in a vague pseudoalveolar, paragangliomalike pattern; however, more conventional spindle cell areas, where the smooth mus-

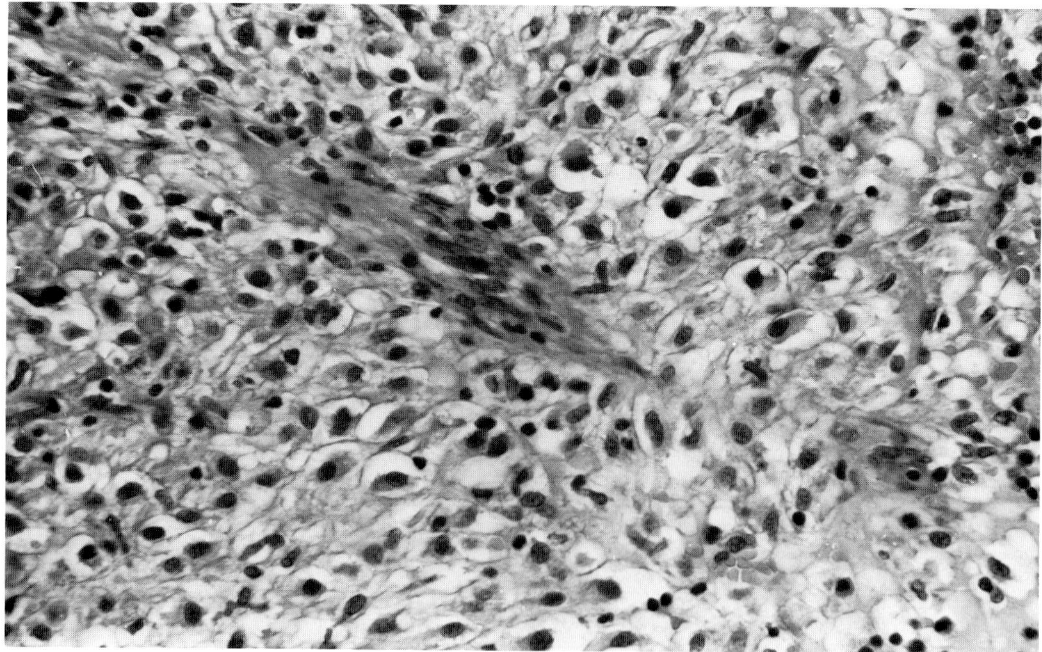

Fig. 4-11. Epithelioid leiomyosarcoma. Diffuse sheaths of large, polygonal, epithelial-like cells with clear cytoplasm, condensed in a thin perinucler eosinophilic rim. (H&E, × 160.)

cle nature of the cells is more easily identified, are frequently observed. Ultrastructurally the typical features of a smooth muscle cell are observed,[38] but myofilaments are less well represented.[40] Desmin is frequently observed in tumor cells, confirming the primitive origin of the lesion.[7]

Differential Diagnosis

Owing to their signet ring cell appearance, epithelioid smooth muscle tumors may be easily mistaken for carcinoma or liposarcoma; however, PAS, mucin, and fat stains are usually negative.

Prognosis

Like all other smooth muscle tumors, prognosis is largely based on the number of mitoses and the size of the lesion. Tumors larger than 6 cm in diameter and with more than 4 or 5 mitoses per 50 hpf should be considered malignant.[41]

TUMORS OF STRIATED MUSCLE

RHABDOMYOMA

Rhabdomyoma is a rare benign neoplasm, accounting for about 2 percent of all striated muscle tumors.[42] It presents as a slow-growing mass, and two variants, fetal and adult, may be distinguished microscopically.[43] The fetal type of rhabdomyoma mainly affects children under 3 years of age, occurring mostly in the head and neck regions.[42, 44] Histologically the tumor is composed of rhabdomyocytes arranged in parallel bundles, and separated by thin strands of highly vascular connective tissue. Nuclei are round or oval with rare nucleoli; the eosinophilic, fibrillar cytoplasm infrequently shows distinct cross-striations (Fig. 4-12). Mitotic fig-

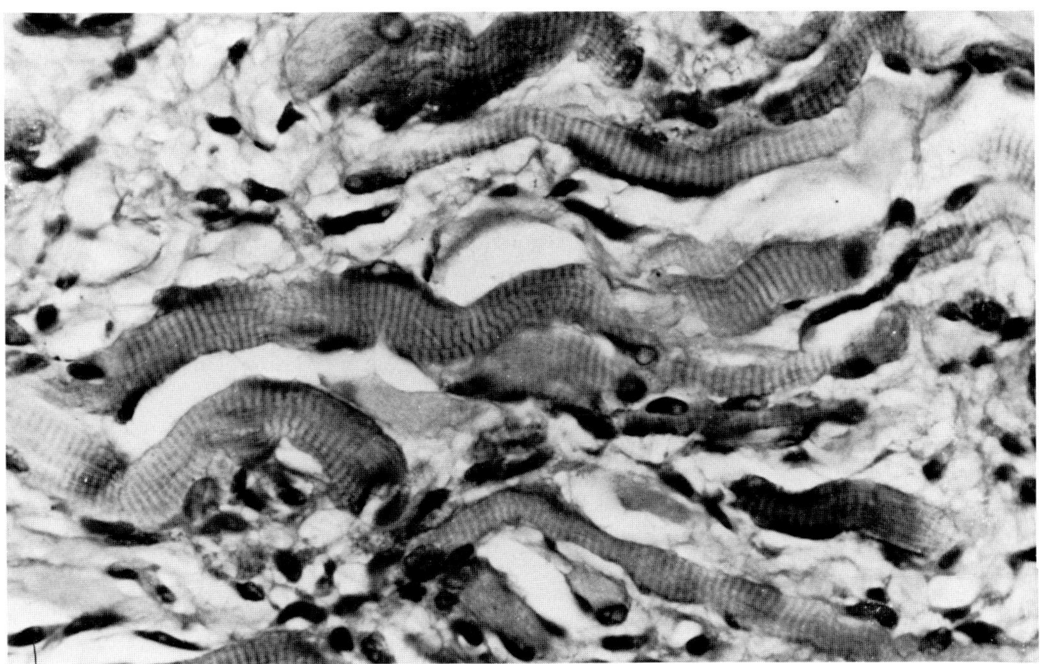

Fig. 4-12. Fully differentiated rhabdomyoblasts with evident cross-striations characterize the adult type of rhabdomyoma. (H&E, × 250.)

ures are rare and the tumor periphery is well outlined by surrounding normal tissue. Similar lesions have also been described in the vulvovaginal region of adult women.[45] The differential diagnosis primarily involves the most differentiated form of embryonal rhabdomyosarcoma. However, the absence of nuclear polymorphism and mitoses and the presence of a clear peripheral demarcation favor the diagnosis of rhabdomyoma.

Adult-type rhabdomyoma is more frequent in patients over 40 years of age; in fact, the mean age at diagnosis is 52 years,[44] with a clear male predominance (M:F 5:1). About 90 percent of the cases occur in the head and neck region, with the mouth, tongue, pharynx, and larynx constituting the favored sites. Histologically this tumor is composed of round or polygonal large cells, ranging from 15 to 150 μm in diameter, separated by thin fibro-vascular septa. The cells have an intensely acidophilic, finely granular cytoplasm, and a vesicular nucleus with a small nucleolus; large cytoplasmic vacuoles and distinct cross-striations are also observed. Granular cell tumor is the main differential diagnosis problem, but it may be ruled out by the absence of large cytoplasmic vacuoles and cross-striations, and the presence of a strong immunocytochemical positivity to S-100 protein.

Both fetal and adult forms of rhabdomyoma are invariably benign tumors, and do not recur after excision.

Rhabdomyosarcoma

Rhabdomyosarcoma (RMS) is the most frequent malignant soft tissue tumor in infancy and adolescence, accounting for more than 50 percent of all childhood sarcomas.[46] In the first 5 years of life, RMS outnumbers all other sarcomas by a ratio of 3.1:1,[46] and constitutes 5 to 15 percent of all solid childhood tumors.[47] The annual incidence of RMS in children is estimated at 3.7 to 5 new cases per million.[48, 49] Conversely, RMS is extremely rare after the fourth decade of life,[50–52] and a relative frequency of

11.8 percent among all soft tissue sarcomas has been reported in adults.[53]

RMS can arise virtually anywhere in the body, but the most common sites are the head and neck, extremities, and genitourinary tract (Table 4-2). Twenty percent of the patients present with metastatic disease at diagnosis.[54] A few cases of systemic RMS with diffuse bone marrow involvement and no discernible primary lesion have also been reported.[55–57]

Classification and Histologic Subtypes

Although four major histopathologic classifications have been developed for RMS[58–61] (Table 4-3), their reproducibility and prognostic significance are currently under investigation.[62] Despite the complex terminology employed in the different classifications, four main RMS subtypes may be recognized on the basis of their peculiar cytoarchitectural aspects: embryonal, botryoid, alveolar, and pleomorphic.

Embryonal RMS

Embryonal RMS (ERMS) accounts for about 70 percent of all RMS,[63, 64] and almost exclusively affects children in the first decade of life, and shows a predilection for the head and neck and the genitourinary tract.

Histologically ERMS is characterized by a proliferation of spindle cells embedded in a loose

Table 4-2. Anatomic Distribution of Rhabdomyosarcoma*

Site	%
Head and neck	37
Genitourinary tract	22
Extremities	19
Retroperitoneum and pelvis	9
Others (paravertebral, thorax, abdomen, etc.)	13

*Data from 2,731 cases reported in the literature.[7, 64, 72, 149]

Table 4-3. Proposed Classifications of RMS

Conventional	Cytohistological	SIOP	NCI
Embryonal	Monomorphous round cell	Embryonal sarcoma	Classic embryonal
Botryoid	Anaplastic	Embryonal	Embryonal
		Loose, botryoid	With areas of aggressive
Alveolar	Mixed	Loose, nonbotryoid	cytology
		Poorly differentiated	Leiomyomatous
Pleomorphic	Undifferentiated round cell	dense	Pleomorphic
		Well-differentiated	
		dense	Alveolar
		Biphasic embryonal	Ewing's-type cells
			Pleomorphic cells
		Alveolar	Monomorphic cells
		Myoblastic	Solid variant
		Round cell	
		Intermediate	Pleomorphic
		Adult (pleomorphic)	

SIOP, International Society of Paediatric Oncology; NCI, National Cancer Institute.

myxoid stroma. A wide spectrum of cellular differentiation is commonly observed, and undifferentiated stellate mesenchymal cells with hyperchromatic nuclei and scarce cytoplasm are intermixed with a variable number of rhabdomyoblasts (Fig. 4-13). The latter are characterized by a glossy eosinophilic cytoplasm, which at times shows typical cross-striations (strap cells), or an angular, broken shape (Fig. 4-14). Cells with eccentric nuclei and elongated, eosinophilic "comma-shaped" cytoplasm (tadpole cells) and larger polygonal cells are usually scattered in the stroma. These cytologic aspects correlate with the expression of muscle markers, such as vimentin, desmin, and myoglobin.[65–67] Undifferentiated spindle cells almost exclusively express vimentin, whereas desmin (Fig. 4-15) and myoglobin are commonly found in larger cytoplasm-rich cells. Depending on the relative percentage of rhabdomyoblasts, ERMS has been classified into several histologic subgroups, each with a prognostic significance. Well-differentiated ERMS (greater than 50 percent rhabdomyoblasts) has a better prognosis than poorly differentiated ERMS (less than 10 percent rhabdomyoblasts).[67]

Hypercellular areas made up of round and/or pleomorphic cells are occasionally observed in otherwise typical ERMS; although worrisome, they do not affect the final prognosis. Multinucleated syncytial giant cells are rarely observed.

Short bundles of eosinophilic spindle cells are occasionally observed in ERMS. Tumors composed almost exclusively of bundles of elongated spindle cells arranged in a storiform or leiomyomatous pattern can also be found (Fig. 4-16). This variant of ERMS has been tentatively named *spindle cell RMS*.[68] It occurs chiefly in the genital areas (paratesticular and parauterine), and predominantly in males (M:F 3:1). At the light microscope, it may be confused with a leiomyosarcoma or a fibrosarcoma if the presence of cross-striations is overlooked. Mitoses and areas of necrosis or hemorrhage are rare. Muscular markers (desmin, skeletal-muscle myosin, myoglobin, and titin) are all highly expressed in most tumor cells, a finding that denotes a high degree of tumor differentiation, reminiscent of terminal stages of skeletal muscle development.

Botryoid RMS

A distinctive variant of ERMS, termed *botryoid*, is found in hollow organs such as the vagina, nasal sinuses, and bladder. Macroscopically this variant displays a characteristic exophytic grapelike growth. The histologic diagnosis rests on the recognition of a discrete

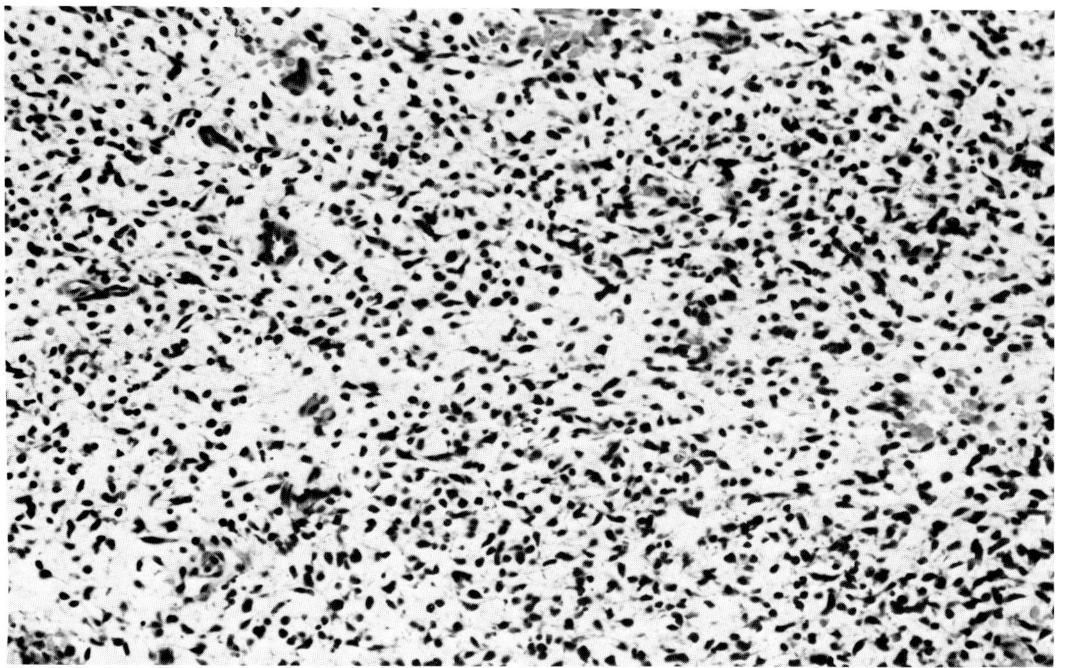

Fig. 4-13. ERMS. Primitive spindle and stellate mesenchymal cells embedded in a loose myxoid stroma. Tumors entirely composed of these cells without morphologic evidence of myogenesis have been also referred to as *embryonal sarcomas* (H&E, × 160.)

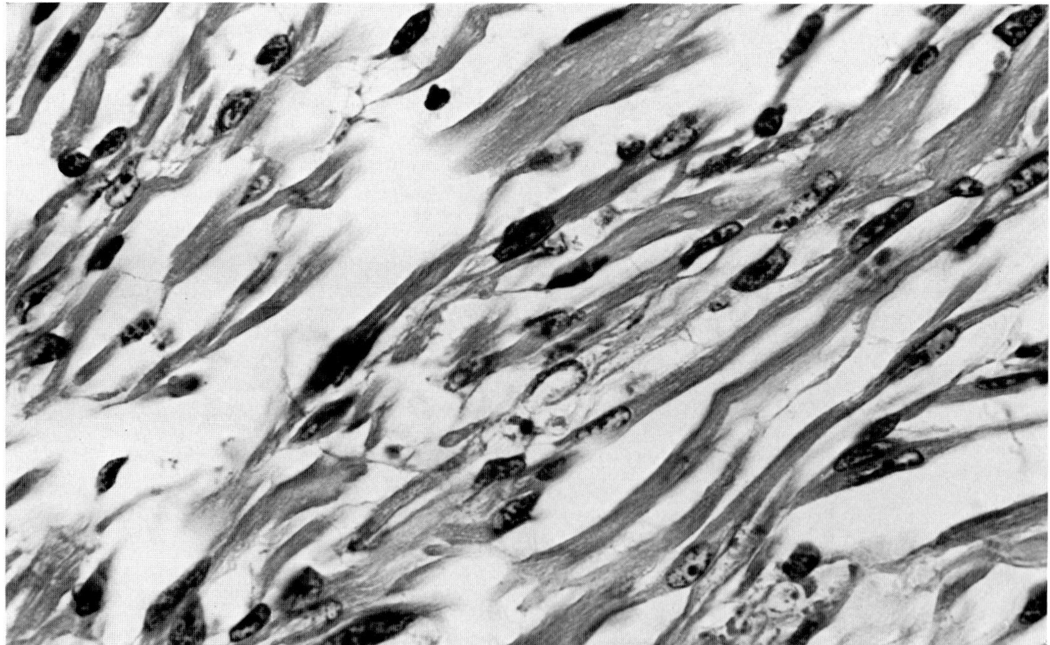

Fig. 4-14. Elongated strap-shaped rhabdomyoblasts are diagnostic hallmarks of embryonal RMS. Cross-striations are easily detected in these cells. (H&E, × 250.)

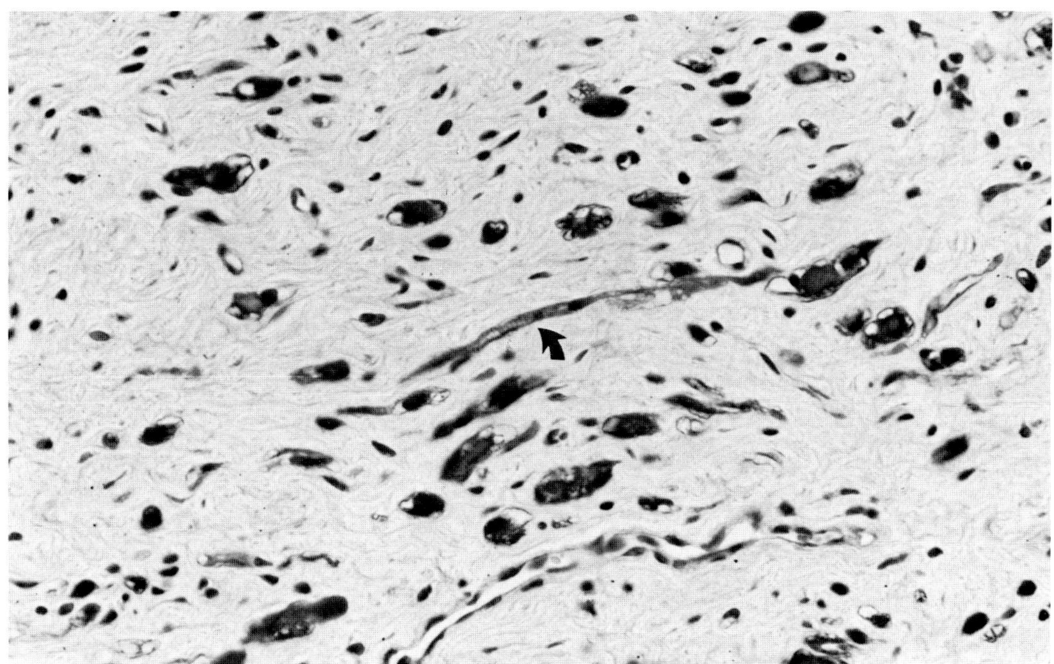

Fig. 4-15. A strong desmin positivity is more often observed in strap cells (arrow) and in cytoplasm-rich myoblasts. (ABC method; × 160.)

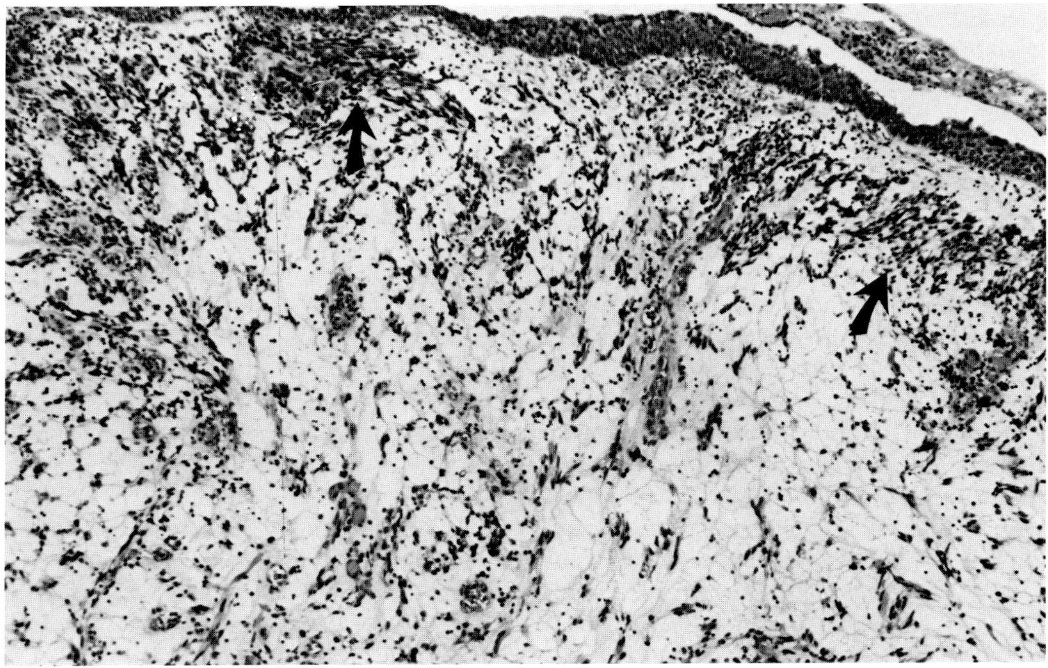

Fig. 4-16. Spindle cell RMS. Fusiform cells are arranged in a fasciculated pattern closely resembling a leiomyosarcoma. (H&E, × 160.)

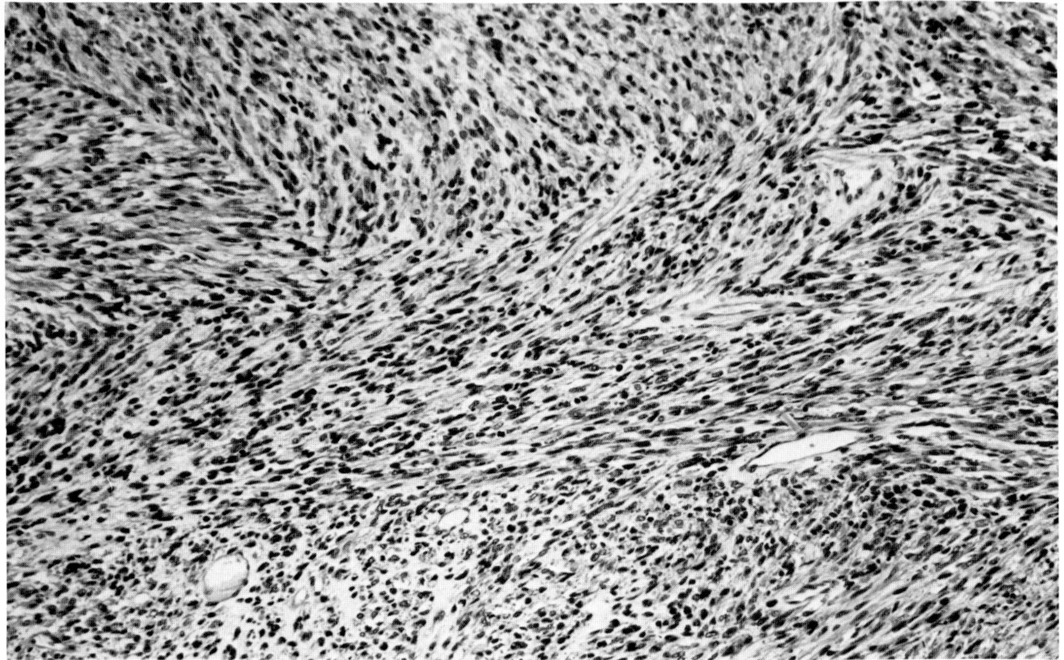

Fig. 4-17. Botryoid RMS of the bladder. Note the presence of a distinct hypercellular zone (cambium layer) (arrow) beneath the epithelium. (H&E, × 160.)

hypercellular zone (''cambium layer'') composed of tightly packed, rather undifferentiated myoblasts that are condensed just beneath the epithelium (Fig. 4-17).

Alveolar RMS

Alveolar RMS (ARMS) accounts for 15 to 30 percent of all RMS[63, 64] and is more common in the second and third decade of life. Extremities, retroperitoneum, pelvis, mediastinum, paravertebral, chest, and head and neck are the most commonly involved sites. Microscopically ARMS is characterized by the presence of alveolar spaces lined by a single row of small or intermediate-sized cells with dark hyperchromatic nuclei, evident nucleolus, and a rim of eosinophilic cytoplasm (Fig. 4-18). Multinucleated giant cells are common; cross-striations are rare, and are usually absent in the cells lining the alveolar spaces,[69] which are divided by collagenous, at times sclerotic septa containing dilated blood vessels. Hemorrhagic and necrotic areas, as well as atypical mitoses, are frequent findings.

The term *mixed type RMS* was proposed for RMS in which embryonal and/or pleomorphic areas are intermixed with alveolar spaces.[70, 71] Consequently, it was suggested that only tumors consisting at least of 70 percent of alveolar spaces should be classified as ARMS[72]; however, the number of alveolar spaces is not significantly correlated with prognosis. Therefore tumors showing even a *single* alveolar space should be classified as ARMS.[46]

As originally observed,[73, 69] solid areas of closely packed round cells occasionally are present at the periphery of ARMS. Tsokos et al.[74] proposed that tumors consisting almost entirely of these solid areas should be considered a *solid variant* of ARMS, and accordingly classified. Microscopically this variant shows a compact proliferation of round tumor cells with hyperchromatic nuclei, evident nucleoli, and scant cytoplasm (Fig. 4-19). A few cells with larger, bright eosinophilic cytoplasm are constantly encountered, but cross-striations are notably absent. Mitoses are numerous, and often atypical. Sin-

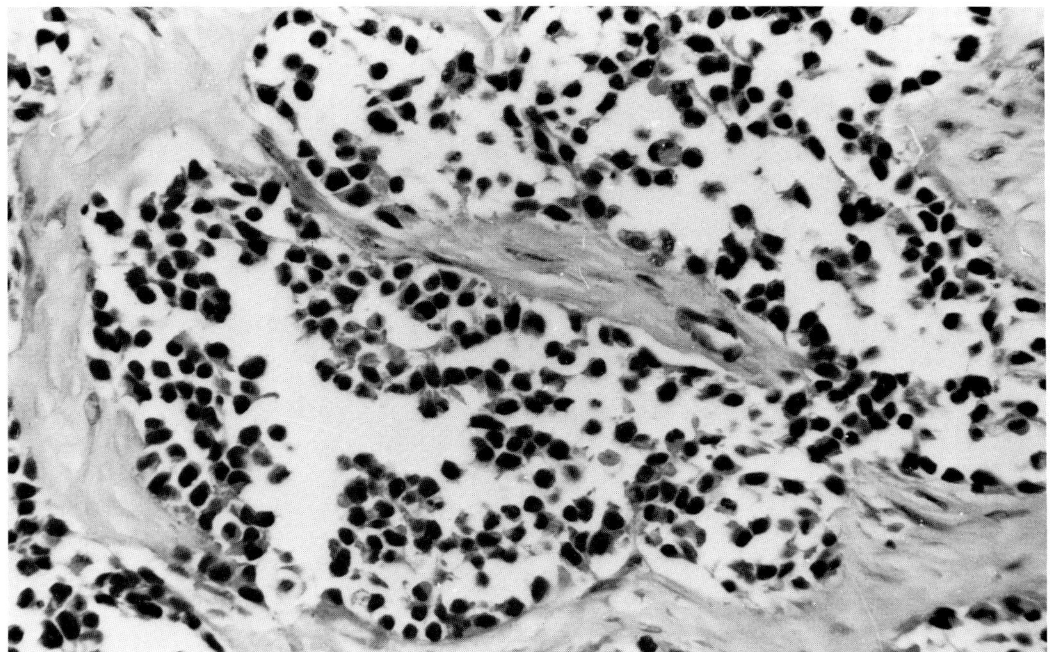

Fig. 4-18. ARMS. Alveolar spaces are lined by small hyperchromatic cells with eosinophilic cytoplasm. No cross-striations are discerned. Note the presence of highly sclerotic septa. (H&E, × 200.)

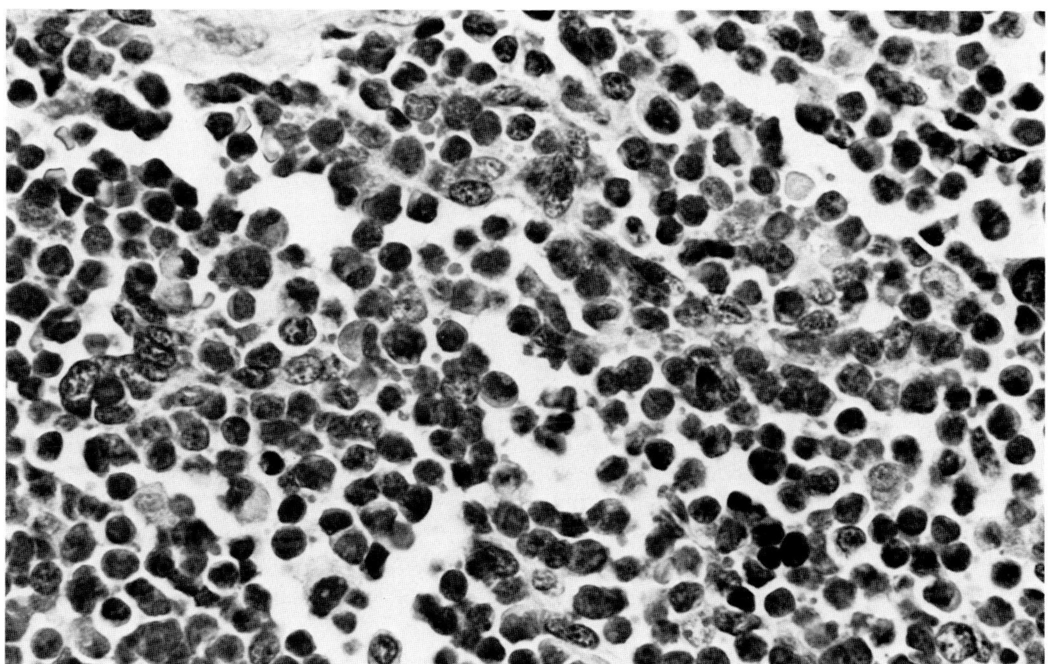

Fig. 4-19. Hypercellular areas composed of tightly packed roundish cells with scarce cytoplasm, hyperchromatic nuclei, and prominent nucleoli characterize the solid variant of ARMS. (H&E, × 250.)

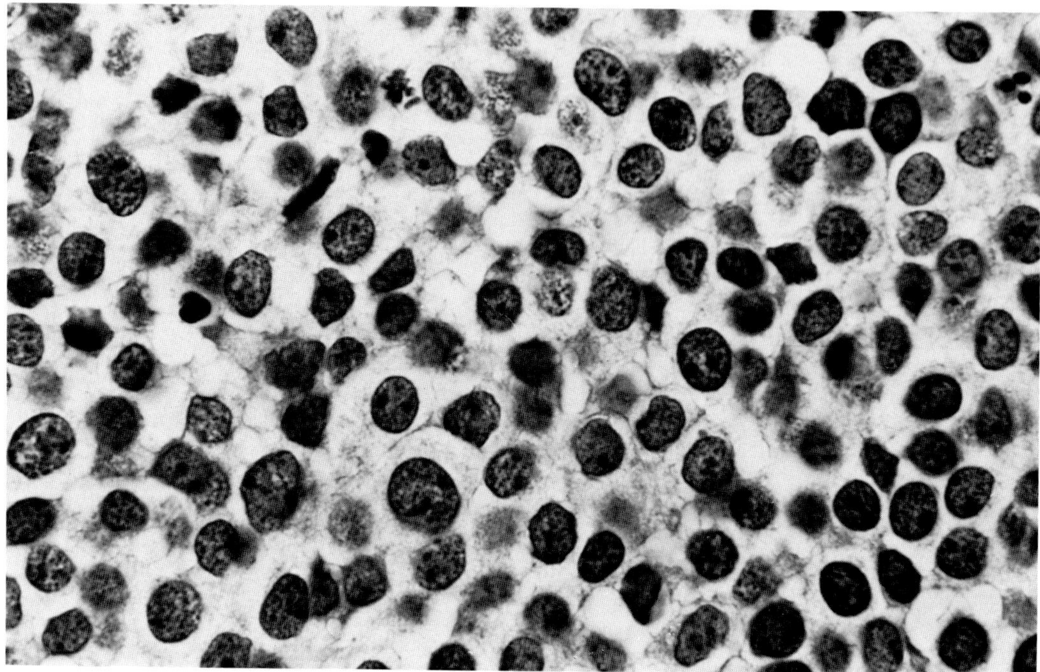

Fig. 4-20. So-called monomorphous RMS. Note the marked nuclear uniformity. Although a certain degree of similarity is apparent between the solid variant of ARMS and the monomorphous variant, the latter is recognized by its greater cellular uniformity. (H&E, × 600.)

gle cell necrosis and nuclear pyknosis are frequently observed. Some reticulin fibers interspersed between the tumor cells, and a vague alveolar pattern are occasionally seen. Despite the minimal and barely detectable morphologic differentiation, however, the rhabdomyoblastic origin of this tumor is documented by its positivity to muscle markers, such as desmin, myosin, and actin.[75]

In a similar manner, Palmer and Foulkes[60] noted that 10 percent of RMS in the second Intergroup Rhabdomyosarcoma Study were composed of a homogeneous population of round cells with scant cytoplasm and a distinctive nuclear morphology. The nuclei were uniform in shape and size and characterized by a peripherally distributed chromatin, one or two prominent nuclear folds, and a single evident paracentral nucleolus (Fig. 4-20). The name, monomorphous RMS, was proposed for this variant.

Both the solid variant of ARMS and mono-morphous RMS show a very aggressive clinical course with an unfavorable prognosis.

Pleomorphic RMS

Pleomorphic RMS (PRMS) is the rarest variety of RMS, accounting for 1 to 5 percent of pediatric RMS,[46, 64] and was once considered the main type of RMS in adults.[7, 76] However, after MFH was accepted as a distinct entity,[77] many adult PRMS were reclassified as MFH; retrospective immunocytochemical studies confirmed the initial diagnosis of PRMS only in 8 to 10 percent of these cases,[50, 78, 79] thus indicating that PRMS is exceptional in adults, if it exists at all.[52, 80, 81] At the light microscope, PRMS closely mimics pleomorphic MFH owing to its extreme cellular pleomorphism. The giant cells have a syncytial appearance with marginated nuclei and a pear-shaped cytoplasm, reminiscent of abortive myotubule formation (Fig. 4-21); perinuclear tangles of filaments and cross-striations are occasionally observed in the cytoplasm of larger cells.

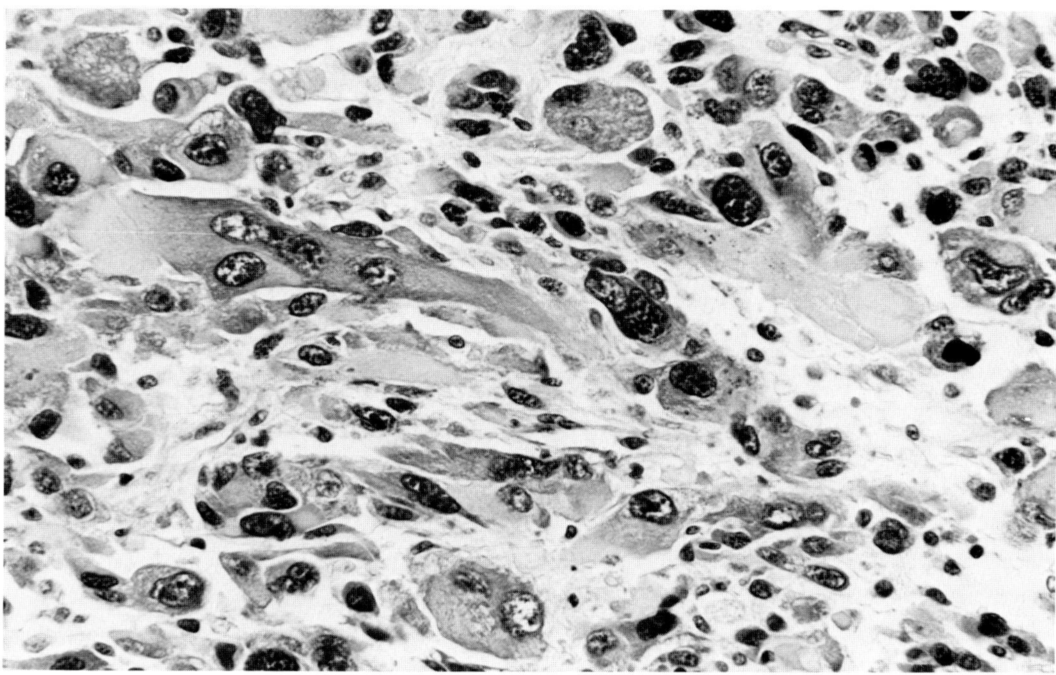

Fig. 4-21. Large multinucleated giant cells with bright eosinophilic cytoplasm are observed in pleomorphic RMS. (H&E, × 500.)

Ultrastructural Findings

Conclusive morphologic evidence of skeletal muscle differentiation consists of thin and thick filaments arranged in typical 6 + 1 sarcomeric fashion, and ordinately organized in parallel rows by a rather flocculent, transversely oriented, electron-dense structure (Z band) (see Fig. 4-2). This regular arrangement of contractile filaments is not frequently observed in RMS and a variety of ultrastructural features have been described depending on the degree of tumor differentiation.[82–85]

A fibroblastlike, primitive spindle cell appearance is frequently observed, particularly in ERMS. These cells are characterized by few profiles of rough endoplasmic reticulum, numerous free ribosomes, and a moderate amount of glycogen. Intermediate vimentin-type and thin filaments are commonly observed, but myofilaments are notably absent.

The presence of myosin filaments, alone or in association with actin filaments, denotes a more differentiated phenotype. Bundles of thick filaments with ribosomes arranged in "Indian file" (ribosome/myosin complexes) (Fig. 4-22) were proposed as minimal criteria for the ultrastructural diagnosis of RMS.[83] Although a complete sarcomere is a rather rare finding, focal densities or rodlike structures composed of Z-band material are frequently encountered also in poorly differentiated tumors (Fig. 4-23).[85, 86] Nuclei show irregular borders with marked nuclear folds and roughly distributed chromatin; nucleoli are generally prominent. A discontinuous basal lamina surrounds the rhabdomyoblasts, and rudimentary cell junctions may be seen. Collagen fibers are frequently observed in the extracellular spaces.[86]

Immunocytochemistry

In the past few years a large number of polyclonal and monoclonal antibodies to muscle-specific proteins have been developed and em-

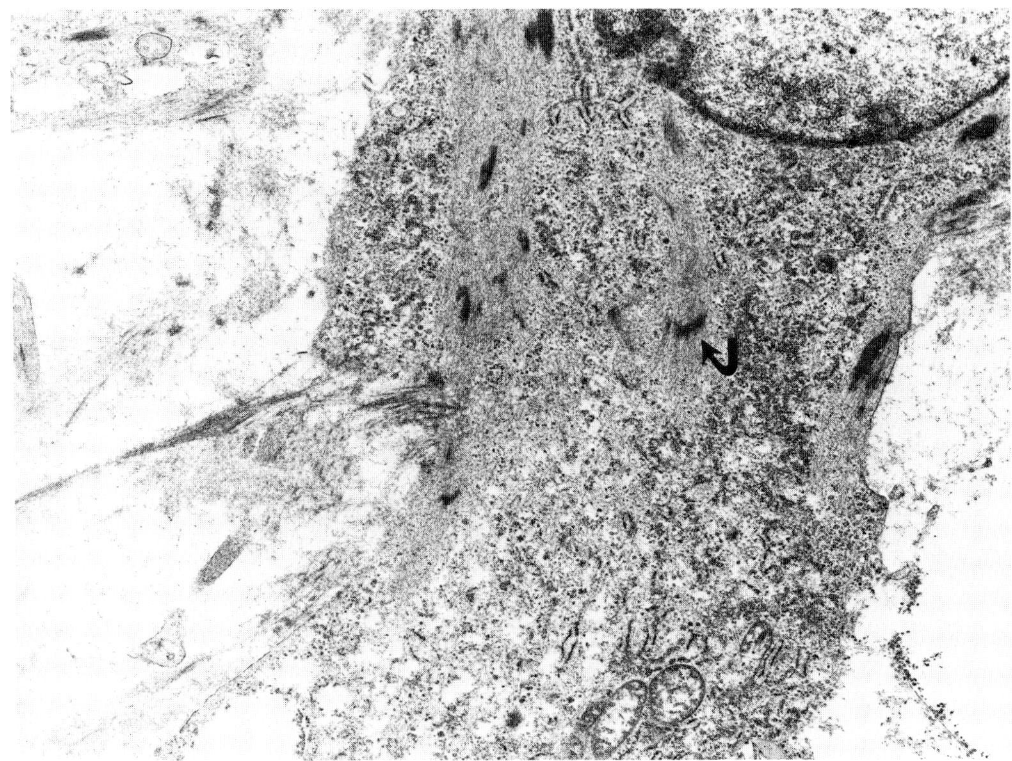

Fig. 4-22. Thick filaments with ribosomes arranged in ''Indian file'' represent a highly characteristic ultrastructural finding of rhabdomyoblastic differentiation. ($\times$ 20,000.) (Courtesy of Dr. A. Parenti.)

ployed in the immunodiagnosis of RMS (Table 4-4).

Vimentin, an intermediate filament with a molecular weight of 57,000 constitutes the major cytoskeletal component of all mesenchymal cells and derived tumors.[87] Although vimentin is not a specific marker of muscle differentiation, it is expressed by myoblasts in the early stages of development, and is later replaced by desmin.[88, 89] Vimentin is absent in normal adult skeletal muscle, but it is almost uniquely expressed by undifferentiated spindle or round cells; vimentin and desmin are commonly coexpressed by cytoplasm-rich neoplastic rhabdomyoblasts.[65, 90, 91]

Myoglobin, a simple heme protein with a molecular weight of 17,800 is usually present in developing embryonic striated muscle, and is absent in smooth muscle. Although the latter characteristic ensures that myoglobin expression has a 100 percent specificity for skeletal muscle tumors, its sensitivity, however, ranges from 100 to 30 percent,[92–98] according to the extent of the tumor's cytological differentiation; undifferentiated round cells are the least reactive.[98] Finally, great care must be taken to avoid interpretative pitfalls: a false-positive may result from diffusion or phagocytosis of muscle myoglobin from disrupted muscle cells into the cytoplasm of reactive histiocytes or lymphomatous cells invading normal skeletal muscles.[99]

Desmin, an intermediate filament with a molecular weight of 53,000 is found in both smooth and striated muscle.[87] With synemin[100] and filamin,[101] desmin constitutes the peripheral domain of the Z bands in adult striated muscle,[102] and forms an interconnecting network that ensures the proper myofibril alignment during the contraction-relaxation cycle.[103] Although its sensitivity is almost 100 percent,[104, 105] desmin-

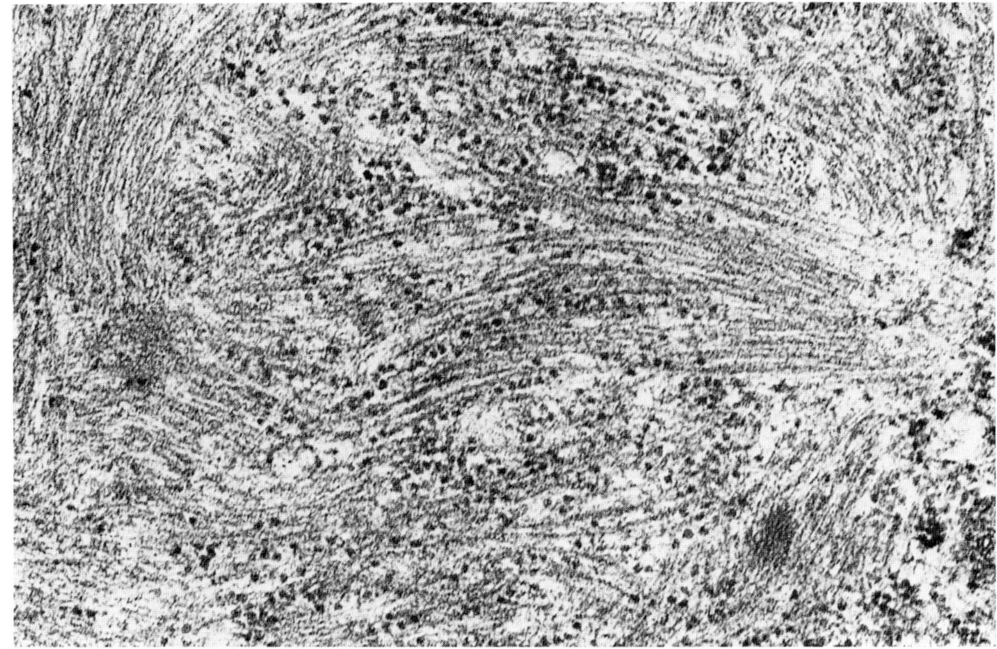

Fig. 4-23. In ERMS, primitive sarcomeres (arrow) are occasionally observed in the cytoplasm. ($\times$ 4000) (Courtesy of Prof. M.L. Valente.)

Table 4-4. Markers in Immunodiagnosis of RMS

Marker	Specificity
Vimentin	Mesenchymal cells[52, 65, 67, 78, 90, 98, 104, 106, 108, 112]
Desmin	Smooth and skeletal muscles[29, 52, 65, 67, 78, 90, 104–106, 108, 112, 114]
Skeletal muscle myosin	Skeletal muscle[78, 97, 105, 117]
Fetal myosin	Skeletal muscle[118, 119]
Muscular actin	Smooth and skeletal muscles[29, 78, 98, 114]
α-Sarcomeric actin	Skeletal muscle[106, 108, 113]
Myoglobin	Skeletal muscle[52, 67, 78, 90, 92, 95, 97, 98, 105, 112]
Titin	Skeletal muscle[68, 124]
Z-band protein	Skeletal muscle[127]
Tropomyosin	Skeletal muscle[117]
α-Actinin	Skeletal muscle[117]
Creatin-kinase MM	Skeletal muscle[78, 98]
β-Enolase	Smooth and skeletal muscles[126]

negative RMS have also been reported.[29, 106] Desmin is extremely sensitive to fixatives, particularly formalin,[106] and is of little value in distinguishing smooth from striated muscle tumors.[107, 108] Furthermore, desmin positivity in a variety of cells, including myofibroblasts, glial cells, astrocytes, and endothelial cells, has been occasionally reported.[107, 109–111] Nevertheless, desmin appears the most reliable *single* marker in the immunodiagnosis of RMS.[75, 90, 104, 105, 112]

Muscular isoforms of actin have been proven to be even more highly sensitive markers of muscle differentiation[29, 98, 106, 113, 114] than desmin.[29, 106] The expression of muscular isoforms of actin in desmin-negative RMS[29, 106] and the resistance of this antigen to a wide range of fixatives[29] make the presence of antibodies to muscular actins a valid alternative to desmin in the immunodiagnosis of RMS.

Skeletal muscle myosin has also been proposed as a useful marker for RMS.[96, 97, 105] The myosin molecule consists of two heavy and four light chains. Multiple forms of myosin heavy chains are encoded by different genes, whose expression is tissue specific and developmentally regulated.[115 116] The sensitivity of antibodies to fast myosin heavy chain ranges from 85 percent[97] to 75 percent.[96, 117] Recently developed monoclonal antibodies to the embryonic form of skeletal muscle myosin heavy chain[118] seem to provide better results in detecting early skeletal muscle differentiation in RMS.[119]

Titin (also known as connectin) is a protein with a very high molecular weight (1,400,000 to 2,800,000) that makes up about 10 percent of the myofibrillar mass of sarcomeric muscle.[120, 121] It appears late during myogenesis in postmitotic myoblasts and myotubes,[122] and plays an important role in passive elasticity of muscle fibers.[123] Its unique expression in skeletal muscle is helpful in distinguishing rhabdomyosarcoma from other myogenic and nonmyogenic tumors,[124] although its expression seems restricted to well-differentiated rhabdomyoblasts (strap cells and myotubes) (Fig. 4-24).[68]

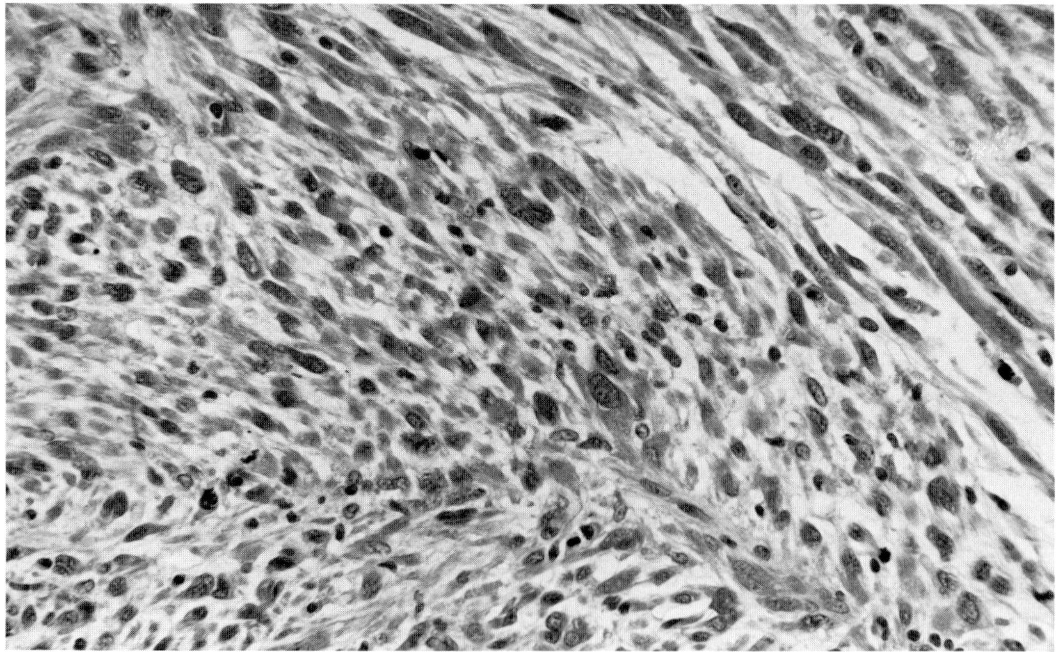

Fig. 4-24. Titin positivity in spindle cell RMS. The majority of rhabdomyoblasts show an intense cytoplasmic positivity. (Peroxidase-antiperoxidase technique, × 160.)

Therefore, antibodies to titin should be used in conjunction with other muscle markers to allow unequivocal identification of RMS.

Other muscle markers, including creatine-kinase MM,[66, 125] β-enolase,[126] tropomyosin,[117] α-actinin[117] and Z-band protein,[127] have been employed for the immunocytochemical diagnosis of RMS. Unfortunately no single marker can consistently recognize every RMS, and a panel of antibodies is required; in this sense, myoglobin, desmin, and muscle-specific actins seem to provide the most satisfactory results.

Antibodies to extracellular matrix components, including collagen IV, laminin, and fibronectin, may also provide useful information in the differential diagnosis between RMS and other small round cell tumors.[128–130] RMS, Ewing's sarcoma, neuroblastoma, small cell osteosarcoma and primitive neuroectodermal tumors may be differentiated on the basis of their extracellular matrix;[95] ERMS stains positively for collagen IV, laminin, and fibronectin, whereas ARMS, neuroblastoma, and primitive neuroectodermal tumors are all negative. Ewing's sarcoma is positive for collagen IV and laminin, whereas small cell osteosarcoma is positive only for fibronectin.

Neuron-specific enolase,[98, 131] S-100 protein,[132] keratin, and neurofilaments[132, 133] have all been occasionally reported positive in RMS; an awareness of these unexpected findings will help avoid diagnostic errors.

Diagnostic Criteria

A morphologic diagnosis of RMS can be achieved in about 90 percent of cases, and only a few will require additional ultrastructural and/or immunocytochemical studies. A confident diagnosis of RMS rests on the recognition of cytoplasmic cross-striations, which are detected in 30 percent[71] to 60 percent[58] of cases. Special stains, such as PTHA or ferric-hematoxylin, generally facilitate the search for this feature. Strap cells, reminiscent of the early stages of myotube development, and tadpole cells are highly characteristic of RMS. They are fre-quently observed and easily recognized in the embryonal and botryoid variants of RMS, whereas they are scarce or absent in ARMS and PRMS.

In the absence of cross-striations or strap and tadpole cells, other cytoarchitectural features can help in establishing the diagnosis. A loose myxoid or alveolar pattern is recognized in most cases, whereas fasciculated or solid growths are less frequent. Furthermore, a bright eosinophilic, slightly granular, and PAS-positive, diastase-sensitive cytoplasm is highly indicative of a rhabdomyoblastic differentiation. Therefore, the finding of spindle or round cells with bright, eosinophilic cytoplasm, arranged in an alveolar pattern or embedded in a loose myxoid stroma, points to a rhabdomyoblastic origin of the tumor. The presence of Z bandlike material associated with bundles of thin and thick filaments at the ultrastructural level and positivity to one or more of the above muscle markers will definitely corroborate the diagnosis of RMS.

An alternative diagnostic approach is offered by the use of genetic markers.[134, 135] When immunocytochemistry and electron microscopy fail to provide conclusive results, the myogenic nature of undifferentiated tumors can be ascertained by the expression of skeletal muscle-specific genes, such as MYOD1.[136] Furthermore, the loss of chromosome 11 heterozygosity identifies and distinguishes ERMS from ARMS,[137] as the latter is often associated with a reciprocal chromosomal translocation t(2;13) (q37; q14).[138–140]

Differential Diagnosis

RMS can mimic a variety of soft tissue tumors and pseudotumors. Inflammatory processes in hollow organs, pseudosarcomatous lesions, and benign tumors such as myxomas can be misdiagnosed as ERMS; however, findings such as cellular hyperchromasia, atypical mitoses, and the presence of cross-striations in strap-shaped cells help to identify ERMS. Proliferative myositis and fascitis can also enter the differential diagnosis, but the presence of typical ganglionlike cells and a checkerboard pattern are diagnostic of the former.

Leiomyosarcoma and infantile fibromatosis may be involved in the differential diagnosis of the spindle cell variant of ERMS. Since leiomyosarcoma is exceedingly rare in childhood,[141] a spindle cell RMS should always be considered when dealing with a fasciculated tumor located in a paragenital area. On the other hand, the presence of cross-striations and positivity to muscle markers rule out fibrous proliferations.

An alveolar pattern suggests but is not conclusive for ARMS; other neoplasms, such as alveolar soft part sarcoma and pigmented neuroectodermal tumor of infancy (retinal anlage tumor or melanotic progonoma) may display the same pattern. Alveolar soft part sarcoma however, shows larger polygonal cells with PAS-positive diastase-negative cytoplasm containing the diagnostic rodlike inclusions, whereas melanic pigment is readily demonstrated in pigmented neuroectodermal tumor.

The differential diagnosis between a solid variant of ARMS and other small round cell tumors is probably the most thought-provoking and difficult task, and often requires additional investigations. Extraosseous Ewing's Sarcoma displays a more densely packed and regular cellular proliferation than RMS, where cellular molding or a typical biphasic light and dark cellular pattern are rarely observed. On the other hand, prominent nucleoli and irregular nuclear profiles are rarely seen in extraosseous Ewing's sarcoma. Recently, nucleolar organizer regions were proposed as useful markers to differentiate extraosseous Ewing's sarcoma from RMS,[142] nucleolar organizer regions being significantly less numerous in RMS. Peripheral neuroectodermal tumors at times may be confused with RMS. The large eosinophilic gangliar cells found in ganglioneuroblastoma are occasionally mistaken for rhabdomyoblasts; the perinuclear basophilia reminiscent of Nissl's tigroid substance of gangliar cells and the neurofibromatous stroma will facilitate distinction from RMS. Difficulty can be encountered in the differential

diagnosis with a PNET. The absence of Homer-Wright rosettes at the light microscope, the presence of neuritic extensions with dense-core granules at the electron microscope, and/or positivity to neural markers, such as neuron-specific enolase, S-100 protein, chromogranin, synaptophysin, and neurofilaments, however, favor a neuroectodermal rather than a muscular origin of the tumor (Table 4-5).

Rhabdoid tumor may be misdiagnosed as RMS owing to its intense cytoplasmic eosinophilia. Nonetheless, rhabdoid tumor has a homogeneous cellular appearance, with characteristic cytoplasmic hyalin globules and typical grooved nuclei.

Pleomorphic sarcomas, including MFH, pleomorphic liposarcoma, and pleomorphic leiomyosarcoma, have often been confused with PRMS in the past.[50, 78] Ultrastructural and/or immunocytochemical evidence of skeletal muscle differentiation are often required to support the diagnosis of PRMS.

A category of soft tissue tumors showing heterologous elements with a focal rhabdomyoblastic differentiation, such as the malignant triton tumor, malignant mesenchymoma, and ectomesenchymoma, deserve special mention. In these rare cases, diagnosis is based on the recognition of multiple lines of differentiation (i.e., schwannian, osteoblastic, lipoblastic, etc.) present in the tumor.

Prognosis

RMS is a highly aggressive tumor. In the prechemotherapy era, overall survival was 20 percent,[58, 69, 143–146] however, multimodal therapy has dramatically improved this figure in the last two decades.[147, 148] Several prognostically significant parameters have been identified (Table 4-6). The head and neck, orbit, and genitourinary tract are the most favorable sites (greater than 90 percent survival at 3 years), whereas tumors in the retroperitoneum and extremities have a far less favorable outcome (less than 65 percent survival);[54] recently, 44 percent

Table 4-5. Undifferentiated RMS: Differential Diagnosis

	RMS	ES	PNET
Ultrastructure			
Nuclei	Irregular	Regular	Regular
Nucleoli	Prominent	Absent or small	Prominent
Glycogen	+ +	+ + +	+/−
5–7-nm filaments	Present	Present	Present
10-nm filaments	Present	Present	Present
15-nm filaments	Present	Absent	Absent
Ribosome/myosin complexes	Present	Absent	Absent
Z-band material	Present	Absent	Absent
Dense-core granules	Absent	Absent	Present
Cell junctions	Present	Rare	Rare
Basement membrane	Present	Rare	Occasional
Extracellular matrix	Present	Absent	Rare
Immunocytochemistry			
Vimentin	+ +	+	+
Desmin	+ +	−	−
Keratin	+/−	+/−	+/−
Muscle-specific actin	+ +	−	−
Neurofilaments	−	−	+ +
Neuron-specific enolase	+	−	+ +
S-100	+/−	−	+
Chromogranin	−	−	+
Synaptophysin	−	−	+

RMS, rhabdomyosarcoma; ES, Ewing's sarcoma; PNET, primitive neuroectodermal tumor.

survival at 5 years was reported for RMS of the extremities.[149] Extent of disease at diagnosis greatly affects the final prognosis regardless of the anatomic site.[54, 149] Patients with disseminated disease at diagnosis (stage IV) have lower 3-year survival rates (30 percent) than patients with localized disease or a completely excised tumor (stage I) (80 percent survival).[54] The histologic subtype is another important parameter. Spindle cell RMS and the botryoid variant fare better than typical ERMS,[64, 68] whereas patients with ARMS have the poorest prognosis.[45, 71, 150] The combination of nuclear gigantism, hyperchromasia, and abnormal mitoses (anaplastic RMS) has also been associated with an unfavorable outcome.[60, 151]

Regional lymph nodes, lungs, liver, bone, and brain are the most commonly involved sites of metastases.

Table 4-6. Prognostic Factors in RMS

	Favorable	Unfavorable
Stage	I–II	III–IV
Type	Embryonal, botryoid, spindle cell	Alveolar, solid and monomorphous variants, pleomorphic
Site	Orbit, genitourinary tract	Retroperitoneum, pelvis, parameningeal, extremities
Sex	Male	Female

REFERENCES

1. Landon DN: Skeletal muscle—normal morphology, development and innervation—In Mastaglia FL, Walton J (eds)L: Skeletal Muscle Pathology. Churchill Livingstone, Edinburgh, 1987

2. Stout AP: Solitary cutaneous and subcutaneous leiomyoma. Am J Cancer 29:435, 1937

3. Fisher WC, Helwig EB: Leiomyomas of the skin. Arch Dermatol 88:510, 1963

4. Duhig JJ, Ayer IP: Vascular leiomyoma: a study of 61 cases. Arch Pathol Lab Med 68:424, 1959

5. Hachisuga T, Hashimoto H, Enjoji M: Angioleiomyoma: a clinicopathologic reappraisal of 562 cases. Cancer 54:126, 1984

6. Ekestrom S: Comparison between glomus tumour and angioleiomyoma. Acta Pathol Microbiol Scand 27:86, 1950

7. Enzinger FM, Weiss SW: Soft Tissue Tumors. 2nd ed. CV Mosby, St. Louis, 1988

8. Russell WO, Cohen J, Enzinger FM, et al: A clinical and pathological staging system for soft tissue sarcomas. Cancer 40:1562, 1977

9. Hashimoto H, Daimaru Y, Tsuneyoshi M, et al: Leiomyosarcoma of the external soft tissues. A clinicopathologic, immunohistochemical and electron microscopic study. Cancer 57:2077, 1986

10. Yannopoulos K, Stout AP: Smooth muscle tumors in children. Cancer 15:958, 1962

11. Kempson R, Bari W: Uterine sarcomas: classification, diagnosis and prognosis. Hum Pathol 1:331, 1970

12. Appelman HD: Smooth muscle tumors of gastrointestinal tract: what we know that Stout didn't know. Am J Surg Pathol 10:83, 1986

13. Saul SH, Rast ML, Brooks JJ: The immunohistochemistry of gastrointestinal stromal tumors: evidence supporting an origin from smooth muscle. Am J Surg Pathol 11:464, 1987

14. Shmookler BM, Lauer DH: Retroperitoneal leiomyosarcoma: a clinicopathologic analysis of 36 cases. Am J Surg Pathol 7:269, 1983

15. Dahl L, Angervall L: Cutaneous and subcutaneous leiomyosarcoma: a clinicopathologic study of 47 patients. Pathol Eur 9:307, 1974

16. Fields JP, Helwing BH: Leiomyosarcoma of the skin and subcutaneous tissue. Cancer 47:156, 1981

17. Thomas MA, Fine G: Leiomyosarcoma of veins. Report of 2 cases and review of the literature. Cancer 13:96, 1960

18. Dorfman HD, Fisher ER: Leiomyosarcoma of the greater saphenous vein. Am J Clin Pathol 39:73, 1963

19. Kevoskian S, Cento DP: Leiomyosarcoma of large arteries and veins. Surgery 73:390, 1973

20. Adeyemi E, Sceibal V: Leiomyosarcoma of the inferior vena cava. A case report with review of the literature. Postgrad Med J 58:515, 1982

21. Berlin O, Stener B, Kindblom L-G, Angervall L: Leiomyosarcomas of venous origin in the extremities. A correlated clinical, roentgenologic and morphologic study with diagnostic and surgical implications. Cancer 54:2147, 1984

22. Baker PB, Goodwin RA: Pulmonary artery sarcomas. A review and report of a case. Arch Pathol Lab Med 109:35, 1985

23. Leu HJ, Makek M: Intramural venous leiomyosarcomas. Cancer 57:1395, 1986

24. Mackay B, Ro J, Floyd C, Ordonez NG: Ultrastructural observations on smooth muscle tumors. Ultrastruct Pathol 11:593, 1987

25. Morales AR, Fine G, Pardo V, Horn R: The ultrastructure of smooth muscle tumors with a consideration of the possible relationship of glomangiomas, hemangiopericytomas and cardiac myxomas. Pathol Annu 10:65, 1975

26. Miettinen M, Letho VP, Badley RA, Virtanen I: Expression of intermediate filaments in soft tissue sarcomas. Int J Cancer 30:541, 1982

27. Donner L, de Lanerolle P, Costa J: Immunoreactivity of paraffin-embedded normal tissues and mesenchymal tumors for smooth muscle myosin. Am J Clin Pathol 80:677, 1983

28. Ogawa K, Oguchi M, Yamabe H, et al: Distribution of collagen type IV in soft tissue tumors. An immunohistochemical study. Cancer 58:269, 1986

29. Tsukada T, McNutt MA, Ross R, Gown AM: HHF35, a muscle actin-specific monoclonal antibody. II: reactivity in normal, reactive and neoplastic human tissues. Am J Pathol 127:389, 1987

30. Schurch W, Skalli O, Seemayer TA, Gabbiani G: Intermediate filament proteins and actin isoforms as markers for soft tissue tumor differentiation and origin. I. Smooth muscle tumors. Am J Pathol 128:91, 1987

31. Brown DC, Theaker JM, Banks PM, et al: Cytokeratin expression in smooth muscle and

smooth muscle tumours. Histopathology 11:477, 1987

32. Norton AJ, Thomas JA, Isaacson PG: Cytokeratin-specific monoclonal antibodies are reactive with tumours of smooth muscle derivation. An immunocytochemical and biochemical study using antibodies to intermediate filament cytoskeletal proteins. Histopathology 11:487, 1987

33. Proppe KH, Scully RE, Rosai J: Postoperative spindle-cell nodules of genitourinary tract resembling sarcomas: A report of eight cases. Am J Surg Pathol 8:101, 1984

34. Ro JY, Ayala AG, Ordonez NG, et al: Pseudosarcomatous fibromyxoid tumor of the urinary bladder. Am J Clin Pathol 86:583, 1986

35. Wile AG, Evans HL, Romsdahl MM: Leiomyosarcoma of soft tissue: a clinicopathologic study. Cancer 48:1022, 1981

36. Lavin P, Hajdu SI, Foote FW: Gastric and extragastric leiomyoblastomas. Cancer 29:305, 1972

37. Pizzimbono CA, Higa E, Wise L: Leiomyoblastoma of the lesser sac: case report and review of the literature. Am Surg 39:692, 1973

38. Salazar H, Totten RS: Leiomyoblastoma of the stomach. An ultrastructural study. Cancer 25:176, 1970

39. Brooks JJ: Short Course 1: Surgical Pathology of Soft Tissue Tumors. Case 8. United States and Canadian Academy of Pathology. Washington, DC, 1988

40. Weiss RA, Mackay B: Malignant smooth muscle tumors of gastrointestinal tract. Ultrastruct Pathol 2:231, 1981

41. Appelman HD, Helwig EB: Gastric epithelioid leiomyoma and leiomyosarcoma (leiomyoblastoma). Cancer 38:708, 1976

42. Dehner LP, Enzinger FM, Font RL: Fetal rhabdomyoma. An analysis of nine cases. Cancer 30:160, 1972

43. Stout AP, Lattes SR: Tumors of the soft tissues. p. 35. Atlas of Tumor Pathology. Series II, Fascicle I. Armed Forces Institute of Pathology, Washington, DC, 1967

44. Di Sant'Agnese PA, Knowles DM: Extracardiac rhabdomyoma: a clinicopathologic study and review of the literature. Cancer 46:780, 1980

45. Gold JH, Bossen EH: Benign vaginal rhabdomyoma: a light and electron microscopic study. Cancer 37:2283, 1976

46. Harms D, Schmidt D, Treuner J: Soft-tissue sarcomas in childhood. A study of 262 cases including 169 cases of rhabdomyosarcoma. Z Kinderchir 40:140, 1985

47. Maurer H, Ragab AH: Rhabdomyosarcoma. In Sutow WW, Fernbach DJ, Vietti TJ (eds): Clinical Pediatric Oncology. CV Mosby, St. Louis, 1984

48. Birch JM, Marsden HB, Swindell R: Incidence of malignant disease in childhood: a 24 year review of the Manchester Children's Tumor Registry data. Br J Cancer 42:215, 1980

49. Young JL, Miller RW: Incidence of malignant tumors in U.S. children. J Pediatr 86:254, 1975

50. Miettinen M: Rhabdomyosarcoma in patients older than 40 years of age. Cancer 62:2060, 1988

51. Lloyd RV, Hajdu SI, Knapper WH: Embryonal rhabdomyosarcoma in adults. Cancer 51:557, 1983

52. Seidal T, Kindblom L-G, Angervall L: Rhabdomyosarcoma in middle-aged and elderly individuals. Acta Pathol Microbiol Scand (A) 97:236, 1989

53. Enjoji M, Hashimoto H: Diagnosis of soft tissue sarcomas. Pathol Res Pract 178:215, 1984

54. Lawrence W, Gehan EA, Beltangady M, Maurer HM: Prognostic significance of staging factors of the UICC staging system in childhood rhabdmyosarcoma: a report from the Intergroup Rhabdomyosarcoma Study (IRS-II). J Clin Oncol 5:46, 1987

55. Almanaseer IV, Trujillo YP, Taxy JB, Okuno T: Systemic rhabdomyosarcoma with diffuse bone marrow involvement. Case report of an unusual presentation. Am J Clin Pathol 82:349, 1984

56. Cho KR, Olson JL, Epstein JI: Primitive rhabdomyosarcoma presenting with diffuse bone marrow involvement: an immunohistochemical and ultrastructural study. Mod Pathol 1:23, 1988

57. Henderson DW, Raven JL, Pollard JA, Walter MN: Bone marrow metastases in disseminated alveolar rhabdomyosarcoma: case report with ultrastructural study and review. Pathology 8:329, 1976

58. Horn RC, Enterline HT: Rhabdomyosarcoma: a clinicopathological study and classification of 39 cases. Cancer 11:181, 1958

59. Marsden HB: The pathology of soft-tissue sarcomas with emphasis on childhood tumors. p. 14. In D'Angio GI, Evans AE (eds): Bone Tu-

mours and Soft Tissue Sarcomas. Edward Arnold Ltd, England, 1985

60. Palmer NF, Foulkes M: Histopathology and prognosis in the second Intergroup Rhabdomyosarcoma Study (IRS II). Proc Am Soc Clin Oncol 3:897, 1987

61. Tsokos M, Webber B, Parham D, et al: Rhabdomyosarcoma: a new classification scheme related to prognosis. J Natl Cancer Inst (In press)

62. Newton WA, Triche TJ, Marsden H, et al: International Childhood Soft Tissue Sarcoma Pathology Classification Study. Med Pediatr Oncol 17:308A, 1989

63. Harms D, Schmidt D: Classification of solid tumors in children—the Kiel pediatric tumor registry. Monogr Paediatr 18:1, 1986

64. Newton WA, Soule EH, Hamoudi AB, et al: Histopathology of childhood sarcomas, Intergroup Rhabdomyosarcoma Studies I and II: clinicopathologic correlation. J Clin Oncol 6:67–75, 1988

65. Molenaar WM, Oosterhuis JW, Oosterhuis AM, Ramaekers FCS: Mesenchymal and muscle-specific intermediate filaments (vimentin and desmin) in relation to differentiation in childhood rhabdomyosarcomas. Hum Pathol 16:838, 1985

66. Tsokos M, Howard R, Costa J: Immunohistochemical study of alveolar and embryonal rhabdomyosarcoma. Lab Invest 48:148, 1983

67. Schmidt D, Reimann O, Treuner J, Harms D: Cellular differentiation and prognosis in embryonal rhabdomyosarcoma. A report from Cooperative Soft Tissue Sarcoma Study 1981 (CWS 81). Virchows Arch [A] 409:183, 1986

68. Cavazzana AO, Schmidt D, Ninfo V, et al: Spindle cell (leiomyomatous) rhabdomyosarcoma: an unusual variant of embryonal rhabdomyosarcoma. An anatomo-clinical study of 21 cases. Pathol Res Pract 185:35, 1989

69. Enzinger FM, Shiraki M: Alveolar rhabdomyosarcoma: an analysis of 110 cases. Cancer 24:18, 1969

70. Gonzalez-Crussi F, Black-Schaffer S: Rhabdomyosarcoma of infancy and childhood. Problems of morphologic classification. Am J Surg Pathol 3:157, 1979

71. Jaffe N, Filler RM, Farber S, et al: Rhabdomyosarcoma in children. Improved outlook with multidisciplinary approach. Am J Surg 125:482, 1973

72. Bale PM, Parson RE, Stevens MM: Pathology and behavior of juvenile rhabdomyosarcoma. p. 186. In Finegold M (ed): Pathology of Neoplasia in Children and Adolescents. WB Saunders, Philadelphia, 1986

73. Riopelle JL, Thériault JP: Sur une forme méconnue de sarcome des parties molles: le rhabdomyosarcome alveolaire. Ann Pathol 1:88, 1956

74. Tsokos M, Miser A, Wesley R, et al: Solid variant of alveolar rhabdomyosarcoma: a primitive rhabdomyosarcoma with poor prognosis and distinct histology. Proceedings of the XVIIth Meeting of the SIOP, Venice, Italy, October 1985

75. Tsokos M: The role of immunocytochemistry in the diagnosis of rhabdomyosarcoma. Arch Pathol Lab Med 110:776, 1986

76. Hajdu SI: Tumors of muscles. p. 279. In Pathology of Soft Tissue Tumors, Lea & Fabiger, Philadelphia, 1979

77. Weiss SW, Enzinger FM: Malignant fibrous histiocytoma. An analysis of 200 cases. Cancer 41:2250, 1978

78. De Jong ASH, Van Kessel-Van Vark M, Albus-Lutter CE: Pleomorphic rhabdomyosarcoma in adults: immunohistochemistry as a tool for its diagnosis. Hum Pathol 18:298, 1987

79. Molenaar WM, Oosterhuis AM, Ramaekers FCS: The rarity of rhabdomyosarcomas in the adult. A morphologic and immunohistochemical study. Pathol Res Pract 180:400, 1985

80. Kyriakos ML: Tumors and tumorlike conditions of soft tissue. p. 1642. In Kissane J (ed): Anderson's Pathology. 8th Ed. CV Mosby, St. Louis, 1985

81. Rosai J: Soft Tissues. p. 1547. In Ackerman's Surgical Pathology. CV Mosby, St. Louis, 1989

82. Morales AR, Fine G, Horn RC Jr: Rhabdomyosarcoma: an ultrastructural appraisal. Pathol Annu 7:81, 1972

83. Erlandson RA: The ultrastructrual distinction between rhabdomyosarcoma and other undifferentiated "sarcomas." Ultrastruct Pathol 11:83, 1987

84. Ghadially FN: Is it a myosarcoma? p. 186. In FN Ghadially (ed): Diagnostic Electron Microscopy of Tumours. 2nd Ed. Butterworths, London, 1985

85. LaValle Bundtzen J, Norback DH: The ultrastructure of poorly differentiated rhabdomyosarcomas: a case report and literature review. Hum Pathol 13:301, 1982

86. Dickman PS, Triche TJ: Extraosseous Ewing's sarcoma versus primitive rhabdomyosarcoma: diagnostic criteria and clinical correlation. Hum Pathol 17:881, 1986
87. Osborn M, Weber K: Biology of disease. Tumor diagnosis by intermediate filament typing: a novel tool for surgical pathology. Lab Invest 48:372, 1983
88. Bennett GS, Fellini SA, Toyama Y, Holtzer H: Redistribution of intermediate filament during skeletal myogenesis and maturation in vitro. J Cell Biol 82:577, 1979
89. Tokuyasu KT, Maher PA, Singer SJ: Distribution of vimentin and desmin in developing chick myotubes in vivo. I. Immunofluorescence study. J Cell Biol 98:1961, 1984
90. Seidal T, Kindblom L-G, Angervall L: Myoglobin, desmin and vimentin in ultrastructurally proven rhabdomyomas and rhabdomyosarcomas. An immunohistochemical study utilizing a series of monoclonal and polyclonal antibodies. Appl Pathol 5:201, 1987
91. Kodet R: Rhabdomyosarcoma in childhood. An immunohistological analysis with myoglobin, desmin and vimentin. Pathol Res Pract 185:207, 1989
92. Brooks JJ: Immunohistochemistry of soft tissue tumors. Myoglobin as a tumor marker for rhabdomyosarcoma. Cancer 50:1757, 1982
93. Kindblom L-G, Seidal T, Karlsson K: Immunohistochemical localization of myoglobin in human muscle tissue and embryonal and alveolar rhabdomyosarcoma. Acta Pathol Microbiol Scand (A) 90:167, 1982
94. Kahn HJ, Yeger H, Kassim O, et al: Immunohistochemical and electron microscopic assessment of childhood rhabdomyosarcoma. Increased frequency of diagnosis over routine histologic methods. Cancer 51:1897, 1983
95. Leader M, Patel J, Collins M, Henry K: Myoglobin: an evaluation of its role as marker of rhabdomyosarcomas. Br J Cancer 59:106, 1989
96. Tsokos M, Triche TJ: Immunocytochemical and ultrastructural study of primitive "solid variant" rhabdomyosarcoma. Lab Invest 54:65A, 1986
97. de Jong ASH, van Vark M, Albus-Lutter Ch E, et al: Myosin and myoglobin as tumor markers in the diagnosis of rhabdomyosarcoma. A comparative study. Am J Surg Pathol 8:521, 1984
98. Schmidt RA, Cone R, Haas JE, Gown AM: Diagnosis of rhabdomyosarcomas with HHF35, a monoclonal antibody directed against muscle actins. Am J Pathol 131:19, 1988
99. Eusebi V, Bondi A, Rosai J: Immunohistochemical localization of myoglobin in nonmuscular cells. Am J Surg Pathol 8:51, 1984
100. Granger BL, Lazarides E: Synamin: A new high molecular weight protein associated with desmin and vimentin in muscle. Cell 22:727, 1980
101. Gomer RH, Lazarides E: The synthesis and deployment of filamin in chicken skeletal muscle. Cell 23:524, 1981
102. Granger BL, Lazarides E: Desmin and vimentin coexist at the periphery of the myofibril Z-disc. Cell 18:1053, 1979
103. Lazarides E: Intermediate filaments as mechanical integrator of cellular space. Nature 283:249, 1980
104. Altmannsberger M, Weber K, Droste R, Osborn M: Desmin is a specific marker for rhabdomyosarcomas of human and rat origin. Am J Pathol 118:85, 1985
105. Eusebi V, Ceccarelli C, Gorza L, et al: Immunocytochemistry of rhabdomyosarcoma. The use of four different markers. Am J Surg Pathol 10:293, 1986
106. Skalli O, Gabbiani G, Babai F, et al: Intermediate filament proteins and actin isoforms as markers for soft tissue tumor differentiation and origin II. Rhabdomyosarcomas. Am J Pathol 130:515, 1988
107. Wick M: Antibodies to desmin in diagnostic pathology. p. 93. In Wick M, Siegal GP (eds): Monoclonal Antibodies in Diagnostic Immunohistochemistry. Clinical and biochemical analysis. N. 24. Marcel Dekker, New York, 1988
108. Schurch W, Skalli O, Seemayer TA, Gabbiani G: Intermediate filament proteins and actin isoforms as markers for soft tissue tumor differentiation and origin. I. Smooth muscle tumors. Am J Pathol 128:91, 1987
109. Dahl D, Bignami A: Immunohistological localization of desmin, the muscle-type 100 A filament protein, in rat astrocytes and Müller glia. J Histochem Cytochem 30:207, 1982
110. Dahl D, Zapatka S, Bignami A: Heterogeneity of desmin, the muscle type intermediate filament, in blood vessels and astrocytes. Histochemistry 84:145, 1986
111. Fujimoto T, Singer SJ: Immunocytochemical studies of endothelial cells in vivo. I. The pres-

ence of desmin only, or desmin plus vimentin, or vimentin only, in the endothelial cells of different capillaries of adult chicken. J Cell Biol 103:2775, 1986

112. Dodd S, Malone M, McCulloch W: Rhabdomyosarcoma in children: a histological and immunocytochemical study of 59 cases. J Pathol 158:13, 1989

113. Cintorino M, Vindigni C, Del Vecchio MT et al: Expression of actin isoforms and intermediate filament proteins in childhood orbital rhabdomyosarcomas. J Submicrosc Cytol Pathol 21:409, 1989

114. Miettinen M: Antibody specific to muscle actins in the diagnosis and classification of soft tissue tumors. Am J Pathol 130:205, 1988

115. Whalen R, Sell S, Butler-Browne G: Three myosin heavy-chain isoenzymes appear sequentially in rat muscle development. Nature 292:805, 1981

116. Bandman E, Matsuda R, Strohman RC: Developmental appearance of myosin heavy and light chain isoforms in vivo and in vitro in chicken skeletal muscle. Develop Biol 93:508, 1982

117. Scupham R, Gilbert EF, Wilde J, Wiedrich TA: Immunohistochemical studies of rhabdomyosarcoma. Arch Pathol Lab Med 110:818, 1986

118. Schiaffino S, Gorza L, Sartore S, et al: Embryonic myosin heavy chain as a differentiation marker of developing human skeletal muscle and rhabdomyosarcoma. A monoclonal antibody study. Exp Cell Res 163:211, 1986

119. Eusebi V, Rilke F, Ceccarelli C, et al: Fetal heavy chain skeletal myosin. An oncofetal antigen expressed by rhabdomyosarcoma. Am J Surg Pathol 10:680, 1986

120. Maruyama K, Yoshioka T, Higuchi H, et al: Connectin filaments link thick filaments and Z lines in frog skeletal muscle as revealed by immunoelectron microscopy. J Cell Biol 101:2167, 1985

121. Trinick J, Knight P, Whiting A: Purification and properties of native titin. J Mol Biol 180:331, 1984

122. Hill C, Weber K: Monoclonal antibodies distinguish titins from heart and skeletal muscle. J Cell Biol 102:1099, 1986

123. Horowits R, Kempner ES, Bisher ME, Podolsky RJ: A physiological role for titin and nebulin in skeletal muscle. Nature 323:160, 1986

124. Osborn M, Hill C, Altmannsberger M, Weber K: Monoclonal antibodies to titin in conjunction with antibodies to desmin separate rhabdomyosarcomas from other tumor types. Lab Invest 55:101, 1986

125. de Jong ASH, van Kessel-van Vark M, Albus-Lutter CE, Voute PA: Creatine kinase subunits M and B as markers in the diagnosis of poorly differentiated rhabdomyosarcomas in children. Hum Pathol 16:924, 1985

126. Royds JA, Variend S, Timperley WR, Taylor CB: An investigation of beta enolase as a histological marker of rhabdomyosarcoma. J Clin Pathol 37:905, 1984

127. Mukai M, Hisami I, Torikata C, et al: Immunoperoxidase demonstration of a new muscle protein (Z-protein) in myogenic tumors as a diagnostic aid. Am J Pathol 114:164, 1984

128. Autio-Harmainen H, Apaja-Sarkkinen M, Martikainen J, et al: Production of basement membrane laminin and type IV collagen by tumors of striated muscle: an immunohistochemical study of rhabdomyosarcomas of different histologic types and a benign vaginal rhabdomyoma. Hum Pathol 17:1218, 1986

129. Scarpa S, Modesti A, Triche TJ: Extracellular matrix synthesis by undifferentiated childhood tumor cell lines. Am J Pathol 129:74, 1987

130. Stracca-Pansa V, Dickman PS, Zamboni G, et al: Extracellular matrix of small round cell tumors of childhood: an immunohistochemical study of 80 cases. XVII International Congress of the International Academy of Pathology. Abstract 394, 1988

131. Tsokos M, Linnoila RI, Chandra RS, Triche TJ: Neuron-specific enolase in the diagnosis of neuroblastoma and other small, round-cell tumors in children. Hum Pathol 15:575, 1984

132. Coindre J-M, De Mascarel A, Trojani M, et al: Immunohistochemical study of rhabdomyosarcoma. Unexpected staining with S-100 protein and cytokeratin. J Pathol 155:127, 1988

133. Miettinen M, Rapola J: Immunohistochemical spectrum of rhabdomyosarcoma and rhabdomyosarcoma-like tumors. Am J Surg Pathol 13:120, 1989

134. Scrabe HJ, Witte DP, Lampkin BC, Cavenne WK: Chromosomal localization of the human rhabdomyosarcoma locus by mitotic recombinant mapping. Nature 329:645, 1987

135. Koufos A, Hansen MF, Copeland NG, et al: Loss of heterozygosity in three embryonal tu-

mors suggests a common pathogenetic mechanism. Nature 316:330, 1985
136. Davis RL, Weintraub H, Lassar AB: Expression of a single transfected cDNA converts fibroblasts to myoblasts. Cell 51:987, 1987
137. Scrable H, Witte D, Shimada H, et al: Molecular differential pathology of rhabdomyosarcoma. Genes Chromos Cancer 1:23–35, 1989
138. Turc-Carel C, Izard-Nacol S, Justrabo E, et al: Consistent chromosomal translocation in alveolar rhabdomyosarcoma. Cancer Genet Cytogenet 19:361, 1986
139. Douglass EC, Valentine M, Etcubanas E, et al: A specific chromosomal abnormality in rhabdomyosarcoma. Cytogenet Cell Genet 45:148, 1987
140. Wang-Wuu S, Soukup S, Ballard E, et al: Chromosomal analysis of sixteen human rhabdomyosarcomas. Cancer Res 48:983, 1988
141. Jenkin D, Sonley M: Soft-tissue sarcomas in the young. Medical treatment advances in perspective. Cancer 46:621, 1980
142. Egan MJ, Raafat F, Crocker J, Smith K: Nucleolar organizer regions in small cell tumours of childhood. J Pathol 153:275, 1987
143. Mackenzie AR, Whitmore WF Jr, Melamed MR: Myosarcomas of the bladder and prostate. Cancer 22:833, 1968
144. Soule EH, Geitz M, Henderson ED: Embryonal rhabdomyosarcoma of the limbs and limbgirdles: a clinicopathologic study of 61 cases. Cancer 23:1336, 1969
145. Lawrence W Jr, Jeege G, Foote FW: Embryonal rhabdomyosarcoma. A clinicopathological study. Cancer 17:361, 1964
146. Bale PM, Reye RDK: Rhabdomyosarcoma in childhood. Pathology 7:101, 1975
147. Flamant F, Hill C: The improvement in survival associated with combined chemotherapy in childhood rhabdomyosarcoma. A historical comparison of 345 patients in the same center. Cancer 53:2417, 1984
148. Raney RB, Hays DM, Tefft M, Triche TJ: Rhabdomyosarcoma and undifferentiated sarcomas. p. 635. In Pizzo PA, Poplack DG (eds): Principles and Practice of Pediatric Oncology. JB Lippincott, Philadelphia, 1989
149. Ghavimi F, Mandell LR, Heller G, et al: Prognosis in childhood rhabdomyosarcoma of the extremity. Cancer 64:2233, 1989
150. Gaiger AM, Soule EH, Newton WA: Pathology of rhabdomyosarcoma: experience of the Intergroup Rhabdomyosarcoma Study, 1972–78. p. 19. In Natl Cancer Inst Monogr 56, 1981
151. Hawkins HK, Camacho-Velasquez JV: Rhabdomyosarcoma in children. Correlation of form and prognosis in one institution's experience. Am J Surg Pathol 11:531, 1987

5

Tumors and Tumorlike Lesions of Blood Vessels

Lennart Angervall and Lars-Gunnar Kindblom

Tumors and tumorlike lesions of the blood vessels of soft tissues include a wide variety of reactive and neoplastic lesions as well as malformations and hamartomas, the latter being characterized histologically by an increase in vessels with a normal or abnormal appearance. These lesions are heterogeneous in terms of clinical presentation, significance, and clinical course. At one end of the spectrum are some of the most common and often harmless soft tissue lesions, such as pyogenic granuloma and capillary hemangioma. At the other end are syndromes with widespread hemangiomas and vascular ectasias involving two or more tissues or large parts of the body, and the highly malignant angiosarcomas. The distinction between neoplastic and either reactive or malformative lesions is not always easy to make. The question of benignity or malignancy may, at times, be difficult, and interposed is a group of borderline lesions. There is a large body of literature that deals with the problems of classifying blood vessel tumors. It is obvious that it has been especially difficult to make a simple and logical classification of this group based on light-microscopic findings. The clinical presentation and radiologic findings that provide information about growth pattern, extension, and topographic anatomy and type of vessel and its function (e.g., arteriovenous shunting) may be essential for interpretation and classification. For most of these lesions, blood vessel differentiation is obvious on light-microscopy and often from its gross appearance. Endothelial differentiation is more difficult to recognize in some lesions; in such instances, special stainings (e.g., reticulin staining), electron microscopy, and immunohistochemistry may be helpful.

The classification includes vasoformative lesions, which are entirely or predominantly composed of the principal cell types of vessel, endothelium, and pericytes. Lesions in which the vascular component constitutes only a part, as in such classic tumors as angiolipoma, angiomyelolipoma, angiomyolipoma, and nasal angiofibroma, and the recently described aggressive angiomyxoma of pelvic soft parts[1,2] are excluded. Tumors originating from other cells in the vessel wall, such as angioleiomyoma and leiomyosarcoma of venous origin, are also not included in the classification. The nature of the so-called proliferating angioendotheliomatosis has been greatly debated. Immunohistochemical findings have demonstrated lymphocyte properties of the tumor cells and thus the term *angiotrophic lymphoma* has been proposed,[3] as it most likely represents a malignant lymphoma with a peculiar tendency to grow within vessels.[4] Based on immunohistochemical analysis, two distinct clinicopathologic entities can be distinguished: a reactive and a malignant form, for which the term *intravascular lymphomatosis* has been suggested. This lesion has, therefore, not been included in the classification of vascular tumors.

A classification of tumors and tumorlike lesions of blood vessels is presented in Table 5-1.

BENIGN VASCULAR TUMORS

Hemangioma is broadly defined as a lesion with an increased number of newly formed blood

Table 5-1. Histologic Classification of Tumors and Tumorlike Lesions of Blood Vessels

Benign
  Capillary hemangioma
    Juvenile hemangioendothelioma (immature type)
    Capillary hemangioma (mature type)
    Senile hemangioma
  Cavernous hemangioma
  Venous hemangioma
  Arteriovenous hemangioma (racemose or cirsoid hemangioma)
  Angiolymphoid hyperplasia (epithelioid hemangioma)
  Pyogenic (telangiectatic) granuloma; granuloma gravidarum; intravascular pyogenic granuloma
  Intramuscular hemangioma
    Small vessel type (capillary type)
    Large vessel type (cavernous and venous type)
    Mixed type
    Concomitant arteriovenous vascular malformation in skeletal muscle
  Other deep hemangiomas of soft tissue
    Synovial hemangioma
    Neural hemangioma
  Diffuse (systemic) hemangiomatosis
  Hemangiopericytoma
    Infantile type
  Glomus tumor
    Glomangioma
    Glomangiomyoma
  Papillary endothelial hyperplasia (Masson's pseudoangiosarcoma)
  Vascular ectasias
    Nevus flammeus; port-wine stain
    Arterial spider

Syndromes with hemangiomas and vascular ectasias
  With cavernous hemangiomas
    Kasabach-Merritt syndrome
    Blue rubber bleb nevus syndrome
    Maffucci syndrome
  With vascular ectasias
    Hereditary hemorrhagic telangiectasia (Rendu-Osler-Weber syndrome)
    Sturge-Weber syndrome
    Klippel-Trenaunary syndrome
    Park-Weber syndrome

Intermediate Malignancy
  Epithelioid (atypical) hemangioendothelioma
  Spindle cell hemangioendothelioma
  Kaposi's sarcoma
  Malignant endovascular papillary angioendothelioma (Dabska's tumor)

Malignant
  Angiosarcoma (hemangiosarcoma)
  Malignant hemangiopericytoma
  Malignant glomus tumor (glomangiosarcoma)

vessels. It is a frequent and ubiquitous tumor in humans, especially in infants and children in whom it has been considered the most common of all tumors.[5] Hemangiomas are usually solitary and well-delineated lesions but they may be extensive and involve two or more tissue types and large parts of the body. The greatest number of hemangiomas are situated on the body surfaces.[6]

CAPILLARY HEMANGIOMA

A large number of capillary hemangiomas are present at birth or occur during the first months of life. Capillary hemangiomas of infancy have a predilection for the skin and mucous membranes of the head and neck region, and the parotid gland. These hemangiomas have a tendency to disappear spontaneously; two-thirds have been found to show spontaneous regression before 7 years of age. Histologically the *juvenile hemangioendothelioma* (immature capillary hemangioma) are cellular lesions characterized by proliferating plump endothelial cells that only partly form vascular spaces (Fig. 5-1). Scattered mitotic figures are frequently found in these early lesions. In the solid, cellular, early lesions, the vascular differentiation may be overlooked. As these hemangiomas mature, the vessels widen and attain the appearance of ordinary blood-filled capillaries (Fig. 5-2). Older lesions tend to undergo fibrosis, and eventually they may be completely replaced by scar tissue.[7]

At times, capillary hemangiomas and, occasionally, cavernous hemangiomas that occur during childhood or in young adults, especially those in the lower extremities, may lead to marked hyperplasia and hyperkeratosis of the epidermis, thereby producing a so-called verrucous type of hemangioma. It is believed that these lesions represent a vascular malformation rather than a true neoplasm, and they are considered different from angiokeratoma.[8]

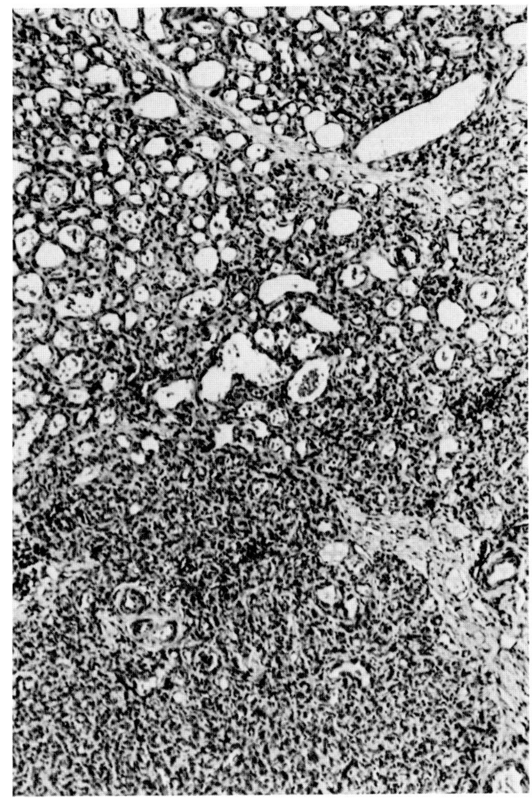

Fig. 5-1. Juvenile hemangioendothelioma (immature capillary hemangioma) with distinct capillary differentiation in some areas (top), whereas other areas consist of proliferating endothelial cells with mostly inconspicuous lumen formation (bottom). (H&E, × 180.)

Senile hemangiomas, or cherry angiomas, are very common lesions that appear as red papules, usually a few millimeters in diameter. They occur most frequently on the trunk and arms of young and middle-aged adults and increase in number and frequency with age. The lesions tend to be slightly elevated and are covered by an atrophic epidermis beneath which are dilated, thin-walled, blood-filled capillaries.

CAVERNOUS HEMANGIOMA

Cavernous hemangioma develops during childhood or, occasionally, later in life. Cavernous hemangiomas often involve both the dermis and subcutis and tend to be larger than capillary hemangiomas. These neoplasms may be well circumscribed or diffuse and poorly delineated. They occur predominantly in the upper part of the body, where they occasionally affect deep structures. Cavernous hemangiomas have a lesser tendency to spontaneous regression than capillary hemangiomas.[7] The subtypes of cavernous hemangioma comprise almost all the hemangiomas of special organs, such as liver, intestine, bone, and skeletal muscle.[5] Light microscopically they are characterized by large dilated vessels with red blood cells. The vessel walls are mostly thin but may contain areas of fibrosis and at times a component of smooth muscle. The endothelial cells tend to be flattened. A capillary component may occur in these lesions, thereby forming a mixed type of capillary and cavernous hemangioma. Cavernous hemangiomas may be a part of various syndromes (Table 5-2).[9–13]

VENOUS HEMANGIOMA

Venous hemangiomas, although rare, occur predominantly in adults and often involve the retroperitoneum, mesentery, or skeletal muscles.[3] These deep, often large lesions are composed of irregular blood-filled vessels whose walls usually have well-developed smooth muscle, though less well organized than in ordinary veins. Thrombosis in various stages of organization is common and, at times, an area with the appearance of a cavernous hemangioma may also be found. Venous hemangioma can be questioned as a distinct histologic subtype, particularly when it occurs in muscle, as the cavernous type of intramuscular hemangioma often contains a prominent component of abnormal veins.

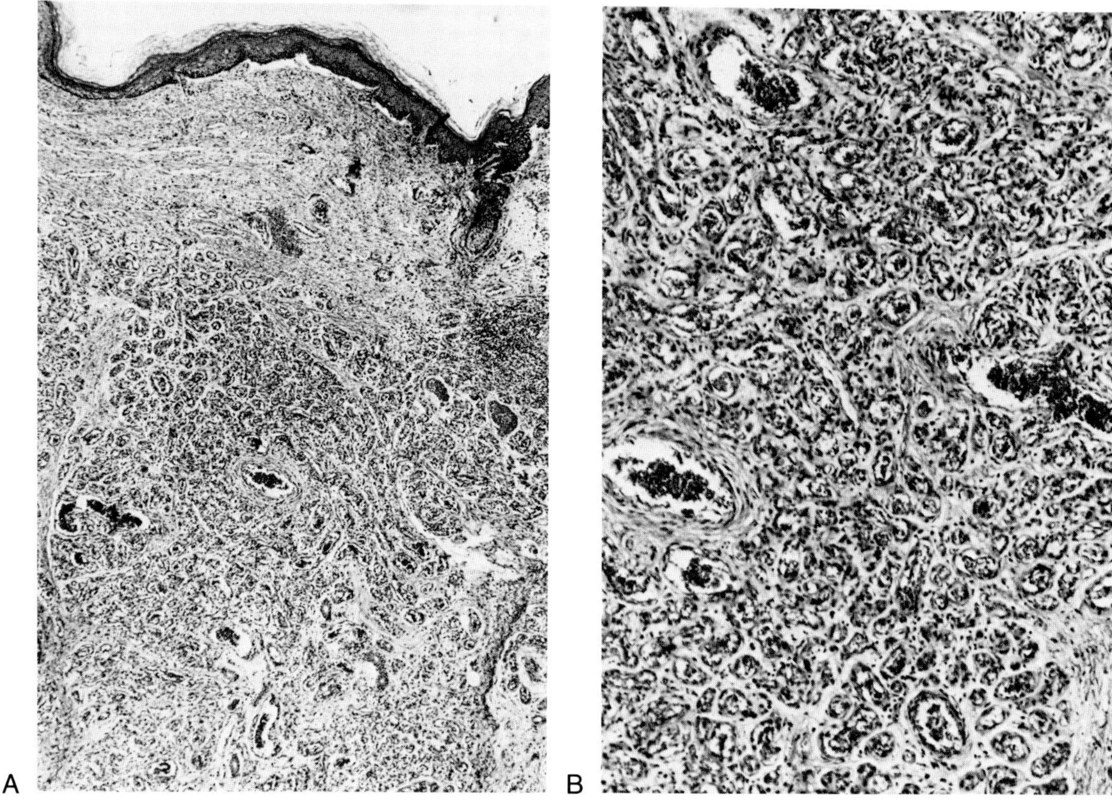

Fig. 5-2. (A & B) Capillary hemangioma of the mature type occurring in the skin. The lesion consists of well-developed capillaries lined by flattened endothelium. (H&E, Fig. A × 60; Fig. B × 180.)

ARTERIOVENOUS HEMANGIOMA

Arteriovenous hemangiomas are unusual lesions that rarely occur in routine histopathologic diagnostic work. The concept of arteriovenous hemangioma includes lesions that are characterized histologically by medium or large arteries with mostly thick walls and veins of variable size. They may have a varicose appearance and may be arterialized when shunting is present. A convolute of proliferating capillary vessels and thickened arterioles may be present together with the arteries and veins (*racemose* or *cirsoid* hemangioma).[5] Arteriovenous hemangioma is not a well-defined entity in terms of its histologic appearance and clinical presentation. The diagnosis of these lesions is based, to a large extent,

on clinical and roentgenologic findings, and only partially on the histopathology. Angiographic examination, in particular, is often essential in order to reveal the nature, extension, and type of circulation in these lesions. Two main types can be recognized: a deep type and a superficial cutaneous type. The deep type, which is usually diagnosed in young individuals and is generally considered to be a congenital malformation, often presents signs of arteriovenous shunting.[14–16] The degree of shunting may vary considerably, from cases with only mild localized symptoms, to cases with severe heart failure. These lesions are located almost exclusively about the face or neck and within the central nervous system, and rarely in the lower extremities. The histopathologic appearance may vary consider-

Table 5-2. Syndromes with Hemangiomas and Vascular Ectasias

Syndrome	Characteristics
With cavernous hemangiomas	
Kasabach-Merritt syndrome	Giant hemangiomas and thrombocytopenic purpura
Blue rubber bleb nevus syndrome	Cavernous hemangioma of skin and gastrointestinal tract
Maffucci syndrome (dyschondroplasia and vascular hamartomas)	Multiple hemangiomas and multiple enchondromas
With vascular ectasia	
Hereditary hemorrhagic telangiectasia (Rendu-Osler-Weber syndrome)	Dominant hereditary disorder with multiple telangiectasias forming tiny reddish-purple spots in skin and mucous membranes
Sturge-Weber syndrome	Port-wine stain of face and vascular malformation in the distribution of the trigeminal nerve, and ipsilateral vascular malformations of leptomeninges, brain, and eye
Klippel-Trenaunary syndrome	Port-wine stain and varicosities causing hypertrophy (local gigantism) of an extremity
Park-Weber syndrome	As Klippel-Trenaunary syndrome but with arteriovenous fistula

ably; a mixture of medium and large arteries, veins, proliferating capillaries, and cavernous vascular space can usually be seen. True arteriovenous fistulas or shunts are usually difficult to demonstrate on light-microscopic examination. With shunting, a proliferation of capillaries and fibroblasts may occur within the overlying dermis and this can mimic a Kaposi's sarcoma (the so-called pseudo-Kaposi's sarcoma).[17–19]

The rare superficial dermal type of arteriovenous hemangioma, which has been named *acral arteriovenous tumor* because it has a predilection for the head and especially the face, is clinically less significant.[20, 21] Most of these lesions present no signs of arteriovenous shunting, although this may occur in occasional cases. They produce only local symptoms.

ANGIOLYMPHOID HYPERPLASIA
(EPITHELIOID HEMANGIOMA)

Angiolymphoid hyperplasia[22] is a rare and peculiar lesion involving skin and subcutaneous tissue. This entity has been described in the literature under different names, such as angiolymphoid hyperplasia with eosinophilia, pseudopyogenic granuloma,[23] and atypical pyogenic granuloma.[24] Those cases described as Kimura's disease[25] in Japan and China differ in clinical and morphologic terms from those described in the European and American literature. Thus, the term *Kimura's disease* should be restricted to Oriental cases whenever possible. In 1979, Rosai and co-workers[26] suggested the term *histiocytoid hemangiomas* for a group of disorders involving the skin, soft tissue, large vessels, bone, lungs, and heart and which share the same basic morphologic features of proliferating "histiocytoid endothelial cells" and conspicuous inflammatory infiltration. They suggest that angiolymphoid hyperplasia with eosinophilia should be included in the general group of these histiocytoid hemangiomas. Due to the wide spectrum of these lesions in terms of clinical presentation and course, Enzinger and Weiss[3] have suggested a subdivision into two main types: epithelioid hemangioma, corresponding to angiolymphoid hyperplasia, and epithelioid hemangioendothelioma, which is a borderline group of lesions. Rare forms of epithelioid angiosarcoma also exist.

Angiolymphoid hyperplasia usually occurs as a cutaneous lesion in the head and neck region of young adults and usually presents as a slightly elevated red plaque, often with excoriation and bleeding. Multiple lesions, which have a ten-

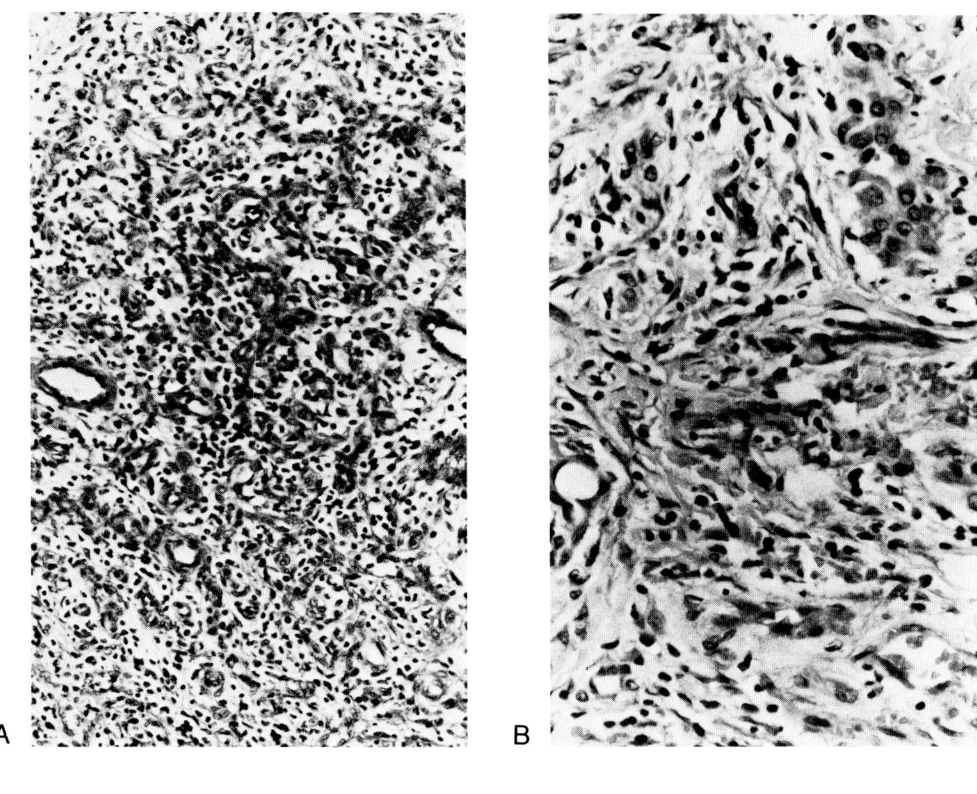

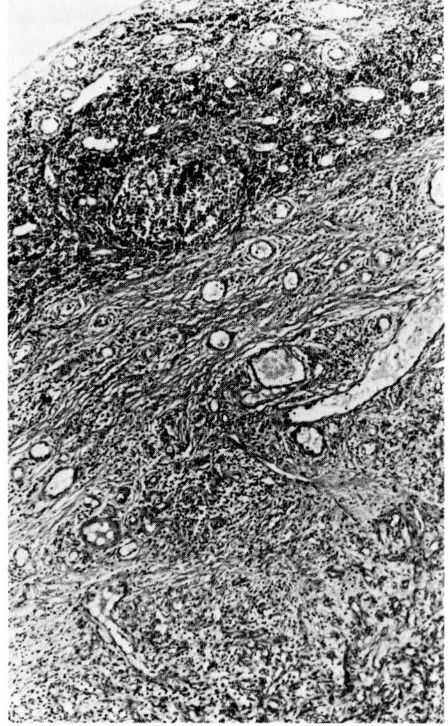

Fig. 5-3. Angiolymphoid hyperplasia. **(A)** Abundant irregular capillaries, some with open lumina, others with inconspicuous lumen formation within a stroma containing a large number of inflammatory cells, many of which are eosinophils. **(B)** Small, solid islands of epithelioid tumor cells, some of which are connected to abortive irregular capillaries. **(C)** Peripheral area with a lymph follicle and many open, small vessels. (H&E, Fig. A × 180; Fig. B × 250; Fig. C × 60.)

dency to coalesce, may occur. Histologically they are characterized by proliferating vessels that are often disposed in a nodular arrangement. The typical spectrum ranges from medium-sized, blood-filled open vessels over capillaries to solid nests of endothelial cells that sometimes present vacuoles, but no true lumen (Fig. 5-3). The endothelial cells are often large and protrude into the vessel lumen presenting epithelial-like features (Fig 5-3B). Groups of vessels are divided by collagen containing a rich inflammatory infiltrate mainly composed of lymphocytes and eosinophils. In the periphery, there may be well-developed lymph follicles (Fig. 5-3C).

At times, reticulin staining may help to disclose the vasoformative nature of the more solid and cellular variants of this lesion. Factor VIII-RAG, by immunohistochemistry, and *Ulex europeus* I lectin binding can be demonstrated within the proliferating cells and may help to establish the vascular nature of these lesions. Immunohistochemical demonstration of collagen IV and laminin within the basal lamina enclosing the endothelial cell nests may also be helpful. Ultrastructurally the endothelial cells of these lesions differ from mature endothelium of ordinary capillaries by their abundance of thin cytofilaments, which partly form elongated densities and a network of intermediate filaments. Moreover, Weibel-Palade bodies are either very rare or cannot be found in these cells.[27] Cytoplasmic vacuoles, probably an early sign of lumen formation, are a frequent finding.

The clinical course of angiolymphoid hyperplasia is benign, but local recurrences occur in about one-third of the cases. Controversy still exists as to whether these lesions should be considered true neoplastic hemangiomas or non-neoplastic reactive lesions. Differential diagnosis includes other lesions characterized by cutaneous or subcutaneous inflammatory reactions and proliferating vessels, such as eosinophilic granuloma, angiomatous lymphoid hamartoma, and persistent reactions to insect bites.[22] The cutaneous and subcutaneous location on the head and face, the occurrence of bleeding, and the vascular structures lined by plump and proliferating endothelial cells may cause problems in differentiating these lesions from angiosarcoma.

PYOGENIC GRANULOMA

Pyogenic granuloma is a common vascular lesion that may occur on any part of the body at any age. A large percentage of these lesions occur on the hands, fingers, lips, and mouth.[28] Cooper and co-workers[29] described subcutaneous and intravenous pyogenic granulomas, and we have also seen a similar case of a lobular capillary lesion in the skeletal muscles of the hand. The distribution in terms of age, sex, and location in a consecutive series of 448 cases diagnosed in our laboratory is presented in Tables 5-3 and 5-4. The relatively high incidence of pyogenic granuloma in young women (Table 5-3) may be related to pregnancy.[30] In our series, about 20 percent of women 20 to 39 years of age were reported to be pregnant. It seems most likely that pyogenic granuloma is a reactive lesion and that minor trauma is a predisposing factor. Pyogenic granuloma can appear in the gingiva during pregnancy (granuloma gravidarum). Characteristically this lesion disappears

Table 5-3. Age and Sex Distribution of 448 Cases of Pyogenic Granuloma

Age (yrs)	No. of Cases		%	
	M	F	M	F
0–09	18	10	8	5
10–19	43	28	19	13
20–29	28	50	12	23
30–39	36	41	16	18
40–49	23	14	10	6
50–59	27	18	12	8
60–69	26	29	11	13
70–79	22	20	10	9
80–	5	10	2	5
Total	228	220	100	100

**Table 5-4. Anatomic Location of 448 Cases
of Pyogenic Granuloma**

Anatomic Location	No. of Cases	%
Hand (incl. fingers)	111	25
Arm	18	4
Foot, leg	23	5
Trunk	109	24
Lips, oral cavity	77	17
Nasal cavity	18	4
Head, neck	79	17
Miscellaneous	13	3
Total	448	100

spontaneously after delivery. Clinically it usually appears as a solitary, soft, sessile, dark red nodule that bleeds easily. Light-microscopically the exophytic lesion often presents a central ulceration of the covering epidermis or mucosal surface. In skin, the epidermis at the periphery of the lesion is often hyperplastic, acanthotic, and hyperkeratotic, forming an epithelial collarette (Fig. 5-4). The tumor consists of lobulated masses of newly formed capillary vessels often lined by prominent endothelium as well as by solid areas of endothelial cells without obvious lumen formation. Characteristically the proliferating capillaries are arranged in a lobular fashion. Medium-sized, blood-filled vessels may be present within these capillary lobules. The number of inflammatory cells, mainly lymphocytes and polymorphonuclear leukocytes, varies considerably from case to case. In early lesions, mitotic activity may be prominent. Occasionally the high mitotic rate, high cellularity, solid appearance of some lesions, and the presence of ulceration and bleeding have led to its confusion with angiosarcoma and Kaposi's sarcoma. The recognition of the fairly sharp delineation of pyogenic granuloma and its characteristic lobular arrangement, in particular, helps to establish the correct diagnosis. These lesions invariably follow a benign clinical course, although they

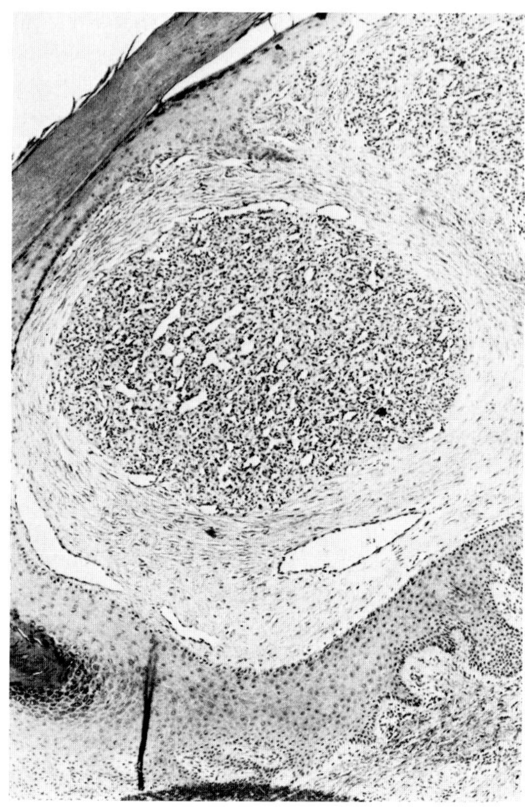

Fig. 5-4. Pyogenic granuloma showing characteristic lobules of proliferating capillaries and a typical collarette of hyperplastic squamous epithelium. (H&E, × 60.)

can recur and satellite nodules may appear.[31–33]

INTRAMUSCULAR HEMANGIOMA

Intramuscular hemangioma is a relatively uncommon tumor that constitutes about 1 percent of all hemangiomas.[5] However, in our experience it is the most common benign deep-seated soft tissue tumor in the extremities apart from intramuscular lipoma and neurilemoma. The distribution in terms of age, sex, and anatomic location in a series of 104 intramuscular hemangiomas examined in the Department of Pathology, Sahlgren Hospital, Göteborg, Sweden during the period of 1960 to 1988 is presented in

Tables 5-5 and 5-6. More than half the cases were located in the lower limbs and most of the others were located in the upper limbs, head and neck, and trunk. Two main types can be recognized on light-microscopy: the small vessel or capillary type and the large vessel or cavernous type.[3, 34] Most cases in the extremities are of the large vessel type, whereas the small vessel type predominates in the head and neck region. Hemangiomas of mixed small and large vessel types can be seen also. A fourth type has been described as a concomitant arteriovenous malformation of skeletal muscle[35] (see below). In the series of 104 cases presented in Table 5-6, 78 percent were of the large vessel type, 10 percent of small vessel type, and 12 percent of the mixed type.

A characteristic clinical feature of the *large vessel type of intramuscular hemangioma* is that pain is provoked when exercising the affected muscle and the tumor increases in size, presumably because the cavernous vessels are distended by blood. At rest, the pain disappears and the tumor size decreases; often it is palpable only after exercise. The clinical symptoms of the small vessel capillary type are usually nonspecific and the vascular nature of the process may not always be evident at the clinical examina-

tion. Radiographic examination is often essential in order to establish the nature of an intramuscular hemangioma. The large vessel type, in particular, presents characteristic radiographic features that make a preoperative diagnosis possible. On plain radiography, spots of adipose tissue can be seen within the muscle in most cases, and sometimes, rounded phleboliths or regular calcifications occur. Contrast-enhanced computed tomography may help to further identify the adipose tissue component as well as the high vascularity of the lesions, and angiography characteristically demonstrates wide, irregular, cavernous vessels with very slow circulation.

On gross examination, intramuscular hemangiomas of the large vessel type are usually easily recognized as vascular lesions since the affected muscle or muscles, characteristically show poorly defined areas with large blood-filled vessels, varying amounts of adipose tissue and fibrosis, and sometimes, thrombosis. Light microscopically the most striking findings in these intramuscular hemangiomas are the abundance of large veins or veinlike vessels with an irregularly distributed and often poorly oriented smooth muscle component, clusters of cavernous thin-walled vessels characteristically filled with erythrocytes, and an abundance of adipose tissue (Fig. 5-5). Other components include

Table 5-6. Anatomic Location of 104 Cases of Intramuscular Hemangioma

Anatomic Location	No. of Cases
Heat and neck	7
Upper extremity	
Hand, lower arm	13
Upper arm, shoulder	12
Lower extremity	
Foot, lower leg	31
Thigh, buttock	32
Trunk	9
Total	104

Table 5-5. Age and Sex Distribution of 104 Cases of Intramuscular Hemangioma

Age (yrs)	No. of Cases		%	
	M	F	M	F
0–09	4	8	8	14
10–19	18	20	37	38
20–29	9	12	19	21
30–39	7	9	14	16
40–49	7	3	14	5
50–59	2	2	4	4
60–	2	1	4	2
Total	49	55	100	100

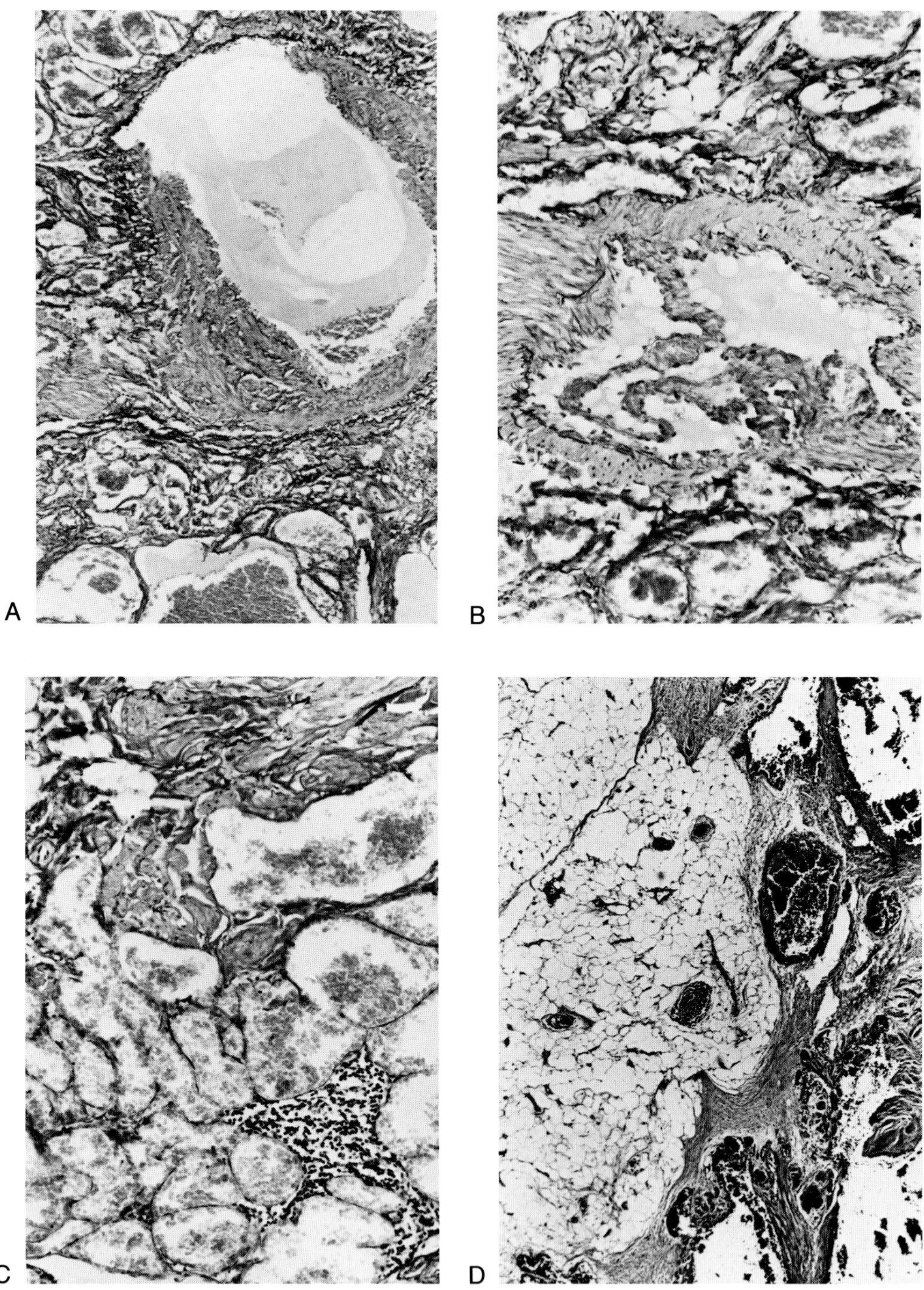

Fig. 5-5. Intramuscular hemangioma of large vessel type. **(A & B)** Large venous-type vessels showing irregular arrangement of the smooth muscle, partly surrounded by groups of thin-walled, blood-filled vessels. **(C)** Thin-walled, cavernous, blood-filled vessels characteristically arranged in groups. **(D)** In this field there is an abundant adipose tissue component. (H&E, Fig. A × 180; Fig. B × 250; Fig. C × 250; Fig. D × 60.)

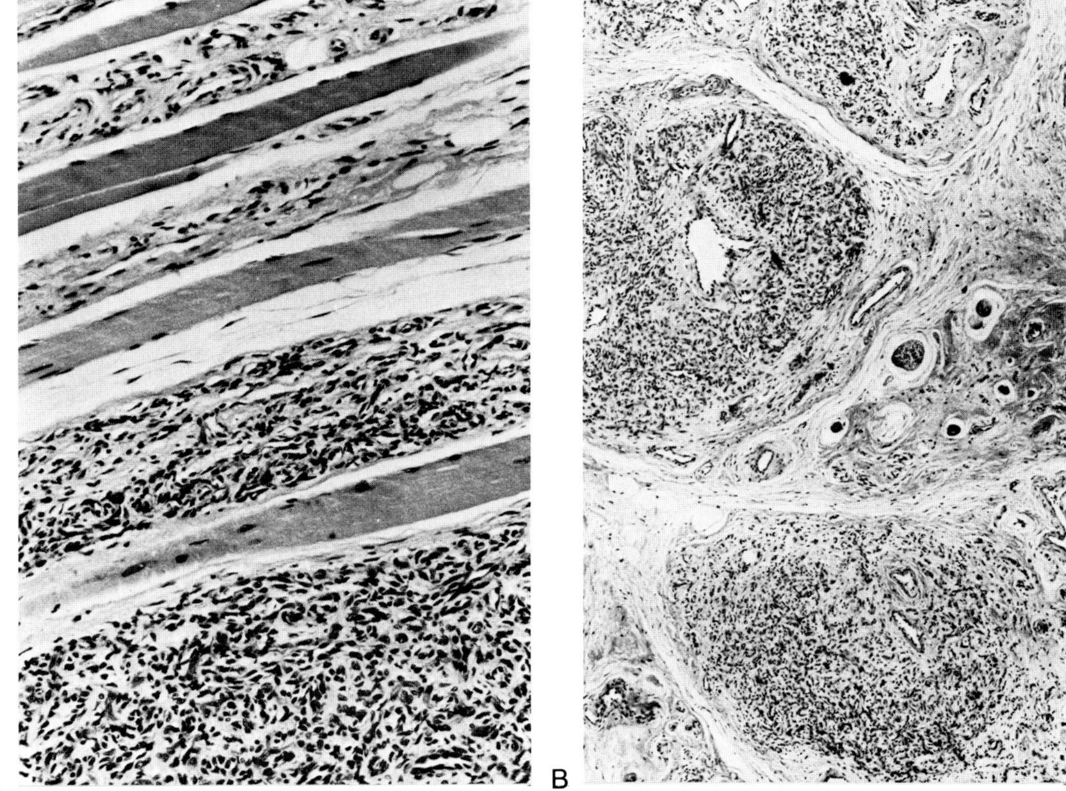

Fig. 5-6. Intramuscular hemangioma of small vessel type. **(A)** An abundance of small proliferating capillaries are seen between muscle fibers. **(B)** Proliferating small capillaries arranged in an unusual lobular fashion within the muscle. (H&E, Fig. A × 250; Fig. B × 60.)

areas of fibrosis, foci of lymphoid tissues, thrombosis, phleboliths, and calcifications. Capillaries may be prominent, especially in adipose tissue. Characteristically these lesions are poorly delineated and sometimes involve not only one or more muscles, but also the muscle fascia and the surrounding subcutaneous adipose tissue.

The *small vessel type of intramuscular hemangioma* usually appears as a solid, poorly delineated, brownish mass and the vascular nature of the lesion normally cannot be recognized macroscopically. Light microscopically these lesions are characterized by abundant proliferating capillaries (Fig. 5-6). There are often solid and highly cellular areas and mitotic figures are quite common. The endothelial cells are prominent and the nuclei may be plump. The occurrence of perineurial infiltration and intraluminal papillations, the prominence of endothelial cells, and mitotic activity may lead to an erroneous diagnosis of angiosarcoma.

Intramuscular hemangiomas are best treated by surgical excision of the involved muscle. Often, due to the poor delineation of these lesions, it is difficult to obtain radical excision of the tumor. Local recurrences are therefore fairly common.

A peculiar and more rare form of intramuscular hemangiomalike lesion is the *concomitant arteriovenous vascular malformation of skeletal muscle,* first described in 1968.[35] All cases reported so far occurred in the lower leg and foot. Light microscopically they are characterized by an abundance of concomitant arteries and veins that are often accompanied by small vessels; the latter have a thicker wall than ordinary capillaries, sometimes containing both smooth muscle and elastic components. The arteries and veins run parallel to the muscle fibers within a somewhat widened space containing small amounts of adipose tissue (Fig. 5-7). Angiography demonstrates the high vascularity of the lesion and contrast medium appears early in draining veins as an indication of arteriovenous shunting. In the angiograms the highly vascularized region shows certain striation owing to the presence of bundles of muscle fibers running between the pathologic vessels. In contrast to the large vessel type of intramuscular hemangioma, these lesions do not cause pain and do not seem to change their size in response to the use of the affected muscle. In contrast to cavernous intramuscular hemangiomas, an increased temperature over the lesions has been noted. These lesions are considered a vascular malformation of the hamartoma type and are not true vascular neoplasms.[35, 36]

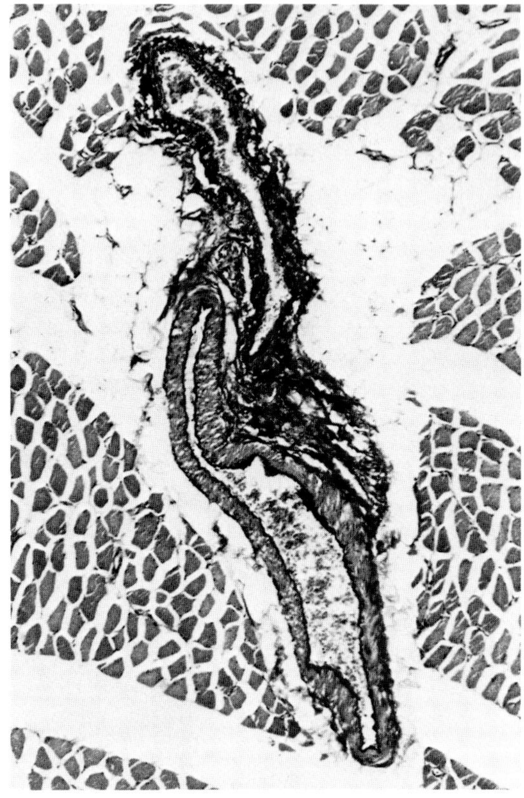

Fig. 5-7. Concomitant arteriovenous vascular malformation of skeletal muscle. A hypertrophic artery and vein, running together within an intramuscular space containing fibrous and adipose tissue. (H&E, × 60.)

OTHER DEEP HEMANGIOMAS OF SOFT TISSUE

Synovial hemangioma is a rare type of cavernous hemangioma that most frequently involves the knee joint and characteristically produces swelling of the affected joint and long-standing recurrent pain. Most cases occur during childhood or adolescence or in young adults. Two types can be recognized: localized and diffuse.[37, 38] The diffuse type is not restricted to the synovia but also involves the surrounding muscles and can be associated with cutaneous and subcutaneous and sometimes visceral hemangiomas.[39] Recurrences frequently occur after attempts at surgical removal of the diffuse type. Angiography and thermography are helpful in the differential diagnosis between the diffuse and localized types and thereby in the treatment protocol. Hemangiomas involving tendon sheaths, peritendinous tissue, and/or tendons have been described.[40, 41]

Neural hemangioma is an extremely rare type of cavernous hemangioma that is confined to the epineurium of medium-sized and large nerves.[42]

DIFFUSE HEMANGIOMATOSIS

The term *diffuse* or *systemic hemangiomatosis* is used to designate rare vascular lesions occurring during infancy and childhood and involving large segments of the body, usually an extremity. From the histologic point of view, it is not a well-defined entity. The vessels of these lesions can be of varying types. The lesions may sometimes be mixed hemolymphangiomas.[5] The distinction between angiomatosis and intramuscular hemangioma and arteriovenous hemangioma is best based on clinical criteria. Arteriovenous shunting has also been described as occurring in cases of angiomatosis. The vascular malformation, which is usually present at infancy and enlarges with general body growth, may result in prominent hypertrophy of adipose tissue, muscle, and bone of the involved body segment. In some infants, the systemic hemangioma is perhaps respresentative of a basic defect in organization and development. It has been associated with neuroectodermal defects of diverse types, thereby constituting various symptom complexes.[43]

HEMANGIOPERICYTOMA

The term *hemangiopericytoma* was first coined by Stout and Murray in 1942.[44] The diagnosis of this tumor is based primarily on the light-microscopic recognition of the characteristic architectural pattern, the so-called pericytoma pattern. Hemangiopericytoma poses several problems for the pathologist. Light microscopically the tumor cells have no unique features and may therefore be difficult to distinguish from several other types of mesenchymal cells. Moreover, the pericytoma pattern may be seen in various types of soft tissue tumors, both benign, such as in myofibromatosis, and malignant, such as synovial sarcoma and malignant fibrous histiocytoma.[45] In our experience, hemangiopericytoma has been much overdiagnosed. On review of 42 tumors diagnosed as hemangiopericytoma in Sweden during the period of 1958 to 1968, only six were accepted as true hemangiopericytomas, whereas the remaining were differently classified as various types of highly vascularized soft tissue tumors often containing areas with a pericytoma pattern.[46] Both sexes are equally involved and about one-third of the tumors occur in the lower

extremities, followed in frequency by the head and neck, trunk, and upper extremities. The rare intracranial tumor, angioblastic meningioma, appears to be impossible to distinguish from hemangiopericytoma by light and electron microscopy. The clinical course of hemangiopericytoma may be difficult to predict. Most hemangiopericytomas are benign. A minority are obviously malignant, but there is also an intermediate group of tumors for which we have suggested the term *atypical hemangiopericytoma*.[47, 48]

Angiography has been most useful in reaching the preoperative diagnosis and in planning treatment. On angiography, hemangiopericytomas are characteristically highly vascular tumors, containing vessels of varying caliber and presenting a prominent diffuse opacification. Despite the high vascularity, the early filling of veins is not usually found. Correlated microangiographic and histologic studies suggest that the irregular vessels seen on angiography correspond to the wide, angulated, thin-walled vessels without muscle coatings or elastic tissue, whereas the diffuse opacification corresponds to a dense network of delicate, branching, slit-like capillaries. Malignant soft tissue tumors are often, but not always, highly vascular masses, whereas benign soft tissue tumors are generally poor in vessels, except for hibernoma,[49, 50] some neurilemomas,[51, 52] and hemangioma. Benign hemangiopericytoma thus seems to be a further exception.[46]

Characteristically hemangiopericytomas are well-circumscribed tumors with a maximum diameter of 5 to 10 cm. The cut surfaces reveal numerous blood-filled vascular spaces of variable size. Although in rare cases, two or more tumor nodules can be observed, this finding is not necessarily indicative of malignancy. Bleeding and necrosis occur in the malignant forms of the tumor.

Characteristically benign hemangiopericytomas are well-circumscribed, as are some malignant hemangiopericytomas. Light microscopically hemangiopericytomas display a wide spectrum of features as far as cellularity, appearance and type of vessels, and degree of fibrosis,

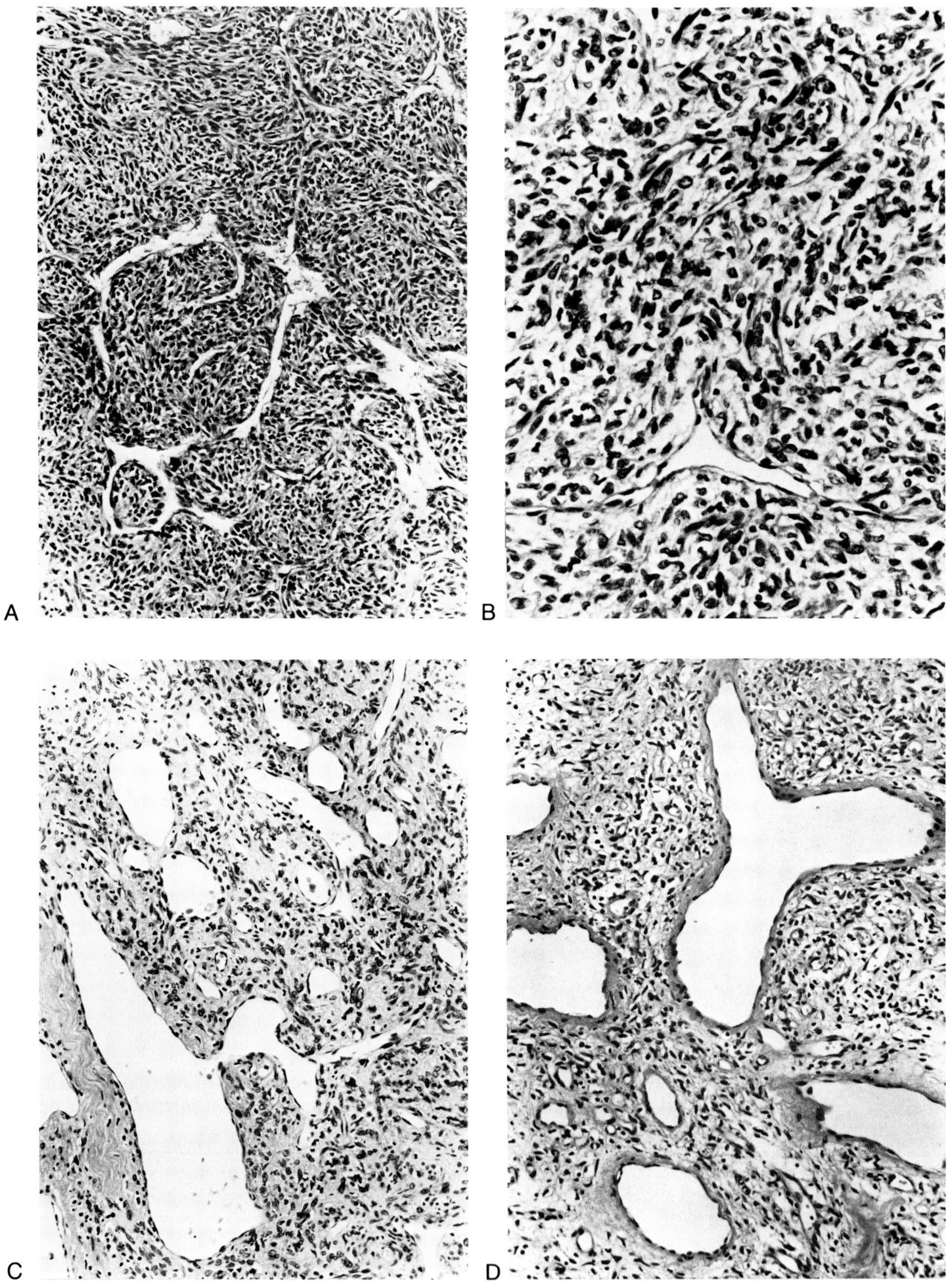
A
B
C
D

are concerned. Smith and Enzinger found that high cellularity, cell atypia, mitotic activity, necrosis, and bleeding were features indicative of malignancy. Most hemangiopericytomas are composed of closely associated, short spindle cells with rounded or oval nuclei and pale-staining, ill-defined cytoplasm. These cells characteristically surround the vascular spaces, which are of varying size (Fig. 5-8A–C). Tumors with a prominent network of irregular branching, slit-like, endothelium-lined capillary spaces have been referred to as *type A* by Battifora.[53] Tumors characterized by somewhat wider, regular, and rounded vessels with a prominent perivascular fibrosis have been referred to as *type B* (Fig. 5-8D).

The differential diagnosis of malignant hemangiopericytoma includes synovial sarcoma, malignant fibrous histiocytoma, and mesenchymal chondrosarcoma. At times, infantile fibrosarcoma may contain richly vascular areas bearing a close resemblance to the infantile type of hemangiopericytoma.[3] Cases of myofibromatosis may be misinterpreted as hemangiopericytoma since they often contain cellular areas with a prominent pericytomalike pattern.[3] The presence of an outer zone of leiomyomatous appearance helps in distinguishing them from hemangiopericytoma. Some hemangiopericytomas contain a prominent myxoid matrix and, occasionally, adipose tissue. Spindle cell lipoma[54, 55] may, therefore, be considered in the differential diagnosis.

Ultrastructurally numerous endothelium-lined vascular slits that are not recognizable on light microscopy, as well as the larger angulated vessels, can be demonstrated (Fig. 5-9). The tumor cells are intimately associated with these vascular slits. A continuous or discontinuous external lamina surrounds the indivdiual tumor cells. Pinocytotic vesicles are frequently found, whereas the cytoplasm is poorly endowed with organelles and displays few characteristic features.[53, 56–59]

Immunohistochemistry and lectin histochemistry may help to identify the myriad of vascular slits that are decorated by factor VIII-RAG (Fig. 5-10A) and *Ulex europeus* I lectin binding. Moreover, the external lamina material can be identified with antibodies to collagen IV and laminin.[60] It is interesting to note that, in contrast to normal pericytes and a single row of pericytes enclosing the vascular slits within the tumor, the vast majority of tumor cells do not express vimentin or α_1-smooth muscle actin (Fig. 5-10B & C). In terms of immunohistochemical properties, tumor cells of hemangiopericytoma thus differ from ordinary pericytes, raising doubts about the true origin and cellular differentiation of this tumor.

An *infantile type of hemangiopericytoma,* which clearly differs clinically and histologically from ordinary hemangiopericytomas, has been recognized.[3, 61] These tumors occur during infancy and almost always have a subcutaneous location. Most tumors are solitary, although a few patients with multiple lesions have also been observed.[61] Light microscopically the lesions present a multilobular growth pattern. They are generally highly cellular with prominent mitotic activity and, at times, contain areas of necrosis.

Intravascular endothelial proliferations are frequently seen, suggesting that there are transitions in the tumor between hemangioendothelioma and hemangiopericytoma.

Almost all cases reported in the literature have followed a benign clinical course.

GLOMUS TUMOR

The glomus tumor is a well-defined vascular lesion with a characteristic light-microscopic ap-

---

Fig. 5-8. Hemangiopericytoma. Characteristic vascular patterns with open angulated, gaping, vascular channels. (**A & B**) Delicate, narrow, vascular slits surrounded by small, short, spindle cells with indistinct cytoplasmic borders. The intimate relationship between the tumor cells and the angulated vessels produces the characteristic pericytoma pattern. (**C & D**) Wide angulated vessels. (**D**) Prominent perivascular fibrosis. (H&E, Fig. A × 180; Fig. B × 250; Fig. C × 180; Fig. D × 180.)

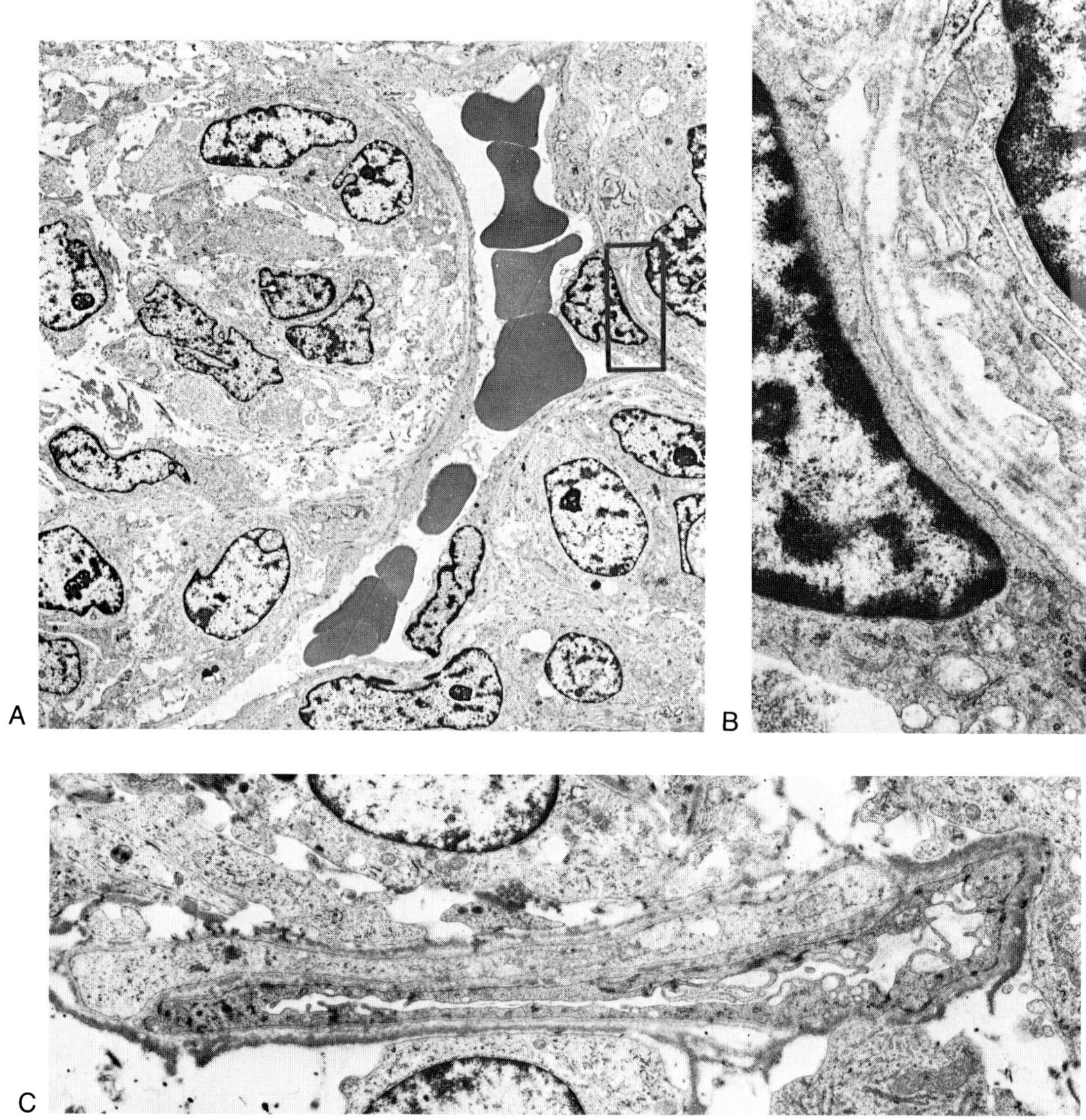

Fig. 5-9. Hemangiopericytoma. **(A)** An angulated, capillarylike vessel containing erythrocytes. The tumor cells which form nests are intimately associated with the endothelium lining the vessel. **(B)** A magnification of the area marked in **A** showing multiple layers of external lamina between a tumor cell (top right) and an endothelial cell (left). **(C)** Ultrastructurally, numerous, delicate, compressed capillaries invested by external laminae, which are not possible to distinguish on light-microscopy, can be observed. (Fig. A × 3,000; Fig. B × 19,000; Fig. C × 9,000.)

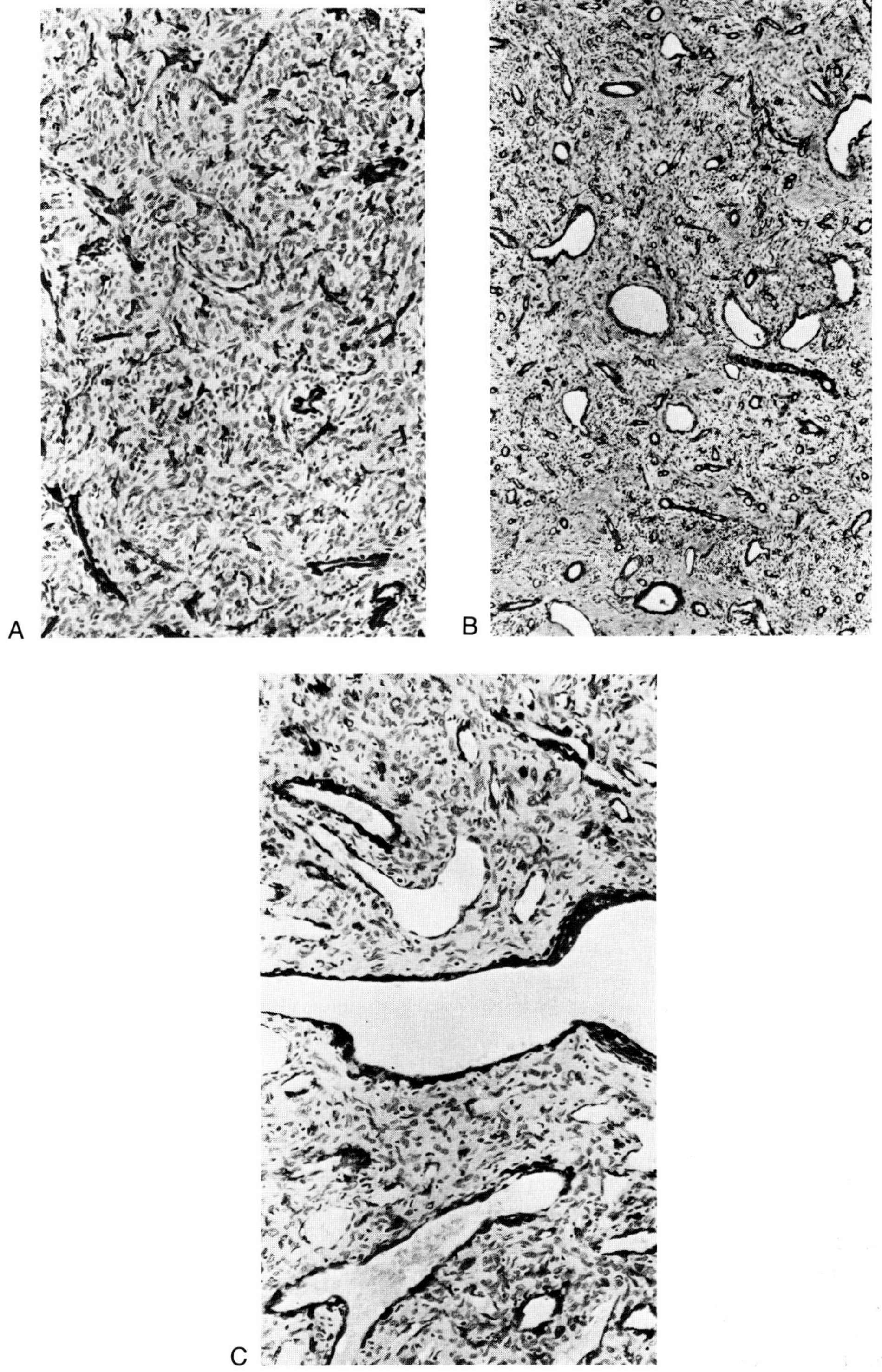

Fig. 5-10. Hemangiopericytoma. The abundance of vessels is demonstrated by factor VIII-RAG positivity **(A)** and vimentin positivity **(B)** of the endothelial cells. The majority of the tumor cells are negative for vimentin **(B).** The pericytes enclosing the larger vascular spaces are positive for α_1-smooth muscle actin **(C),** whereas the tumor cells are negative. (Avidin-biotin-complex method applied to formalin-fixed and paraffin-embedded material, Fig. A × 180; Fig. B × 60; Fig. C × 180.)

pearance. The tumor, as Masson suggested in 1924,[62] is believed to arise from the arterial part of the glomus body. The normal glomus body, located in the dermis, is an arteriovenous shunting structure that regulates blood flow in the distal parts of the extremities. Characteristically paroxysms of radiating pain occur on tactile stimulation. Most glomus tumors are found in young adults and there is a clear predilection for women. Following the distribution of the normal glomus body, glomus tumors usually occur in the hands and feet, the most common location being subungual. Single cases of glomus tumor have been reported in a variety of locations, including deep visceral sites and bone.[3, 63–68]

In rare cases, the maximum diameter of the lesion exceeds 1 cm. On gross examination, it appears as a small, reddish-blue nodule that, when located under the nail, may erode the adjacent bone. Light microscopically the distribution and proportion of the three main components of the glomus tumor (vessels, glomus cells, and smooth muscle) may vary considerably. The most common type consists of capillary-sized vessels enclosed by nests of small, uniform glomus cells, often arranged in concentric rows. Some glomus tumors, referred to as *glomangiomas,* display features similar to a cavernous hemangioma (Fig. 5-11A); the blood-filled, wide vascular spaces are only partly surrounded by a single or double row of glomus cells (Fig. 5-11C). These cases frequently show a marked hyalinization of the stroma. More rarely, glomangioma includes a prominent component of mature smooth muscle cells, referred to as *glomangiomyoma.*[3]

Electron microscopy and immunohistochemistry are of great value in distinguishing the glomus tumor from epithelial tumors such as skin adnexal tumors, for which they may be mistaken. Glomus cells share both immunohistochemical and ultrastructural properties of smooth muscle cells.[69–71] However they differ from ordinary smooth muscle cells in their negativity for desmin. In contrast to the majority of tumor cells of hemangiopericytoma, glomus cells are strongly positive for vimentin and α_1-smooth muscle actin (Fig. 5-11B), as are ordinary pericytes. Immunohistochemical stains for S-100 protein help us to recognize the abundance of very delicate nerve fibers intimately associated with the glomus cells and vascular structures of the glomus tumor (Fig. 5-11C).

Local recurrences may occur following simple excision, but the tumor follows a perfectly benign course. None of the rare cases of so-called glomangiosarcoma, a tumor containing a benign glomus tumor component as well as a spindle cell sarcoma component, has been reported to metastasize.[3, 72]

PAPILLARY ENDOTHELIAL HYPERPLASIA (MASSON'S PSEUDOANGIOSARCOMA)

The papillary endothelial hyperplasia[73, 74] is a fairly common lesion that usually occurs within, or in close association with, a vessel, usually a vein. The lesion often presents as part of an organizing thrombus. These findings strongly suggest that the lesion does not represent a true endothelial tumor but a reactive lesion, as suggested by Henschen.[75] The lesions are commonly found en passant within an organizing thrombus of hemorrhoids or varices. The lesions most commonly detected and excised are those in the head, neck, and hands. The maximum diameter of most of the lesions does not exceed 2 cm, but occasionally larger tumor masses may occur in relation to large veins deeply located in the extremities. Light microscopically the lesions are characterized by a network of vascular channels into which fibrous projections, covered in most cases with a single row of prominent, proliferating, plump endothelial cells, bulge (Fig. 5-12). Ultrastructurally the endothelial cells appear to be well differentiated and a distinct basal lamina can be seen separating the endothelial cells from pericytes,[76] fibroblasts, and abundant myofibroblasts of the stroma of the papillary projections (Figs. 5-13 and Fig. 5-14). Immunohistochemically the endothelial cells are positive for factor VIII-RAG and they bind *Ulex europeus* I lectin.

The recognition of this lesion is important

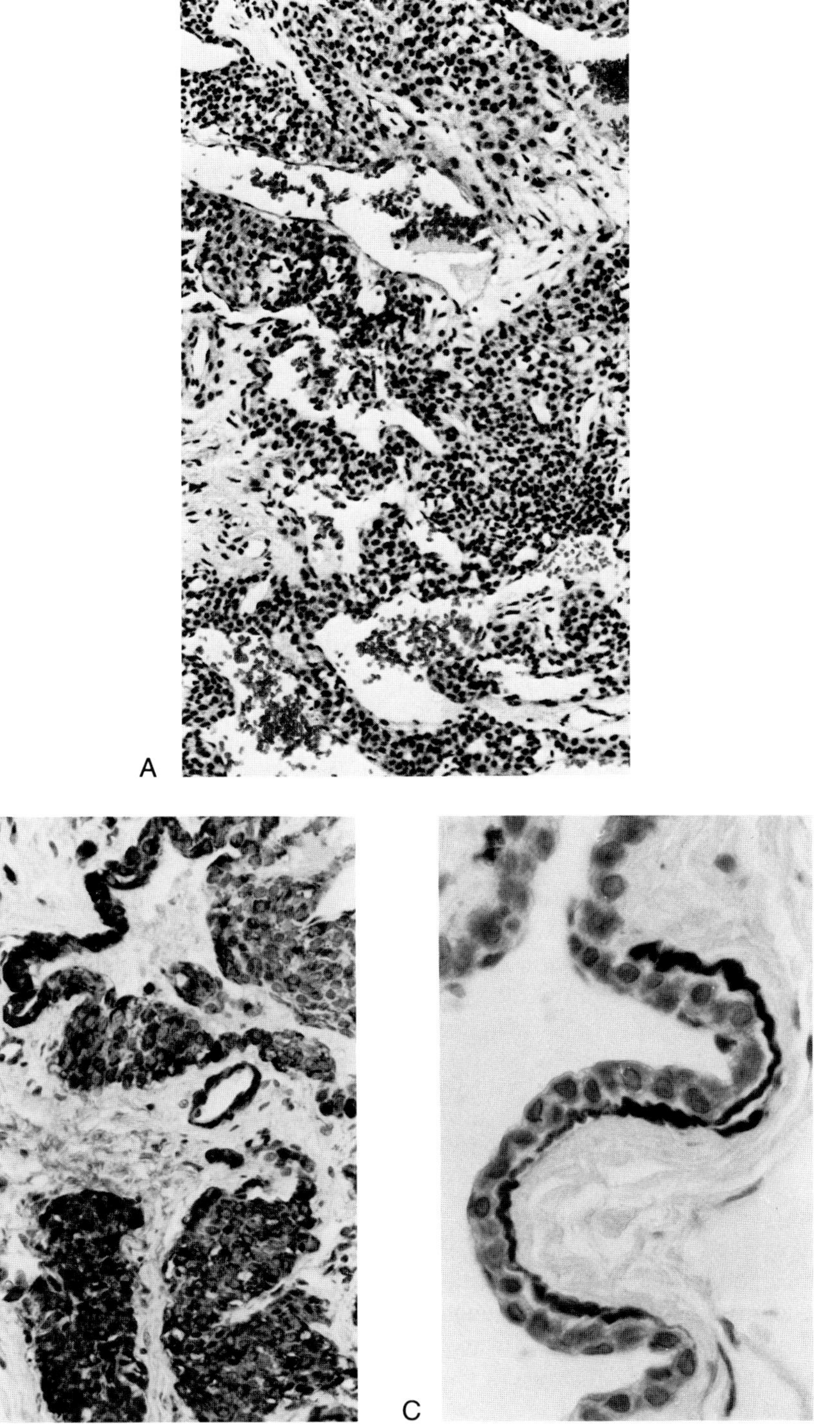

Fig. 5-11. Glomus tumors. **(A)** Glomus tumor with cavernous vessels, so-called glomangioma. **(B)** The glomus cells are positive for α_1-smooth muscle actin. **(C)** A delicate nerve fiber, identified by S-100 protein positivity, is intimately associated with a single layer of glomus cells. (Fig. A, H&E, × 180; Figs. B and C, avidin biotin-complex method applied to formalin-fixed and paraffin embedded material, Fig. B × 250; Fig. C × 500.)

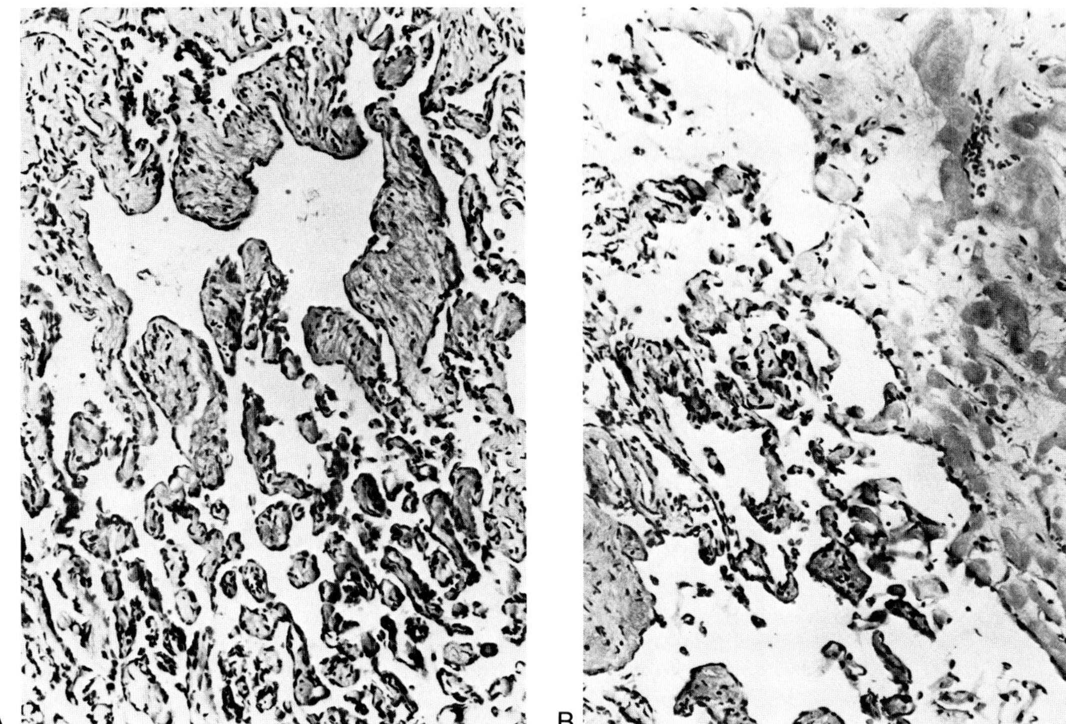

Fig. 5-12. (A & B) Papillary endothelial hyperplasia. Characteristic papillary structures lined by plump endothelial cells bulge into irregular vascular channels. In Fig. B there is part of a thrombus on the right. (H&E, × 250.)

for the pathologist since it may be misdiagnosed as angiosarcoma. The obvious intravascular location and the intimate relationship to a thrombus as well as the lack of anaplasia, abnormal mitotic figures, solid areas, and necrotic foci, which are, in contrast, common findings in angiosarcoma, help in the differential diagnosis.[74]

VASCULAR ECTASIAS

According to Johnson,[7] 50 percent of the normal population presents, at birth, erythematous macular areas often involving the face, and head, and neck, otherwise referred to as the *common birthmark* or *nevus flammeus*. These lesions present a wide spectrum in terms of size, appearance, and course. Many of them, such as those appearing on the forehead and eyelids, have a tendency to fade or disappear completely within a few years, whereas the common birthmark on the neck, the so-called stork bite, often remains throughout life. The special form of nevus flammeus known as the *port-wine stain* also does not fade and the color is more apt to become darker or blue.[43] These lesions, which can become elevated with time, most frequently involve the face and head, but may occur anywhere in the body. Occasionally they appear in mucous membranes (e.g., in the oral cavity). The light-microscopic findings indicate that they are caused by the ectasic dilatation of preformed vessels rather than by newly formed vessels. The port-wine stain type of nevus flammeus, in particular, may be associated with other types of vascular malformations, thereby constituting a component of various syndromes (see Table 5-2).

The *arterial spider*, which has been described in detail by Bean,[16] is characterized clinically

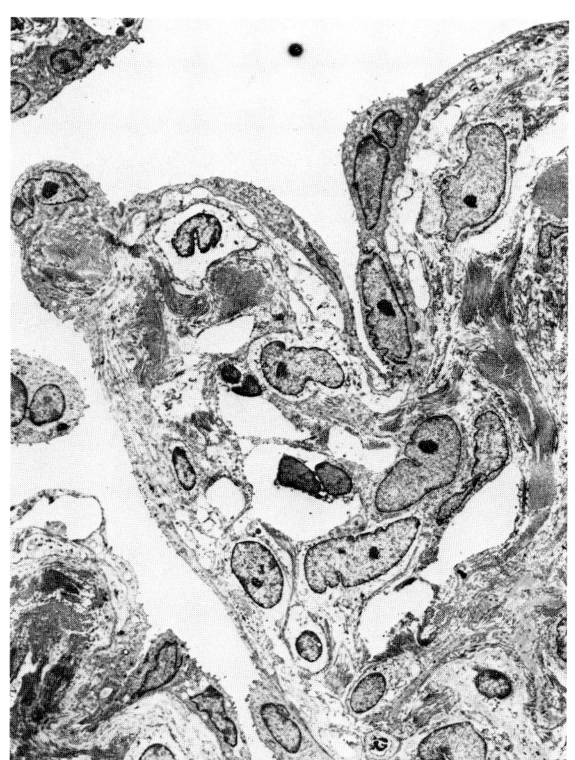

Fig. 5-13. Papillary endothelial hyperplasia. **(A)** A papillary projection in which the central stroma contains collagen and spindle cells and the surface is covered by a single layer of prominent endothelial cells. **(B)** A bulging endothelial cell separated from the stroma by distinct external laminae. (Fig. A × 2,000; Fig. B × 10,000.)

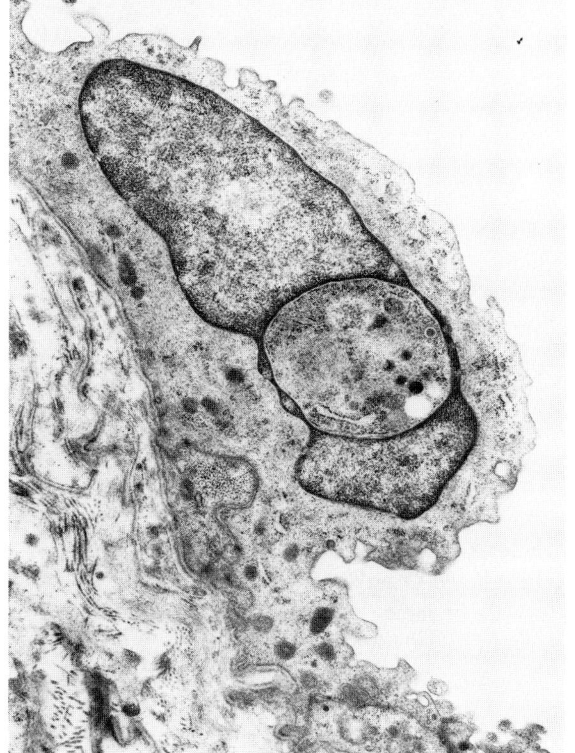

by a central red elevation or punctum that is surrounded by tiny, radial vessels. Pressure over the punctum characteristically bleaches the lesion. The punctum is caused by a thick-walled arteriole that extends into the papillary corium and divides into multiple small vessels that anastomose with capillaries. These lesions are acquired and are usually seen in adults. Arterial spiders may occur in healthy people. But it is of particular interest to note that they more often occur in patients with liver disease (especially cirrhosis) or hyperthyroidism and in pregnant women.

VASCULAR TUMORS OF INTERMEDIATE MALIGNANCY

EPITHELIOID HEMANGIOENDOTHELIOMA

Epithelioid hemangioendothelioma (also referred to as atypical hemangioendothelioma[77]) is a vascular tumor of intermediate malignancy characterized by atypical epithelioid endothelial cells. This lesion belongs to the histiocytoid hemangioma group, as defined by Rosai,[26] which includes lesions that appear to be closely related light microscopically, but show a wide spectrum in terms of biologic potential. Epithelioid hemangioendothelioma occurs in soft tissues and bone as well as in visceral organs, such as liver and lungs. Epithelioid hemangioendotheliomas occurring in the liver and lungs are often multiple and have led to the death of the patient in a fairly high percentage of reported cases. Follow-up studies of epithelioid hemangioendotheliomas of soft tissue, however, indicate an intermediate degree of malignancy. Thus, 6 of the 46 patients reported by Weiss and co-workers[78] died with lymph node and/ or lung metastasis after an average follow-up period of 4 years.

Half of the epithelioid hemangioendotheliomas of soft tissues arise from a medium-sized or large vessel, usually a vein.[78] The involved vessel may be completely obstructed by the tumor or by secondary thrombus formation.[77] The vascular obstruction can be detected preopera-

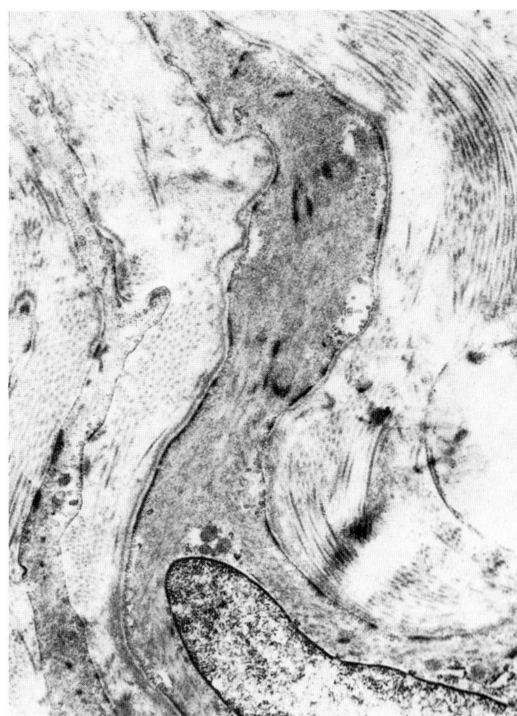

Fig. 5-14. Detail of the papillary stroma showing an abundance of collagen and part of a myofibroblast with an abundance of thin cytofilaments partly forming condensations. The myofibroblast is invested by an external lamina. Numerous pinocytic vesicles are seen along the cytoplasmic border. (× 12,000.)

tively by angiography, which may closely mimic the angiographic findings of a vascular leiomyosarcoma.[77] Typically epithelioid hemangioendotheliomas originating in vessels grow in a centrifugal fashion through the vessel wall into the surrounding soft tissues. The tumor cells are rounded or polygonal and are characteristically arranged in short strands or nests (Fig. 5-15). In some areas, the tumor cells may have less prominent epithelioid features and may even display a spindlelike appearance. Areas in which the tumor cells form distinct vascular channels may be more or less evident. Intracytoplasmic vacuoles representing intracellular lumina can often be found. The usually prominent stroma enclosing the strands and nests of tumor cells varies in appearance from myxoid to hyalin. Mitotic activity and degree of cell atypia varies,

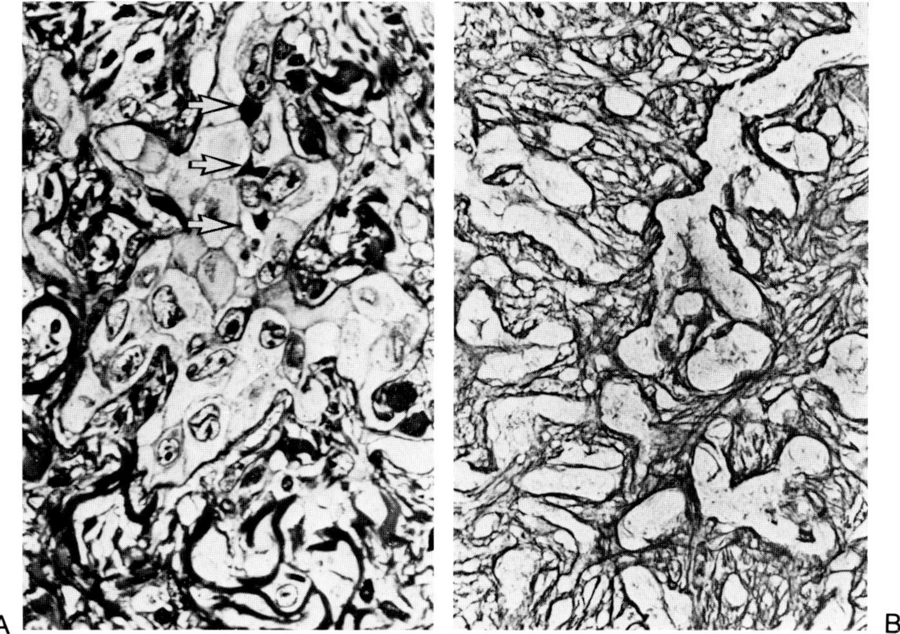

Fig. 5-15. Epithelioid hemangioendothelioma. **(A)** A group of epithelioid tumor cells presenting distinct cytoplasmic outlines and nuclei with an often prominent nucleolus. There are some abortive lumen formations containing erythrocytes (arrows). **(B)** The cordlike solid nests of tumor cells are enclosed by a prominent reticulin network. (Fig. A 1-μm section, toluidine blue, × 600; Fig. B reticulin staining according to Laidlaw, × 250.)

but in most cases in which metastasis has occurred, the tumors have displayed significant cellular and nuclear atypia and brisk mitotic activity.

The differential diagnosis that may be considered include metastatic carcinoma, malignant melanoma, or other types of soft tissue sarcoma with epithelioid features such as epithelioid sarcoma. Immunohistochemistry and electron microscopy may help in solving these differential diagnostic problems. Characteristically the tumor cells of epithelioid hemangioendothelioma are strongly positive for vimentin and express factor VIII-RAG. *Ulex europeus* I lectin, possibly in addition to other markers used in the studies of angiosarcoma (see below) may also help to identify the endothelial nature of the lesion.[77] Some of the immunohistochemical properties of epithelioid hemangioendothelioma and possible differential diagnoses are summarized in Table 5-7. The ultrastructural appear-

ance of the tumor cells very closely resembles that of angiolymphoid hyperplasia, as described above[77, 79] (Fig. 5-16).

SPINDLE CELL HEMANGIOENDOTHELIOMA

Spindle cell hemangioma was described by Weiss and Enzinger[80] as a specific entity among vascular tumors with a very low or intermediate degree of malignancy. Their experience with some 30 cases shows that the lesions predominantly involve the subcutis or dermis of the distal extremities, particularly the hand. The lesions may occur at any age, but one-half of the patients are 25 years of age or younger. Enzinger and Weiss reported three cases of spindle cell hemangioendothelioma in patients with Maffucci's syndrome (Table 5-2). Of the 26 cases of spindle cell hemangioendothelioma reported by Weiss and Enzinger in 1986,[80] local

Table 5-7. Lectin Histochemical and Immunohistochemical Characteristics of Epithelioid Hemangioendothelioma Compared with Epithelioid Sarcoma, Carcinoma, and Malignant Melanoma[a]

	Lectin	Antigen					
Tumor Type	*Ulex europeus* I	Factor VIII-RAG	Cyto-keratins	Vimentin	S-100 Protein	Epithelial Membrane Antigen	Melanoma Antigens
Epithelioid hemangioendo-thelioma	+	+	− +[b]	+	−	−	−
Epithelioid sarcoma	−	−	+	+	−[c]	+	−
Carcinoma	−	−	+	−[c]	−[c]	+	−
Malignant melanoma	−	−	−	+	+	−	+

[a] Epithelioid hemangiendothelioma is included within the concept of histiocytoid hemangiomas, which also encompasses angiolymphoid hyperplasia and low-grade epithelioid angiosarcoma.

[b] Cytokeratin positivity is reported in some cases of both epithelioid hemangiohendothelioma and angiosarcoma.

[c] Occasionally positive.

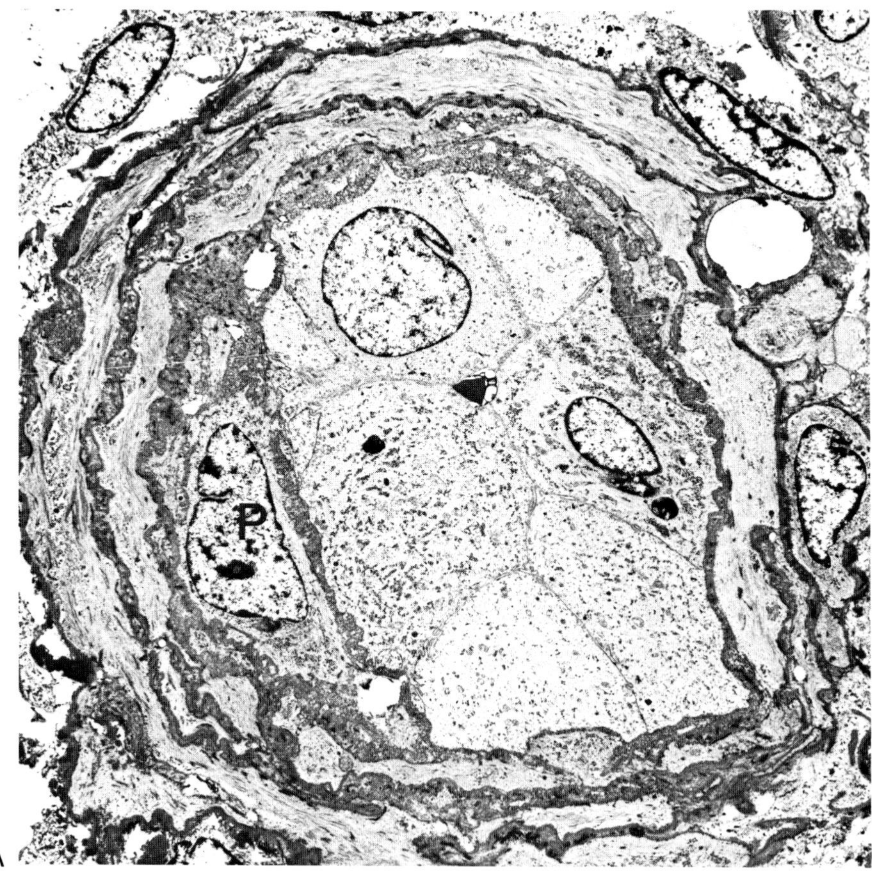

Fig. 5-16. Epithelioid hemangioendothelioma. **(A)** A group of tumor cells, surrounding a central abortive luman enclosed by thick external lamina material, which also ensheaths a pericyte (*P*). (*Figure continues.*)

recurrences occurred in two-thirds of the patients, whereas lymph node metastasis occurred only in one patient, and none of the patients in their series died of the tumor.

The tumors, which produce few symptoms, often appear as small, circumscribed, reddish nodules. The development of multiple nodules, usually in the same area, is quite common. Light microscopically the tumors are characterized by cavernous, blood-filled vascular spaces, often containing organized thrombus material and phleboliths (Fig. 5-17). The cavernous spaces are enclosed by cellular spindle cell tissue (Fig. 5-18A), thereby resembling, to some degree, Kaposi's sarcoma. A continuous spectrum, from the predominating spindle cells to epithelioid cells, can be observed. Intracytoplasmic vacu-

oles can be prominent in the epithelioid cells. According to Weiss and Enzinger's and our own experience, factor VIII-RAG can only be identified within the endothelium lining the vascular spaces and not within the spindle cells (Fig. 5-18B). In a study of two cases, we found the spindle cells to be as strongly positive for vimentin as the endothelial cells. In contrast to the endothelium, the spindle cells were positive for α_1-smooth muscle actin (Fig. 5-18C). Ultrastructurally the cells lining the vascular spaces have endothelial features with an abundance of intermediate filaments. The ultrastructural features closely resemble those of epithelioid hemangioendothelioma and are noticeably different from Kaposi's sarcoma. The spindle cells of Kaposi's sarcoma have the appearance of

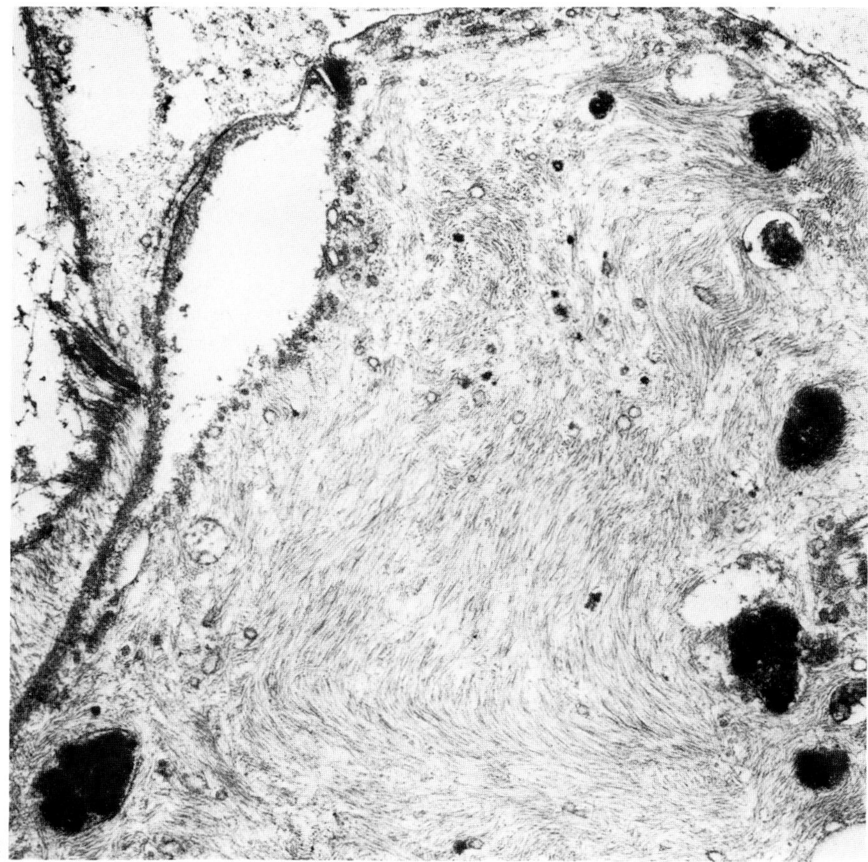

Fig. 5-16 (*Continued*). (**B**) The tumor cells are filled with intermediate filaments. (Fig. A × 3,500; Fig. B × 23,000.)

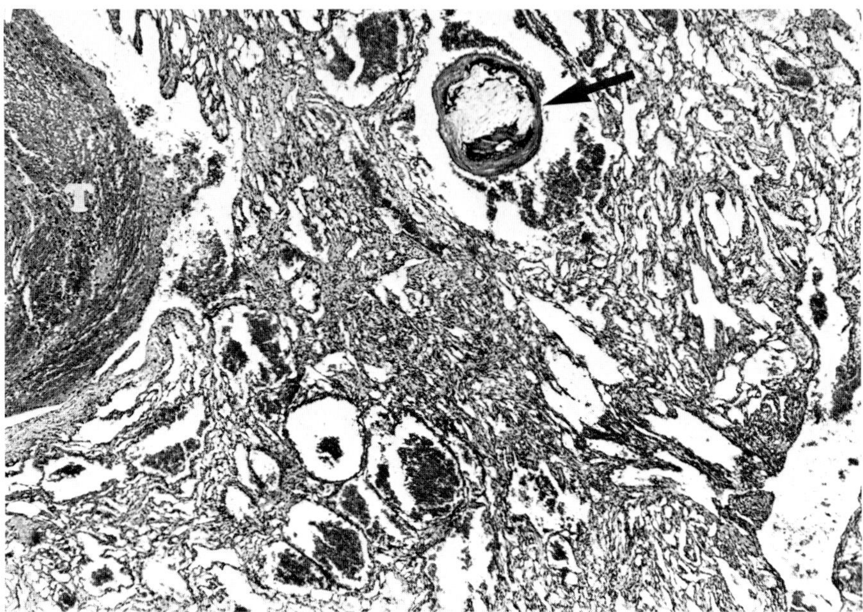

Fig. 5-17. Spindle cell hemangioendothelioma. Cavernous vessels filled with erythrocytes, a thrombus (*T*) and a phlebolith (arrow). (H&E, × 120.)

active proliferating fibroblasts with abundant rough endoplasmic reticulum. The spindle cells of spindle cell hemangioendothelioma are filled, to a large extent, with intermediate and thin filaments, probably corresponding to vimentin and α_1 smooth muscle actin (Fig. 5-19).

Kaposi's Sarcoma

Kaposi's sarcoma is a well-known tumor that is generally included among the vascular neoplasms. The exact cellular differentiation and histogenesis as well as the etiology, especially the etiologic role of virus, is still a much debated topic. Kaposi's sarcoma is most often seen as a cutaneous tumor for which well-established evolutionary steps have been recognized: the early patch lesions, which may be benign in appearance with an inconspicuous proliferation of spindle cells and narrow capillarylike slits; the plaque stage, with more prominent vascular proliferations enclosed within a bland spindle cell component; and the final nodular stage, characterized by slitlike spaces containing erythrocytes within a stroma component that may

resemble a well-differentiated fibrosarcoma (Fig. 5-20A&B). In the nodular stage the degree of cellularity, cell atypia, mitotic activity, and obvious vascular differentiation may vary considerably. Some Kaposi's sarcomas contain angiomatous areas (Fig. 5-20C) that resemble hemangioma, lymphangioma, or angiosarcoma.

Clinically four forms of Kaposi's sarcoma can be distinguished. The chronic or classical form, which mostly afflicts elderly people in Europe and the United States, characteristically presents with one or more cutaneous lesions on the distal extremities, especially the foot and lower leg. A similar type has been recognized in Africa, but it frequently involves younger people. A second lymphadenopathic form of Kaposi's sarcoma occurs primarily in young African children, with the involvement of cervical, inguinal, and hilar lymph nodes. Visceral involvement is quite common and the prognosis is poorer than in the classic chronic form. A third form is the Kaposi's sarcoma that occurs in patients treated with immunosuppressive drugs, especially patients undergoing kidney transplant. The fourth type is the AIDS-related Kaposi's sarcoma, which is characteristically

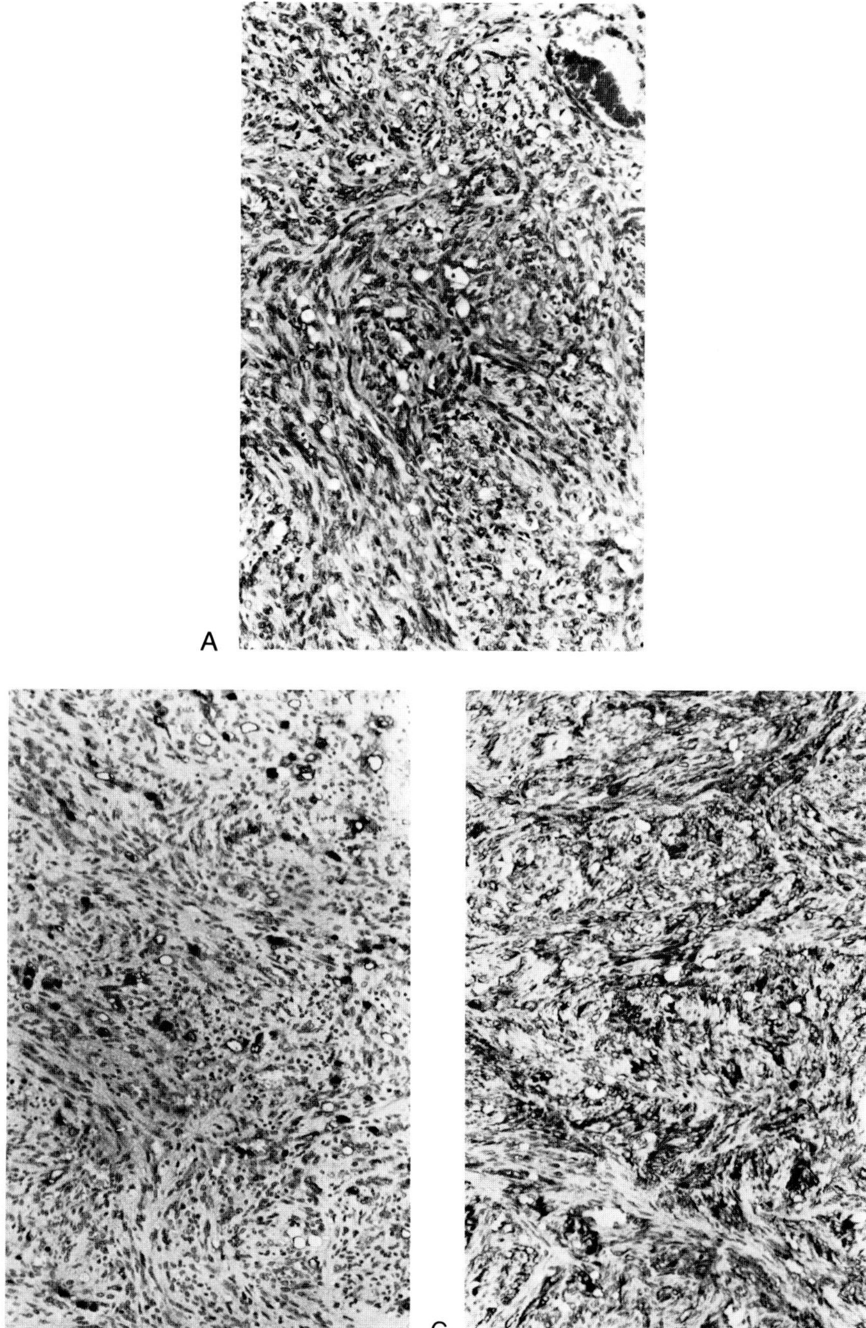

Fig. 5-18. Spindle cell hemangioendothelioma. **(A)** Cellular spindle cell area. **(B)** The delicate vascular spaces within the cellular spindle cell area are identified by the factor VIII-RAG positivity of endothelial cells. **(C)** The spindle cells are positive for α_1-smooth muscle actin. (Fig. A H&E, × 250; Figs. B and C avidin-biotin-complex method applied to formalin-fixed and paraffin-embedded material, × 250.)

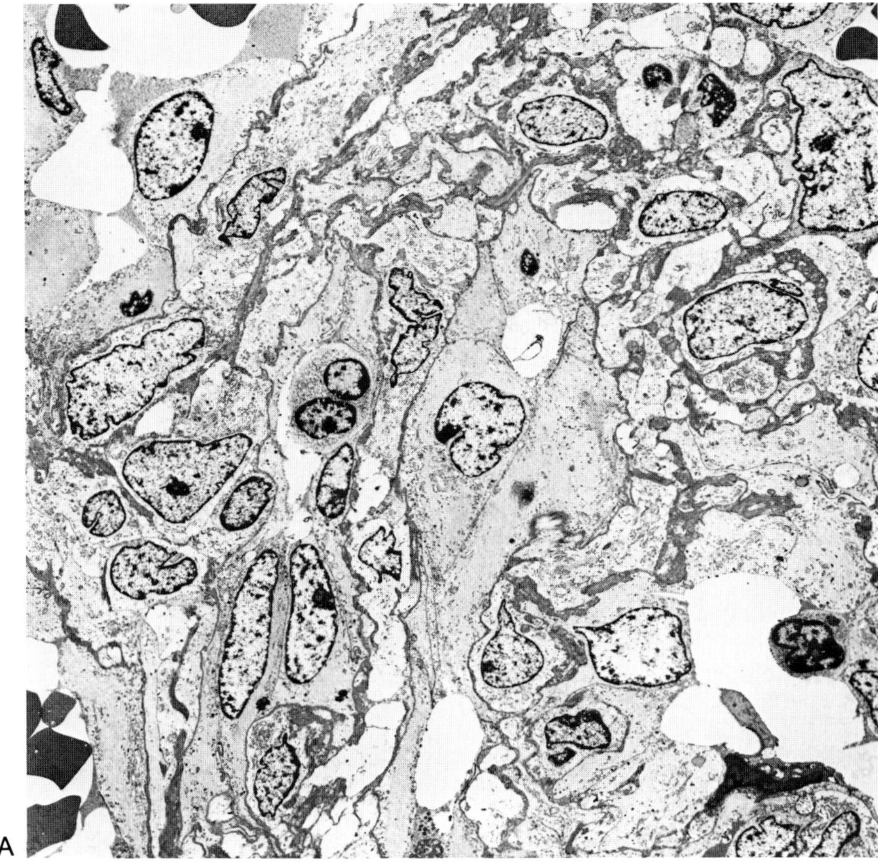

Fig. 5-19. Spindle cell hemangioendothelioma. Irregular vascular slits partly containing erythrocytes **(A)** surrounded by spindle cells which show an abundance of intermediate filaments in the cytoplasm. (*Figure continues.*)

multiple and frequently involves the head region, especially the tip of the nose. A significant proportion of the patients with AIDS-associated Kaposi's sarcoma develop lymph node and gastrointestinal lesions.

Electron microscopy and immunohistochemistry have contributed to the knowledge of the nature of Kaposi's sarcoma although some controversy concerning the endothelial origin of the spindle cell component still exists. Ultrastructurally numerous vascular spaces are seen, some having the appearance of well-developed capillaries with enclosing pericytes and complete external lamina, others being poorly developed and some presenting as solid groups of

proliferating endothelium (Fig. 5-21B). The spindle cells mostly appear as active, proliferating fibroblasts (Fig. 5-21A), and present no obvious features of endothelial differentiation.[81] Factor VIII-RAG has been demonstrated in the endothelial component of the lesions, whereas the spindle cells often are negative. The lack of factor VIII-RAG positivity does not exclude the possibility of an endothelial differentiation of the spindle cells, since the expression of factor VIII-RAG has been found to be highly variable in malignant vascular tumors. Numerous monoclonal antibodies directed against blood vessel and/or lymph vessel endothelium have been applied in recent studies, giving support to the

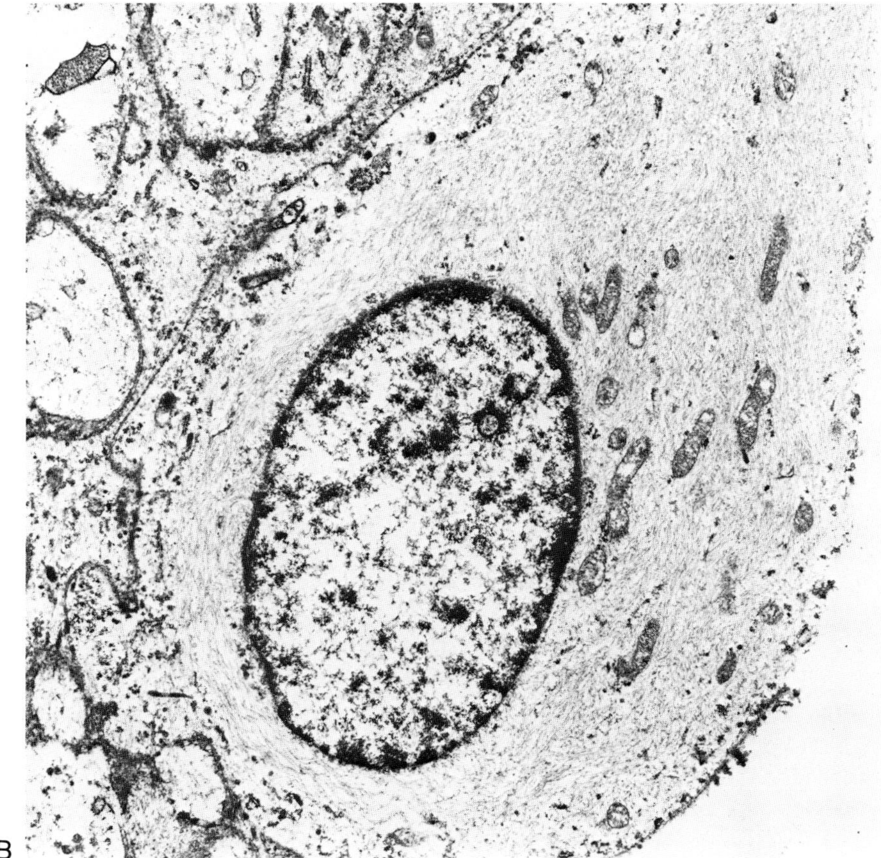

Fig. 5-19 (*Continued*). **(B).** (Fig. A × 2,500; Fig. B × 10,000.)

vascular nature of Kaposi's sarcoma.[82–85] Conflicting opinions still exist as to its origin from blood or lymph vessels.

MALIGNANT ENDOVASCULAR PAPILLARY ANGIOENDOTHELIOMA (DABSKA'S TUMOR)

Malignant endovascular papillary angioendothelioma is a rare vascular tumor that was described by Dabska in 1969.[86] She presented six cases involving the skin or subcutis and occurring during infancy or early childhood. Enzinger and Weiss[3] also report their experience with this tumor in adults. Two of the six cases reported by Dabska developed lymph node metastasis. At low-power light-microscopic examination, the tumor resembles a cavernous hemangioma. The endothelial cells lining the vessels vary from small lymphocytelike cells to cuboidal or columnar cells that form peculiar endovascular papillary structures protruding into the vessel lumina. The papillary projections characteristically have a central hyaline core. In a study of two cases, the tumor cells were labeled by antibodies to factor VIII-RAG, vimentin, and blood group isoantigens; they also bound *Ulex europeus* I lectin, indicating a high degree of endothelial differentiation.[87] Leucocytic determinants were not expressed.

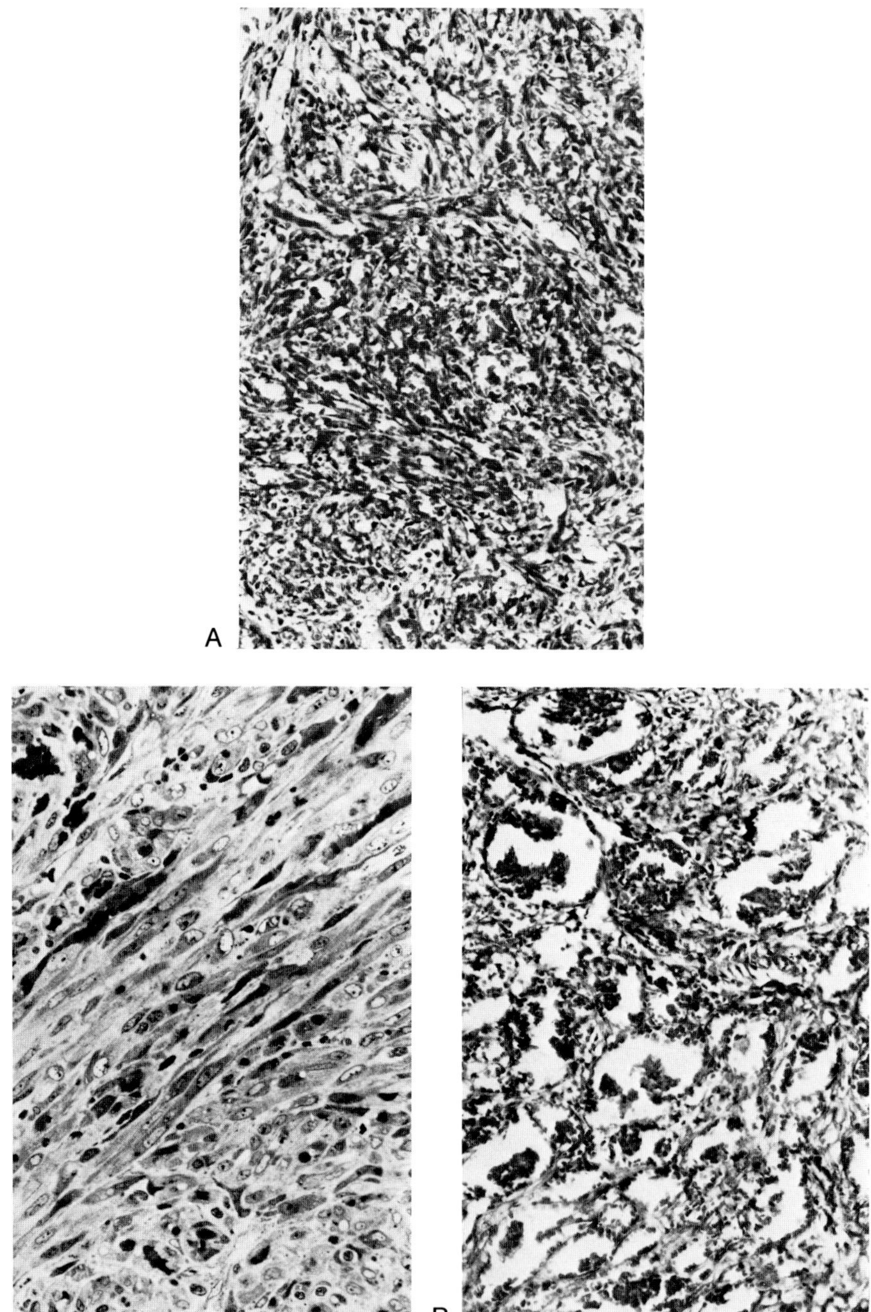

Fig. 5-20. Kaposi's sarcoma. **(A)** The tumor has the appearance of a spindle cell sarcoma with mostly narrow, slitlike lumina and some extravasated erythrocytes. **(B)** Atypical spindle cells are arranged in parallel and there are small nests of endothelial cells. **(C)** Hemangiomatous area with cavernous, blood-filled vessels. (H&E, Fig. A × 250; Fig. B × 500; Fig. C × 250.)

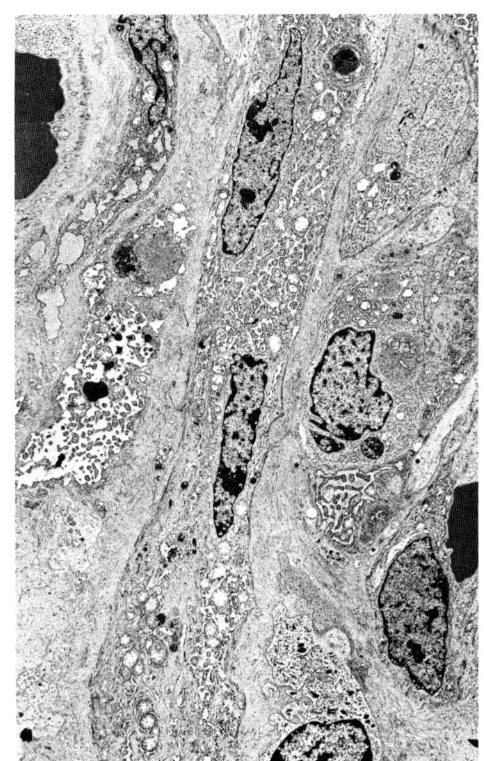

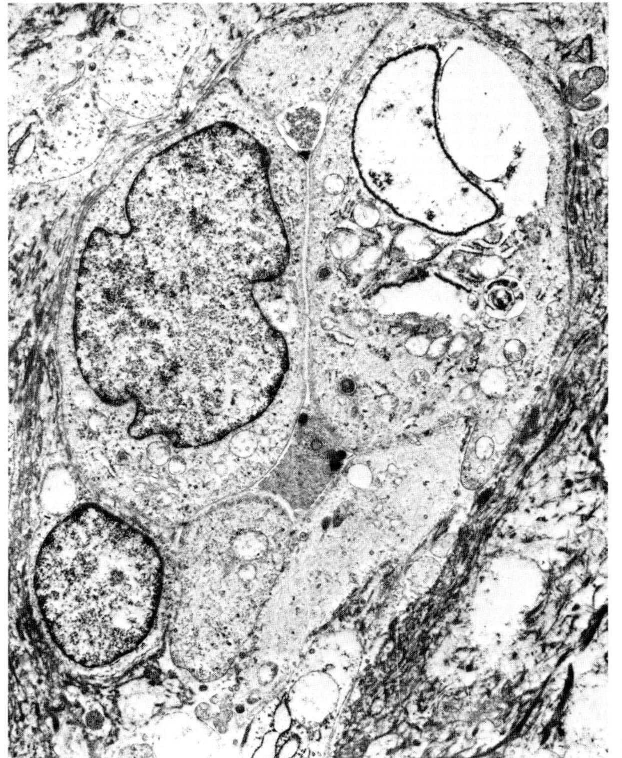

Fig. 5-21. Kaposi's sarcoma. **(A)** Narrow vascular slits containing erythrocytes surrounded by spindle-shaped tumor cells with the features of active fibroblasts with abundant rough endoplasmic reticulum. **(B)** Solid nest of endothelial cells partly enclosed by external lamina and some collagen. (Fig. A × 3,000; Fig. B × 8,000.)

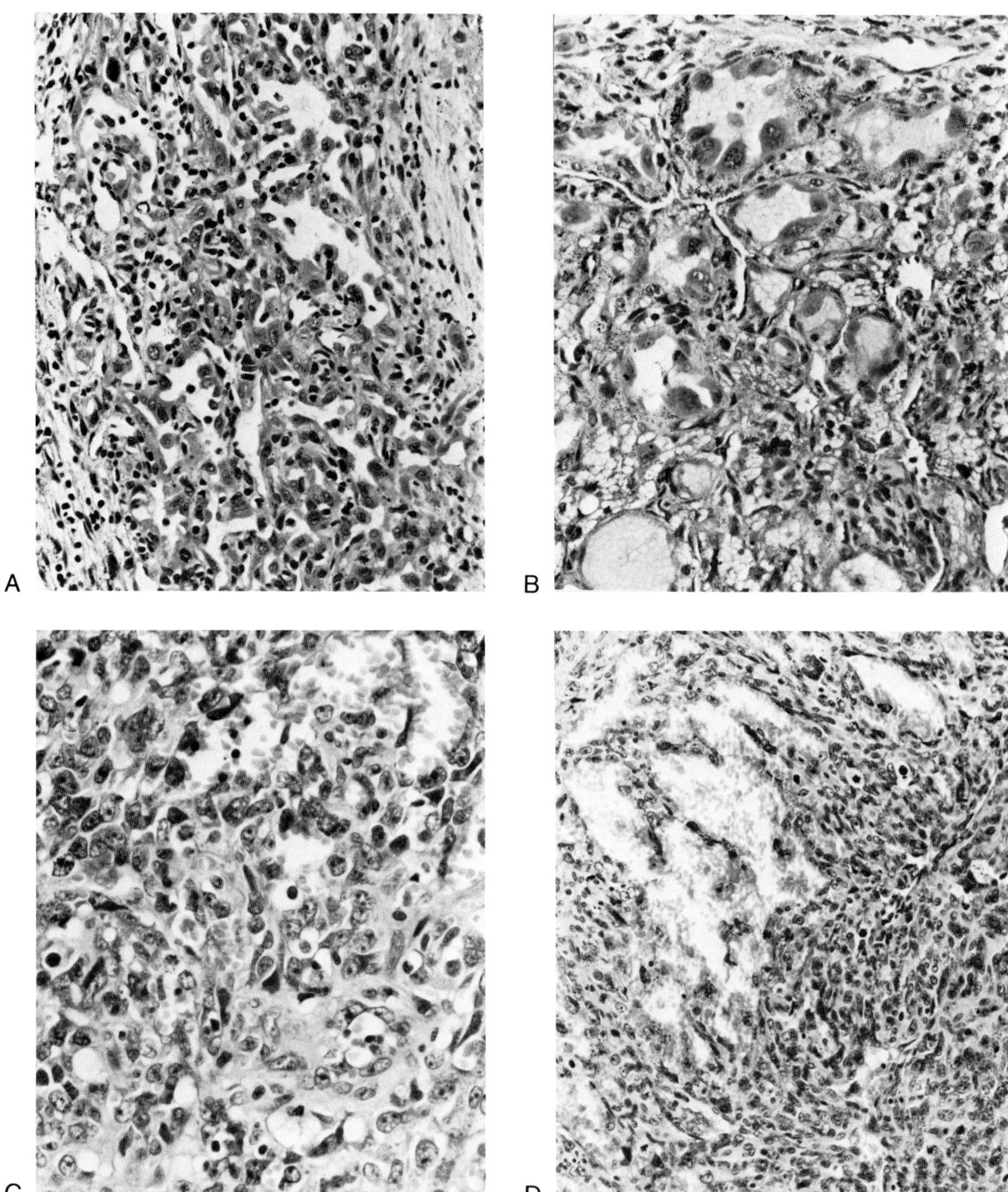

Fig. 5-22. Angiosarcoma with varying degrees of vascular differentiation. **(A & B)** Distinct vascular lumina lined by epithelioid, atypical endothelial tumor cells. **(C & D)** Some solid areas. **(C)** Some intracytoplasmic vacuoles and abortive lumen formations, some of which contain erythrocytes. (H&E, Fig. A × 250; Fig. B × 250; Fig. C × 400; Fig. D × 250.)

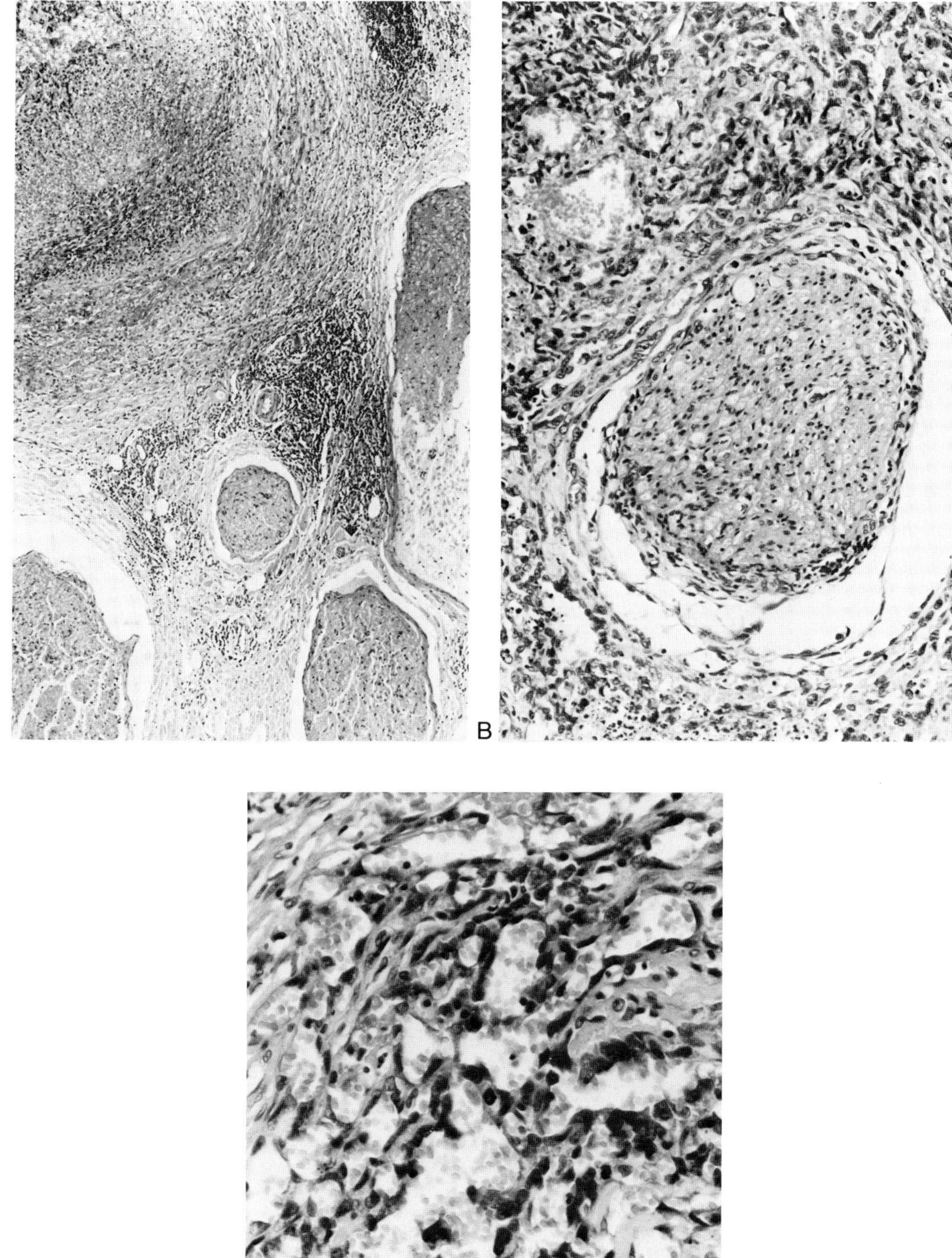

Fig. 5-23. Angiosarcoma occurring in a plexiform neurofibroma of a patient with von Recklinghausen's neurofibromatosis. The angiosarcoma, which encloses the nerve structures **(A & B)**, is characterized by anastomosing, irregular vascular channels lined by hyperchromatic, atypical endothelial tumor cells **(B & C)**. (H&E, Fig. A × 60; Fig. B × 250; Fig. C × 400.)

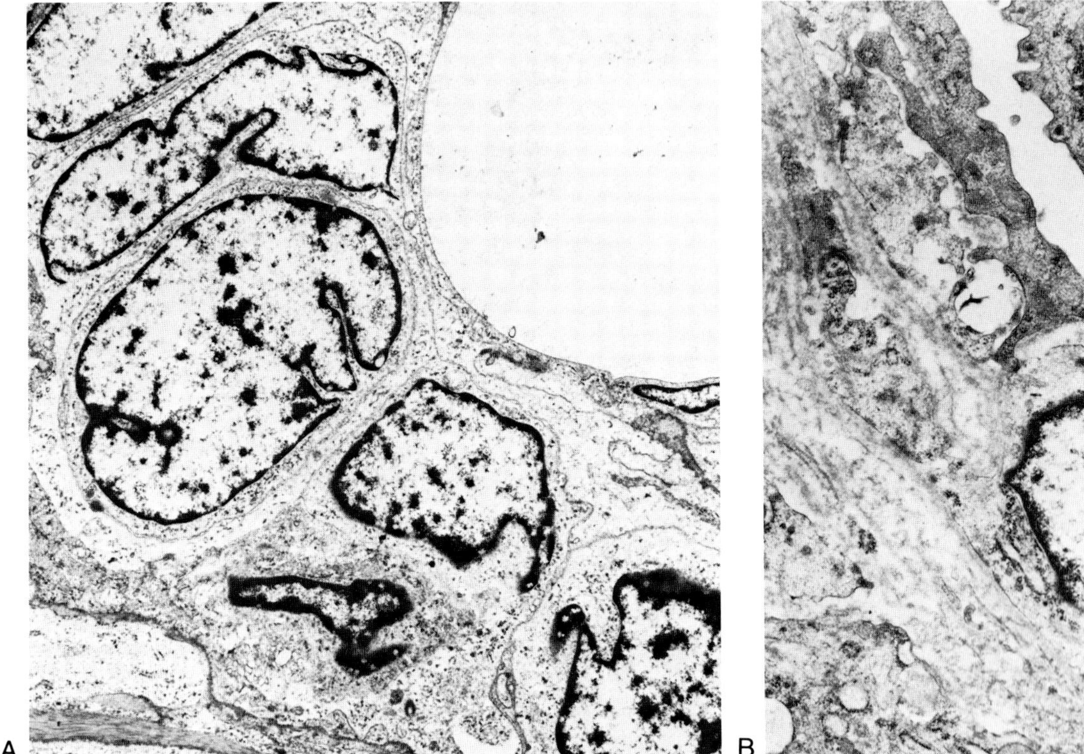

Fig. 5-24. Angiosarcoma. Atypical endothelial tumor cells surround some abortive vascular lumina (**A & C**). Multiple layers of external lamina partly enclose the tumor cells surrounding the vascular slits (**B**). (*Figure continues.*)

MALIGNANT VASCULAR TUMORS

ANGIOSARCOMA

Angiosarcoma is used as a blanket term for malignant tumors presenting blood vessel and/ or lymphatic vessel differentiation. There is a wide spectrum in terms of clinical presentation, localization, histologic appearance, and clinical course. One-third to one-half of all angiosarcomas occur in the skin. Angiosarcomas of the skin develop almost exclusively in the following clinical settings: a lymphoedematous extremity, in most instances secondary to mastectomy; face and skull, usually in elderly individuals; and skin that has been previously irradiated.[88] A highly aggressive form of angiosarcoma occurs in visceral organs, primarily liver and spleen, and in the breast. It is well known that hepatic angiosarcomas may occur in patients who have previously received Thorotrast (thorium dioxide) as a contrast medium in conjunction with cholangiographic examinations. Hepatic angiosarcomas also occur in people employed in the petrochemical industry who are exposed to vinyl chloride and in individuals exposed to arsenic.[89]

Angiosarcoma of soft tissue is not a well-defined group of tumors. It has been estimated to constitute less than 1 percent of soft tissue sarcomas.[90] It is apparent that many of the tumors reported as angiosarcomas in deep soft tissues have occurred primarily[91] in the skin with secondary invasion of underlying soft tissues. Enzinger and Weiss[3] reported 89 cases of angiosarcoma in deep soft tissues. They found the extremities, trunk, and head and neck area to be the most common sites, and also that more often, angiosarcomas of soft tissue tend

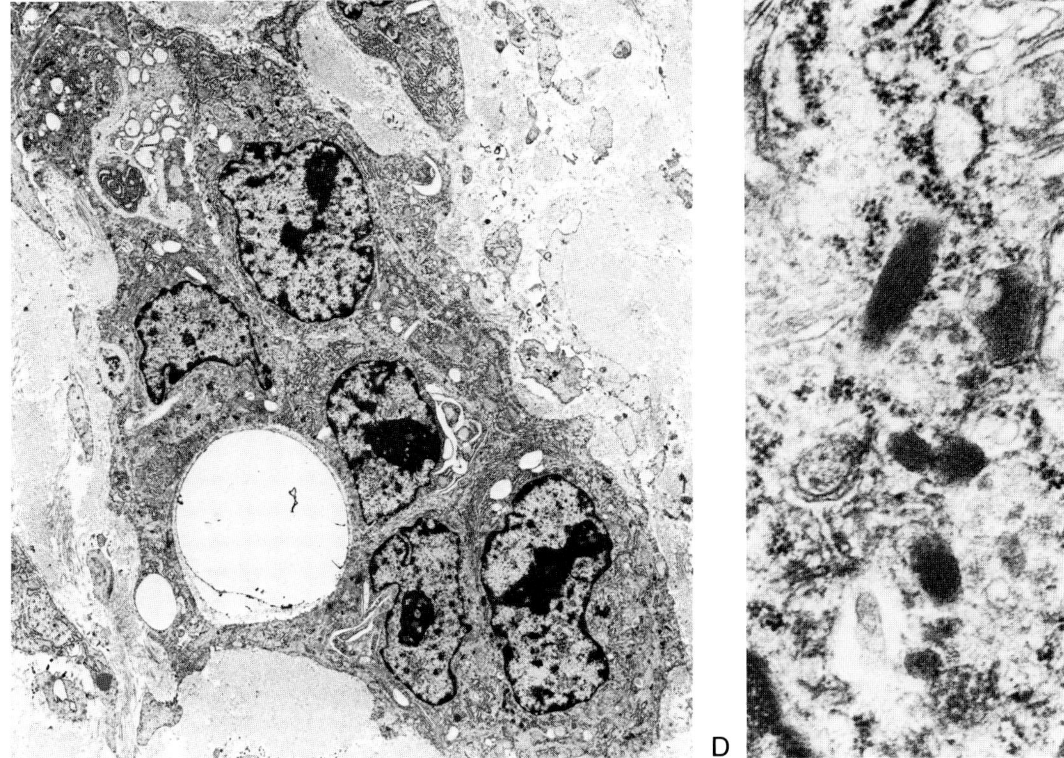

Fig. 5-24 (*Continued*). Scattered Weibel-Palade bodies occur within occasional tumor cells (**D**). (Fig. A × 6,500; Fig. B × 18,000; Fig. C × 4,000; Fig. D × 37,000.)

to be uniformly high-grade lesions than cutaneous angiosarcomas. A detailed knowledge of the prognosis for angiosarcoma of soft tissue is still lacking.

Histologically the diagnosis of angiosarcoma can, in most instances, be based on the capacity of the tumor to form easily recognizable vascular channels. There is, however, a wide spectrum in terms of cellular appearance and degree of polymorphism, mitotic activity, and the tendency to form vascular structures (Fig. 5-22). The most highly differentiated angiosarcomas may be difficult to distinguish from hemangiomas. At times, angiosarcoma cells may present epithelioid features (Fig. 5-22B), which may make it difficult to distinguish them from carcinomas and soft tissue sarcomas with epithelioid features, such as epithelioid sarcoma. Epithelioid and high-grade angiosarcomas may be predominantly solid, mimicking a malignant melanoma, whereas spindle cell angiosarcomas may resemble other types of spindle cell sarcomas.

Angiosarcomas occurring in deep soft tissues may occasionally develop within nerves. A few cases have been described as arising in otherwise healthy patients within medium-sized or large nerves.[92, 93] A few cases have also been reported within plexiform neurofibromas in patients with Recklinghausen's neurofibromatosis (Fig. 5-23)[3, 94, 95] and angiosarcoma may occasionally develop as a component of a malignant peripheral nerve sheath tumor.[96, 97]

The ultrastructural appearance of angiosarcoma is quite variable, depending on the degree of cellular differentiation. In well-differentiated angiosarcomas the tumor cells lining the vascular structures possess many features of normal endothelium, such as tight junctions between

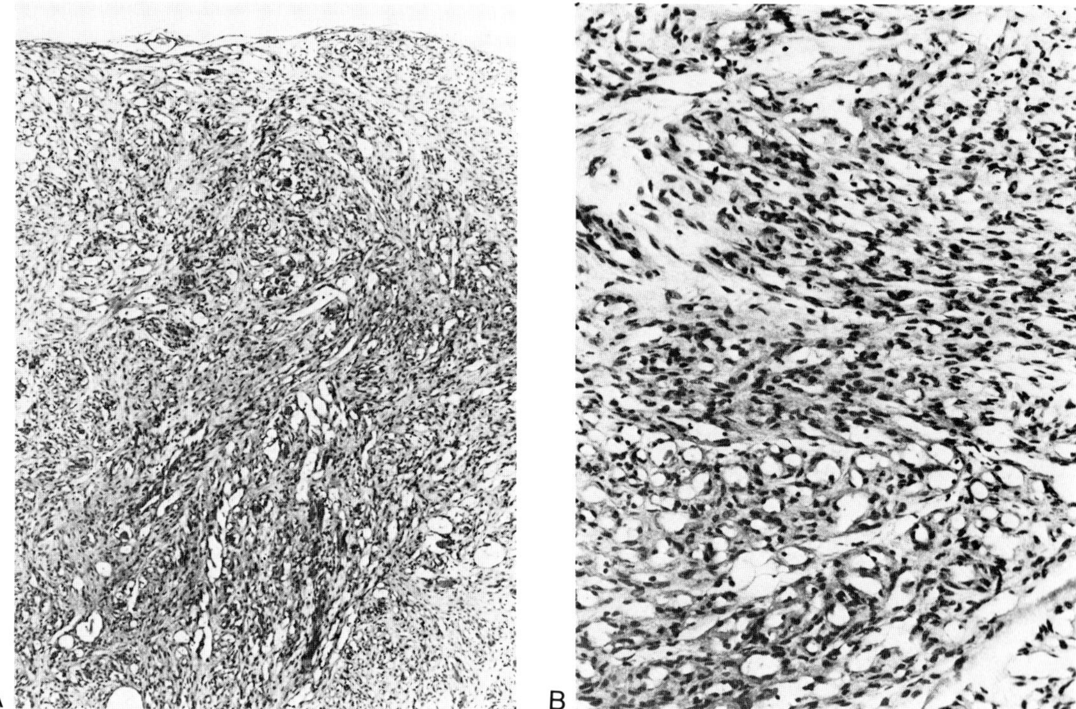

Fig. 5-25. (A&B) An unusually cellular angiolipoma with an inconspicuous adipose tissue component. (H&E Fig. A × 120; Fig. B × 250.)

cells, pinocytic vesicles, intermediate cytofilaments, and external lamina investing the vascular formations. Weibel-Palade bodies can usually be detected in well-differentiated angiosarcomas. In poorly differentiated angiosarcomas, in which the vascular differentiation may not be evident on light microscopy, the electron-microscopic examination may help to disclose abortive vascular slits (Fig. 5-24A–C) and intracytoplasmic lumen formations. Weibel-Palade bodies in convincing neoplastic cells are usually difficult to detect in poorly differentiated angiosarcomas, but they should be carefully sought for, as they are pathognomonic of endothelial differentiation,[81][98][99] (Fig. 5-24D).

Immunohistochemistry may help in the differential diagnosis between angiosarcoma and carcinoma, malignant melanoma, and other types of soft tissue sarcoma. The most specific and widely applied marker of endothelial differentiation available today, appears to be factor VIII-RAG. It is synthesized in endothelial cells and is apparently stored in Weibel-Palade bodies. This marker can be used on formalin-fixed, paraffin-embedded material. In well-differentiated angiosarcomas the expression of factor VIII-RAG is usually easy to detect, whereas it is highly variable in high-grade angiosarcomas. The lectin derived from *Ulex europeus* (*Ulex europeus* I) binds selectively to α-L-fucose residues present on the surface of normal endothelial cells. There are several reports that the binding of this lectin is also found more frequently than the demonstration of factor VIII-RAG in high-grade angiosarcoma. The *Ulex europeus* I lectin is, however, less specific, since it also binds occasionally to carcinomas of various types. Laminin and collagen type IV, components of the external lamina, have been used to identify the external lamina outlining the malignant vascular structures of angiosarcomas. Recent studies have shown that thrombomodulin is a specific and highly sensitive marker for angiosarcomas.[100] The monoclonal antibody BMA 120

Table 5-8. Lesions Simulating Angiosarcoma

Benign vascular lesions that may be mistaken for angiosarcoma
  Juvenile hemangioendothelioma (immature type of hemangioma)
  Small vessel (capillary) type of intramuscular hemangioma
  Angiolymphoid hyperplasia
  Cellular angiolipoma
  Papillary endothelial hyperplasia (Masson's pseudoangiosarcoma)
  Florid forms of granuloma pyogenicum
  Redundant granulation tissue with prominent proliferation of capillaries and endothelium

Vascular lesions of intermediate malignancy that may resemble angiosarcoma
  Spindle cell hemangioendothelioma
  Kaposi's sarcoma—angiomatoid type
  Epithelioid hemangioendothelioma

is another endothelial cell marker that can be applied to routinely prepared tissues.[101] Recently the unexpected expression of cytokeratins has been reported in angiosarcomas. Brooks[102] found that 4 out of 14 angiosarcomas expressed cytokeratins in tumor cells scattered throughout the tumors. Some of these cytokeratin-positive tumors appear to have been angiosarcomas of the epithelioid type. It is of interest to note that cytokeratins may occasionally be expressed not only in malignant endothelial tumors, but in proliferating endothelial cells in reactive lesions and in a few instances, in benign endothelial tumors such as hemangiomas[102] and epithelioid hemangioendothelioma.[103]

Benign vascular lesions (Fig. 5-25) that may be mistaken for angiosarcoma and vascular lesions of intermediate malignancy that should be distinguished from angiosarcoma are summarized in Table 5-8.

REFERENCES

1. Steeper TA, Rosai J: Aggressive angiomyxoma of the female pelvis and perineum. Report of nine cases of a distinctive type of gynecologic soft-tissue neoplasm. Am J Surg Pathol 7:463, 1983
2. Bégin LR, Clement PB, Kirk ME, et al: Aggressive angiomyxoma of pelvic soft parts: a clinicopathologic study of nine cases. Hum Pathol 16:621, 1985
3. Enzinger FM, Weiss SW: Soft Tissue Tumors. 2nd Ed. CV Mosby, St. Louis, 1988
4. Wick MR, Rocamora A: Reactive and malignant "angioendotheliomatosis": a discriminant clinocopathologic study. J Cutan Pathol 15:260, 1988
5. Watson WL, McCarthy WD: Blood and lymph vessel tumors. Surg Gynecol Obstet 71:569, 1940
6. Geshickter CF, Keasbey LE: Tumors of blood vessels. Am J Cancer 23:568, 1935
7. Johnson WC: Pathology of cutaneous vascular tumors. Int J Dermatol 15:239, 1976
8. Imperial R, Helwig EB: Verrucous hemangioma: a clinicopathologic study of 21 cases. Arch Dermatol 96:247, 1967
9. Kasabach HH, Merritt KK: Capillary hemangioma with extensive purpura: report of a case. Am J Dis Child 59:1063, 1961
10. Bean WB: Dyschondroplasia and hemangiomata (Maffucci's syndrome). II. Arch Intern Med 102:544, 1958
11. Osler W: On a family form of recurring epitaxis associated with multiple telangiectases of the skin and mucous membranes. Bull Johns Hopkins Hosp 12:333, 1901
12. Letts RM: Orthopedic treatment of hemangiomatous hypertrophy of the lower extremity. J Bone Joint Surg 59A:777, 1977
13. Lindenaure SM: The Klippel-Trenaunay syndrome: varicosity, hypertrophy and hemangioma with arteriovenous fistula. Ann Surg 162:303, 1965
14. Reid MR: Abnormal arteriovenous communications acquired and congenital. II. The origin and nature of arteriovenous aneurysms, cirsoid aneurysms, and simple angiomas. Arch Surg 10:996, 1925
15. Ward CE, Horton BT: Congenital arteriovenous fistulas in children. J Pediatr 16:746, 1940
16. Bean WB: Vascular Spiders and Related Lesions of the Skin. Charles C Thomas, Springfield, IL, 1958
17. Bluefarb SM, Adams LA: Arteriovenous malformation with angiodermatosis. Stasis dermatitis simulating Kaposi's sarcoma. Arch Dermatol 96:176, 1967
18. Earhart RN, Aeling JA, Nuss DD, et al: Pseudo-Kaposi's sarcoma: a patient with arteriovenous malformation and skin lesions simulating Kapo-

si's sarcoma. Arch Dermatol 110:907, 1974

19. Strutton G, Weedon D: Acro-angiodermatitis: a simulant of Kaposi's sarcoma. Am J Dermatopathol 9:85, 1987

20. Connelly MG, Winkelmann RK: Acral arteriovenous tumor: a clinicopathologic review. Am J Surg Pathol 9:15, 1985

21. Girard C, Graham JH, Johnson WC: Arteriovenous Hemangioma (arteriovenous shunt). A clinicopathologic and histochemical study. J Clin Pathol 1:73, 1974

22. Wells GC, Whimster I: Subcutaneous angiolymphoid hyperplasia with eosinophilia. Br J Dermatol 81:1, 1969

23. Peterson WC, Fusaro RM, Goltz RW: Atypical pyogenic granuloma: a case of benign hemangioendotheliosis. Arch Dermatol 90:197, 1964

24. Wilson Jones E, Bleehen SS: Inflammatory angiomatous nodules with abnormal blood vessels occurring about the ears and scalp (pseudo or atypical pyogenic granuloma). Br J Dermatol 81:804, 1969

25. Kimura T, Yoshimura, S, Ishikawa E: Unusual granulation combined with hyperplastic change of lymphatic tissue. Trans Soc Pathol Jpn 37:179, 1948

26. Rosai J, Gold J, Landy R: The histiocytoid hemangiomas. A unifying concept embracing several previously described entities of skin, soft tissue, large vessels, bone, and heart. Hum Pathol 10:707, 1979

27. Kindblom L-G, Fassina AS: Angiolymphoid hyperplasia with eosinophilia of the skin. Light microscopic and ultrastructural study of 4 cases. Acta Pathol Microbiol Scand [A] 89:271, 1981

28. Kerr DA: Granuloma pyogenicum. Oral Surg 4:158, 1951

29. Cooper HP, McAllister HA, Helwig EB: Intravenous pyogenic granuloma. A study of 18 cases. Am J Surg Pathol 3:221, 1979

30. McDonald RH: Granuloma gravidarum. Pregnancy tumor of the gingiva. Am J Obstet Gynecol 72:1132, 1956

31. Coskey RJ, Mehregan AH: Granuloma pyogenicum with multiple satellite recurrences. Arch Dermatol 96:71, 1967

32. Warner J, Wilson-Jones E: Pyogenic granuloma recurring with multiple satellites. A report of 11 cases. Br J Dermatol 80:218, 1968

33. Zaynoun ST, Juljulian HH, Kurban AK: Pyogenic granuloma with multiple satellites. Arch Dermatol 109:689, 1974

34. Allen PW, Enzinger FM: Hemangiomas of skeletal muscle. An analysis of 89 cases. Cancer 29:8, 1972

35. Angervall L, Nilsson L, Stener B, et al: Angiographic, microangiographic, and histologic study of vascular malformation in striated muscle. Acta Radiol 7:65, 1968

36. Angervall L, Möller Nielsen J, Stener B, et al: Concomitant arteriovenous vascular malformation in skeletal muscle. A clinical, angiographic and histologic study. Cancer 44:232, 1979

37. Bennet GE, Cobey MC: Hemangioma of joints. Report of five cases. Arch Surg 38:487, 1939

38. Cobey MC: Hemangioma of joints. Arch Surg 46:465, 1943

39. McInerney D, Park WM: Thermographic assessment of synovial hemangioma. Clin Radiol 29:469, 1978

40. Lichtenstein L: Tumors of synovial joints, bursae, and tendon sheaths. Cancer 8:816, 1955

41. Burman MS, Milgram JE: Haemangioma of tendon and tendon sheath. Surg Gynecol Obstet 50:397, 1930

42. Wood MB: Intraneural hemangioma: report of a case. Plast Reconstr Surg 65:74, 1980

43. Pack GT, Ariel IM: Tumors of the Soft Somatic Tissues. Hoeber-Harper, New York, 1958

44. Stout AP, Murray MR: Hemangiopericytoma. A vascular tumor featuring Zimmermann's pericytes. Ann Surg 116:26, 1942

45. Tsuneyoshi M, Daimaru Y, Enjoji M: Malignant hemangiopericytoma and other sarcomas with hemangiopericytoma-like pattern. Pathol Res Pract 178:446, 1984

46. Angervall L, Kindblom LG, Moller Nielsen J, et al: Hemangiopericytoma, a clinicopathologic, angiographic and microangiographic study. Cancer 42:2412, 1978

47. Angervall L, Kindblom LG, Rydholm A, et al.: The diagnosis and prognosis of soft tissue tumors. Semin Diagn Pathol 3:240, 1986

48. Angervall L, Kindblom LG: Principles for the pathologic diagnosis of soft tissue sarcomas. Acta Oncol 28 (Suppl 2):9, 1989

49. Angervall L, Nilsson L, Stener B: Microangiographic and histological studies in 2 cases of hibernoma. Cancer 17:685, 1964

50. Kindblom L-G, Angervall L, Stener B, et al: Intermuscular and intramuscular lipomas and hibernomas. A clinical, roentgenologic, histo-

logic and prognostic study of 46 cases. Cancer 33:754, 1974

51. Stener B, Angervall L, Nilsson L, et al: Angiographic and histologic studies of the vascularization of peripheral nerve tumors. Clin Orthop 66:113, 1969

52. Berlin O, Stener B, Lindahl S, et al: Vascularization of peripheral neurilemomas: Angiographic, computed tomographic and histologic studies. Skeletal Radiol 15:275, 1986

53. Battifora H: Hemangiopericytoma: ultrastructural study of five cases. Cancer 31:1418, 1973

54. Enzinger FM, Harvey DA: Spindle cell lipoma. Cancer 36:1852, 1975

55. Angervall L, Dahl I, Kindblom LG, et al: Spindle cell lipoma. Acta Path Microbiol Scand [A] 84:477, 1976

56. Hahn MJ, Dawson R, Esterly JA, et al: Hemangiopericytoma. An ultrastructural study. Cancer 31:255, 1973

57. Pena CE: Meningioma and intracranial hemangiopericytoma. A comparative electron microscopic study. Acta Neuropathol (Berl) 39:69, 1977

58. Nunnery EW, Kahn LB, Reddick RL, et al: Hemangiopericytoma: a light microscopic and ultrastructural study. Cancer 47:906, 1981

59. Batsakis JG, Jacobs JB, Templeton AC: Hemangiopericytoma of nasal cavity: Electron-optic study and clinical correlations. J Laryngol Otol 97:361, 1983

60. Hultberg BM, Daugaard S, Johansen HF, et al: Malignant haemangiopericytomas and haemangioendotheliosarcomas: an immunohistochemical study. Histopathology 12:405, 1988

61. Kauffman SL, Stout AP: Haemangiopericytoma in children. Cancer 13:695, 1960

62. Masson P: Le glomus neuromyoarterial des regions tactiles et ses tumeurs. Lyon Chir 21:257, 1924

63. Bergstrand H: Multiple glomic tumors. Am J Cancer 29:470, 1937

64. Lattes R, Bull DC: A case of glomus tumor with primary involvement of bone. Ann Surg 127:187, 1948

65. Appelman HD, Helwig EB: Glomus tumors of the stomach. Cancer 23:203, 1969

66. Jepson RP, Harris JD: Glomus tumors. Med J Aust 2:452, 1970

67. Smyth M: Glomus cell tumors in the lower extremity: report of two cases. J Bone Joint Surg 53:157, 1971

68. Kanwar YS, Manaligod JR: Glomus tumor of the stomach. An ultrastrucutral study Arch Pathol 99:392, 1975

69. Toker C: Glomangioma: an ultrastructural study. Cancer 23:487, 1969

70. Tsuneyoshi M, Enjoji M: Glomus tumor. A clinicopathologic and electron microscopic study. Cancer 50:1601, 1982

71. Miettinen M, Lehto V-P, Virtanen I: Glomus tumor cells. Evaluation of smooth muscle and endothelial cell properties. Virchows Arch B 43:139, 1983

72. Aiba M, Hirayama A, Kuramochi S: Glomangiosarcoma in a glomus tumor. An immunohistochemical and ultrastructural study. Cancer 61:1467, 1988

73. Masson P: Hemangioendotheliome végétant intravasculaire. Bull Soc Anat (Paris) 93:517, 1923

74. Clearkin KP, Enzinger FM: Intravascular papillary endothelial hyperplasia. Arch Pathol Lab Med 100:441, 1976

75. Henschen F: L'Endovasculite proliferante thrombopoietique dans la lesion vasculaire locale. Ann Anat Pathol (Paris) 9:113, 1932

76. Kreutner A Jr, Smith RM, Trefny FA: Intravascular papillary endothelial hyperplasia. Light and electron microscopic observations of a case. Cancer 42:2305, 1978

77. Angervall L, Kindblom L-G, Karlsson K, et al: Atypical hemangioendothelioma of venous origin. A clinicopathologic, angiographic, immunohistochemical, and ultrastructural study of two endothelial tumors within the concept of histiocytoid hemangioma. Am J Surg Pathol 9:504, 1985

78. Weiss SW, Ishak KG, Dail DH, et al: Epithelioid hemangioendothelioma and related lesions. Semin Diagn Pathol 3:259, 1986

79. Weiss SW, Enzinger FM: Epithelioid hemangioendothelioma. A vascular tumor often mistaken for a carcinoma. Cancer 50:970, 1982

80. Weiss SW, Enzinger FM: Spindle cell hemangioendothelioma. A low grade angiosarcoma resembling a cavernous hemangioma and Kaposi's sarcoma. Am J Surg Pathol 10:521, 1986

81. Henderson DW, Papadimitriou JM, Coleman M: Diagnosis and classification of human neoplasia by electron microscopy. In Ultrastruc-

tural Appearance of Tumours. 2nd Ed. Churchill Livingstone, Edinburgh, 1986

82. Rutgers JL, Wieczorek R, Bonetti F, et al: gens by AIDS-associated Kaposi's sarcoma. Evidence for a vascular endothelial cell origin. Am J Pathol 122:493, 1986

83. Beckstead JH, Wood GS, Fletcher V: Evidence for the origin of Kaposi's sarcoma from lymphatic endothelium. Am J Pathol 119:294, 1985

84. Jones RR, Jones EW: The histogenesis of Kaposi's sarcoma (editorial). Am J Dermatopathol 8:369, 1986

85. Jones RR, Spaull J, Spry C, et al: Histogenesis of Kaposi's sarcoma in patients with and without acquired immune deficiency syndrome (AIDS). J Clin Pathol 39:742, 1986

86. Dabska M: Malignant endovascular papillary angioendothelioma of the skin in childhood. Cancer 24:503, 1969

87. Manivel JC, Wick MR, Swanson PE, et al: Endovascular papillary angioendothelioma of childhood: a vascular lesion possibly characterized by "high" endothelial cell differentiation. Hum Pathol 17:1240, 1986

88. Cooper PH: Angiosarcomas of the skin. Semin Diagn Pathol 4:2, 1987

89. Popper H, Thomas LB, Telles NC, et al: Development of hepatic angiosarcoma in man induced by vinyl chloride, Thorotrast and arsenic. Comparison with cases of unknown etiology. Am J Pathol 92:349, 1978

90. Bardwil JM, Mocega EE, Butler JJ, et al: Angiosarcomas of the head and neck region. Am J Surg 116:548, 1968

91. Maddox JC, Evans HL: Angiosarcoma of skin and soft tissue. A study of forty-four cases. Cancer 48:1907, 1981

92. Conway JD, Smith MB: Hemangio-endothelioma originating in a peripheral nerve (report of a case). Ann Surg 134:138, 1951

93. Bricklin AS, Rushton HW: Angiosarcoma of venous origin arising in radial nerve. Cancer 39:1556, 1977

94. Chadhuri, B, Ronan SG, Manahgod JR: Angiosarcoma arising in a plexiform neurofibroma. Cancer 46:605, 1980

95. Lederman SM, Martin EC, Laffey KT, et al: Hepatic neurofibromatosis, malignant schwannoma, and angiosarcoma in von Recklinghausen's disease. Gastroenterology 92:234, 1987

96. Russel DS, Rubinstein LJ: Pathology of Tumours of the Central Nervous System. 4th Ed. Edward Arnold, London, 1977

97. Macaulay RAA: Neurofibrosarcoma of the radial nerve in von Recklinghausen's disease with metastatic angiosarcoma. J Neurol Neurosurg Psychiatry 41:474, 1978

98. Cartens PHB: The Weibel-Palade body in the diagnosis of endothelial tumors. Ultrastruct Pathol 2:315, 1981

99. Waldo ED, Vuletin JC, Kaye GI: The ultrastructure of vascular tumors: Additional observations and a review of the literature. Pathol Annu 12:279, 1977

100. Yonezawa S, Maruyama I, Sakae K, et al: Thrombomodulin as a marker for vascular tumors. Comparative study with Factor VIII and Ulex europaeus I Lectin. Am J Clin Pathol 88:405, 1987

101. Alles JU, Bosslet K: Immunocytochemistry of angiosarcomas. A study of 19 cases with special emphasis on the applicability of endothelial cell specific marker to routinely prepared tissues.

6

Tumors of Lymph Vessels

Lars-Gunnar Kindblom and Lennart Angervall

As with blood vessel lesions, it is often difficult to distinguish true neoplasms of lymph vessels from malformations and ectasias. A unifying concept linking lymphatic disorders such as lymphangiectasia, different types of lymphangiomas, and lymphangiosarcoma has been proposed in which disturbed lymphangiogenesis and obstruction have a central role.[1,2] Tumors and tumorlike lesions of lymph vessels are rare compared with those of blood vessel origin. Both ultrastructural features and immunohistochemical findings have been reported useful in distinguishing lymph vessels from blood vessels.[3–5] Despite this, it is not always possible to make a clear distinction between lesions of lymph vessel and blood vessel origin. In the early literature, lesions considered to be composed of both blood and lymph vessels were referred to as *hemolymphangiomas*.[6] Lymphangiomas can show secondary hemorrhages, but the diagnosis of hemangiolymphoma should not be based solely on the finding of erythrocytes within the vascular spaces. Lymphangiomas may be associated with such syndromes as Turner's syndrome (gonadal dysgenesis), and in certain cases of Klippel-Trenaunay and Maffucci's syndromes, not only hemangiomas but also lymphangiomas can be a component.[1,7]

A classification of the tumors of lymph vessels is given in Table 6–1.

LYMPHANGIOMA

As with hemangiomas, lymphangiomas show a predilection for the skin, although no tissue or organ is spared. Most lymphangiomas either are congenital or occur during the first 2 years of life. The majority are solitary, but multiple lesions may occur. Lymphangiomas can be divided into three main groups: capillary, cavernous, and cystic.

CAPILLARY LYMPHANGIOMA

The existence of a true, clearly distinguishable capillary type has been questioned. It has been considered to be an early developmental stage of cavernous lymphangioma or a type bordering on simple lymphangiectasia.[8] The term *lymphangioma simplex* has been used to describe single or multiple nodular and mostly superficial lesions within the skin or mucous membranes; they are characterized histologically by thinwalled, generally dilated, lymph vessels. Those rare lesions composed of small capillarylike lymph vessels may be referred to as being of *capillary type* (Fig. 6-1). Characteristically the covering squamous epithelium does not show hypertrophy, as is frequently the case with cavernous lymphangioma of skin and mucous membranes. Flanagan and Helwig[9] have suggested a simple and easily adaptable classification of cutaneous lymphangiomas that divides them into two categories: superficial lymphangioma circumscriptum and deep lymphangioma cavernosum. The lymphangioma circumscriptum[10] is, in its classical form, present at birth or appears soon afterward as a lesion usually larger than 1 cm.[11] Lymphangioma circumscriptum has a tendency to recur after excision.[12]

Age, sex, anatomic distribution, and the his-

163

Table 6-1. Histologic Classification of Tumors of Lymph Vessels

Benign
  Lymphangioma
    Capillary
    Cavernous
      Lymphangiolymphoma
      Lymphangioendothelioma (cellular or hypertrophic
        type)
    Cystic
      Cystic hygroma
    Mixed type (cavernous and cystic)
  Lymphangiomatosis
  Lymphangiomyoma and lymphangiomyomatosis

Malignant
  Lymphangiosarcoma

tologic types of a consecutive series of 100 cases examined in our laboratory (1983 to 1988) are summarized in Tables 6-2 and 6-3.

CAVERNOUS LYMPHANGIOMA

The cavernous type of lymphangioma, which constitutes the majority of lymphangiomas, occurs predominantly within the skin or mucous membranes. The majority of the lesions are fairly superficial, but they may extend deep into muscles when they occur in the head and neck region, for which these tumors have a predilection. They may also involve the deep structures

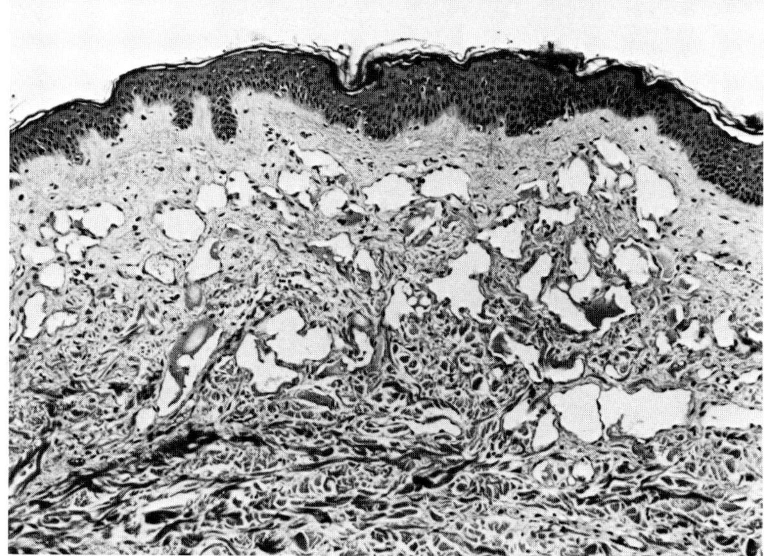

Fig. 6-1. Cutaneous lymphangioma of capillary type, so-called lymphangioma simplex, occurring in the axilla of a woman who was previously operated and irradiated for breast carcinoma. (H&E, × 60.)

Table 6-2. Histologic Type, Age (in Years), and Sex Distribution in 100 cases of Lymphangioma

Type	0–5		6–10		11–20		21–30		>30		Total
	M	F	M	F	M	F	M	F	M	F	
Capillary	0	1	0	0	0	0	0	0	1	2	4
Cavernous	10	10	2	2	6	3	1	3	10	12	59
Cystic[a]	13	10	0	4	1	1	1	2	2	3	37
Total	23	21	2	6	7	4	2	5	13	17	100

[a] Including mixed cavernous/cystic type.

**Table 6-3. Anatomic Location of
100 Cases of Lymphangioma**

Anatomic Location[a]	No. of Cases
Head and neck, including the oral cavity	29
Shoulder and axilla	11
Thoracic wall and mediastinum	11
Other parts of the trunk	6
Upper extremity, including the hand	10
Intra-abdominal	8
Lower extremity, including the hip and groin	22
Vulva	3
Total	100

[a] Six tumors also involved one or more other sites.

of the shoulder and axilla and may extend into the upper arm and mediastinum. Lymphangiomas of the cavernous type also occur within the retroperitoneum and the abdominal cavity, where they may involve the omentum, mesentery, intestine, and mesocolon. The rare intestinal lymphangiomas should be distinguished from lymphangiectasias, which may be part of a more generalized disorder affecting mesenteric lymphatics and lymph nodes and leading to chylous ascites and serious malabsorption.[13] Other sites involved by cavernous lymphangiomas are structures around the eye, foot, and ankle. Three of the cutaneous cavernous lymphangiomas and one of the capillary lymphangiomas of the series in Tables 6-2 and 6-3 occurred after surgery or radiotherapy for breast carcinoma. One lymphangioma developed in the scar after a burn injury. Single cases of superficial cutaneous lymphangioma (lymphangioma circumscriptum) have also been previously observed following radical mastectomy and radiation therapy.[14, 15] Lymphangioma circumscriptum has also occurred spontaneously in a congenitally lymphedematous extremity without prior surgery or radiation.[16] It is interesting to note that three of our cavernous lymphangiomas were located in the vulva, as we have found only four cases previously reported in the literature with or without a history of radiotherapy in this region.[17, 18]

Grossly the cavernous lymphangiomas often have a spongy appearance. When they occur in the skin and mucous membranes of the oral cavity, multiple, brownish-red papules are often observed on the surface. Characteristically the covering squamous epithelium shows acanthosis and hyperkeratosis, as well as some areas of thinning; others present with hypertrophy. Sometimes the lesions have a verrucous appearance (Fig. 6-2). When the tongue is involved,

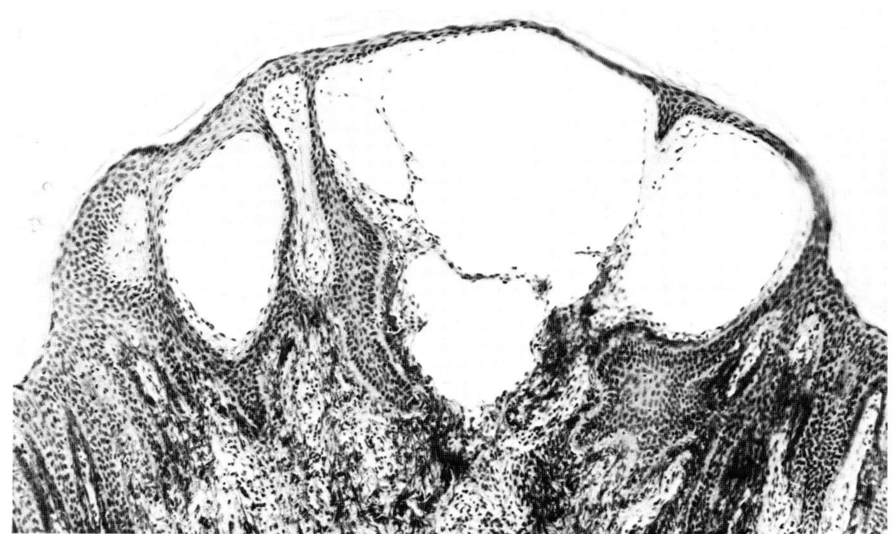

Fig. 6-2. Superficial cutaneous cavernous lymphangioma of so-called verrucous type. (H&E, × 60.)

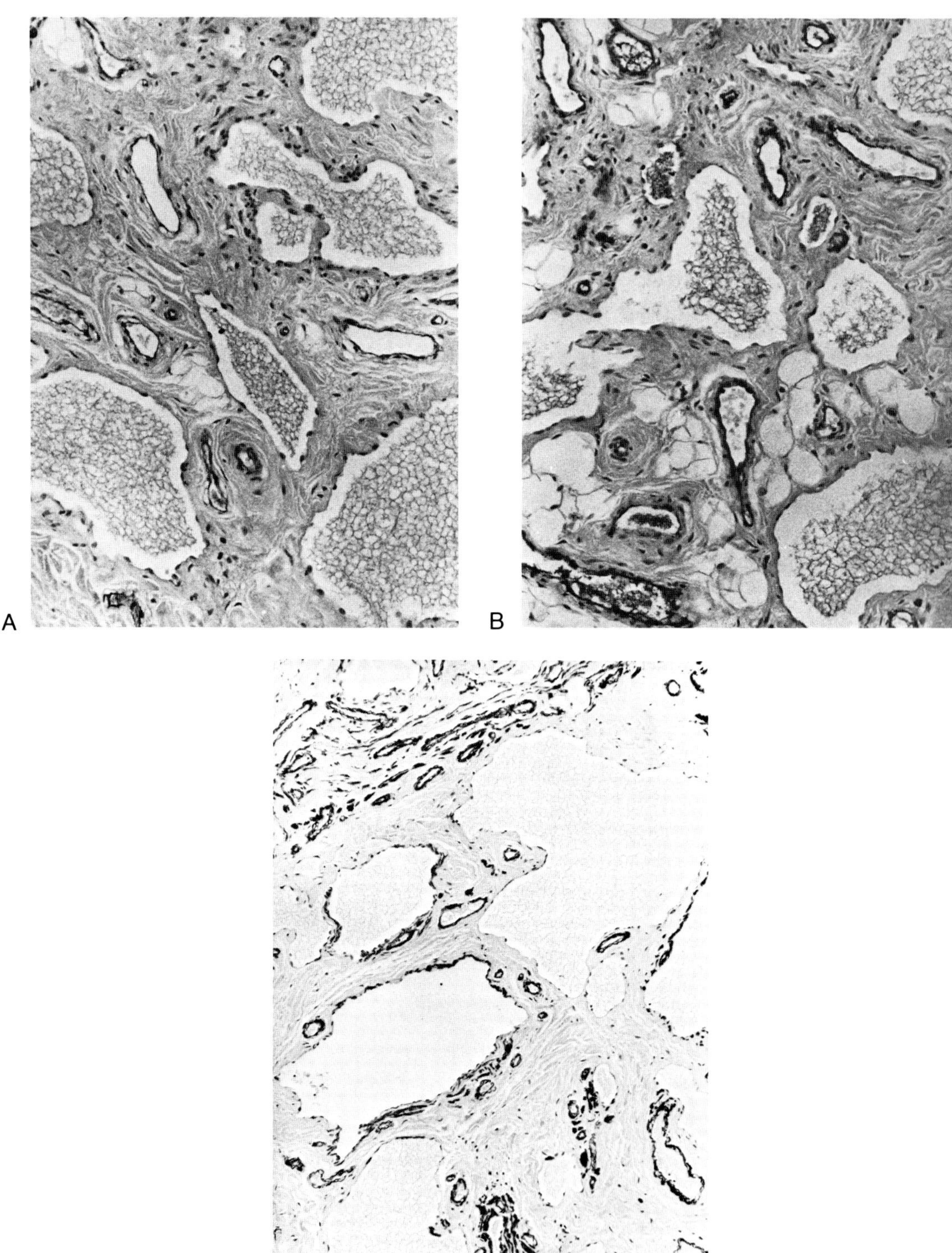

Fig. 6-3. (**A**) Cavernous lymphangioma showing irregular, widely dilated lymphatic spaces filled with lymph. In the fibrous stroma are blood vessels of variable size. (H&E, × 180.) (**B**) Immunohistochemical staining for factor VIII:RAg is positive in the endothelium of blood vessels, whereas the endothelium of the lymph vessels is negative. (**C**) The pericytes of blood capillaries and the smooth muscle of cavernous lymphatic spaces are positively stained for smooth muscle-specific actin. (Figs. B & C, Avidin-biotin complex method. Fig. B × 180, Fig. C × 60.)

macroglossia often develops. Light microscopically cavernous lymphangiomas are composed of communicating open lymph spaces that run in different directions and have highly variable shapes (Fig. 6-3A). The lymph spaces may be empty or filled with lymph; they may also contain lymphocytes and, occasionally, erythrocytes. Lymph thrombus and, more rarely, calcifications may occur. The cavernous lymphangiomas involving the subcutis and deeper structures are frequently composed of vessels having a more or less well-organized mature smooth muscle component (Fig. 6-4). Sometimes the smooth muscle tissue is very abundant and blends with the fibrous stroma (Fig. 6-5). The vessels are lined by one or more layers of flattened endothelium, resembling that of

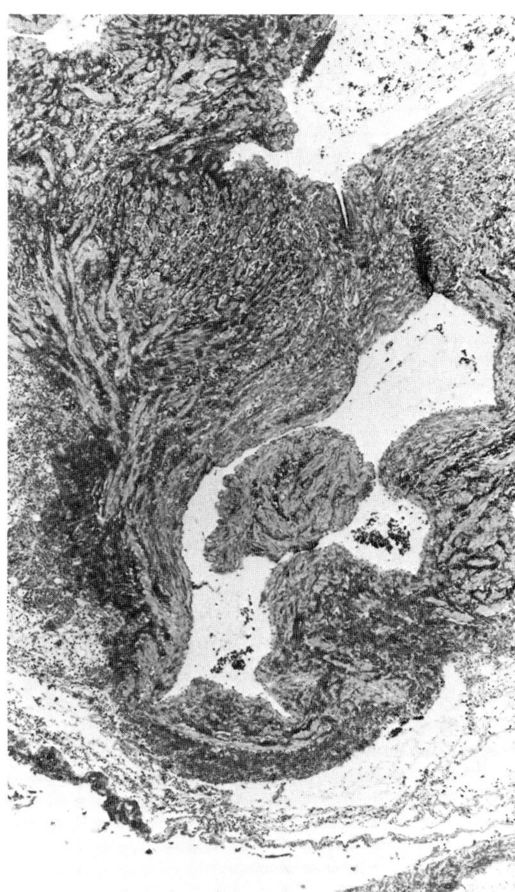

Fig. 6-5. Cavernous lymphangioma with a relatively large vessel having an abundance of smooth muscle fibers that extend into the surrounding stroma. (H&E, × 60.)

normal lymphatics. Occasionally the endothelium may assume a cuboidal or epithelioid appearance. Characteristically there is an abundant fibrous stromal component, which is often most well-developed around the vessels (Fig. 6-6). The lymph vessels of the cavernous lymphangiomas occurring in the subcutis blend with an abundance of adipose tissue sometimes arranged in a lobular fashion and has the appearance of hyperplasia. At times lymphoid tissue is present within the stroma. Rarely the lymphoid component can predominate, giving the lesion the appearance of a cavernous lymphangiolymphoma. Two of the 100 cases of lymphangioma presented in Table 6-2 and 6-3 were of this type

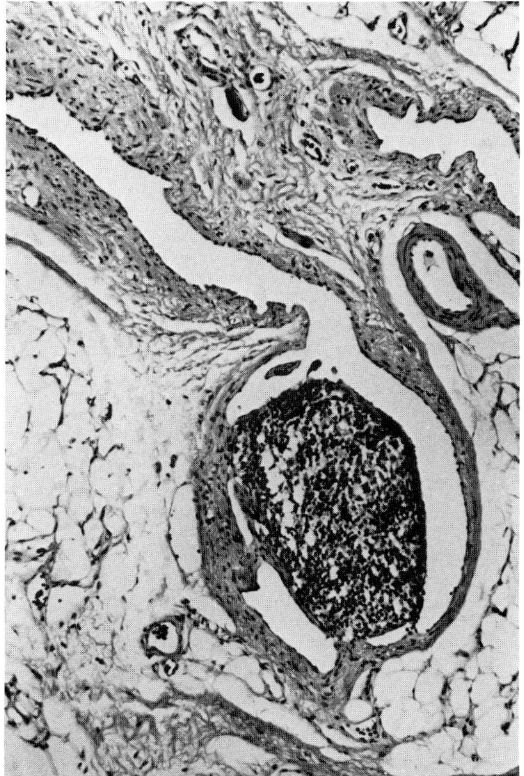

Fig. 6-4. Subcutaneous cavernous lymphangioma with some smooth muscle in the walls of the lymphatic vessels. A papillary projection with an abundance of lymphocytes protrudes into the vessel lumen. Note the rich component of adipose tissue. (H&E, × 120.)

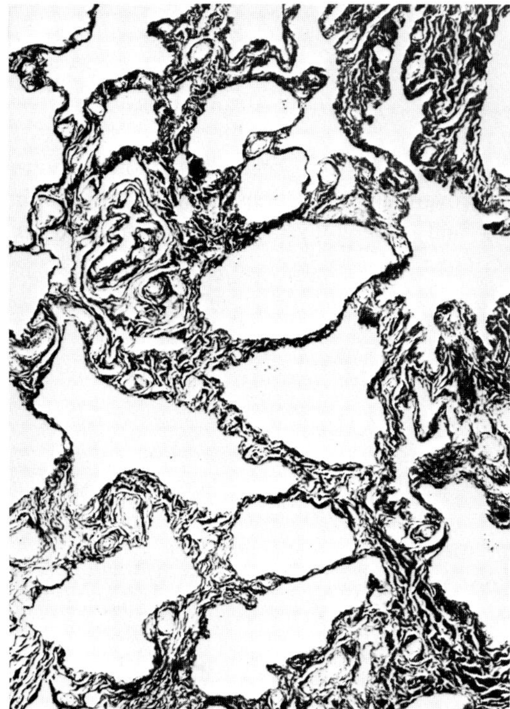

Fig. 6-6. Characteristic cavernous lymphangioma with a rather dense fibrous tissue between the lymph vessels. (van Gieson trichrome, × 60.)

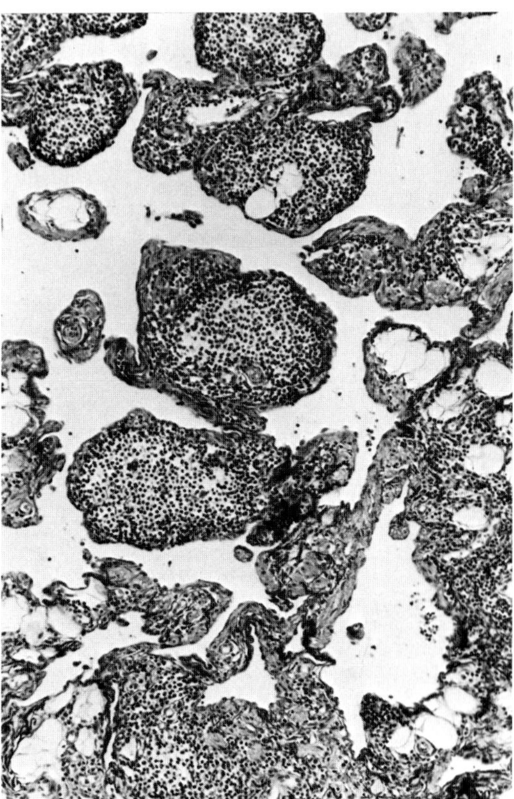

Fig. 6-7. Papillary cavernous lymphangioma with an abundance of lymphoid tissue in the papillary structures, a so-called lymphangiolymphoma. (H&E, × 180.)

(Fig. 6-7). The stroma of the intraperitoneal lymphangiomas is usually more loose and may appear to be edematous. Using blood vessel endothelium as a positive internal control, we have found the factor VIII:RAg to be variably expressed in the endothelium of the lymphatic vessels (Fig. 6-3B). The binding of the *Ulex europeus* lectin is seen more constantly in the lymphatic vessel endothelium. The endothelium of both the lymph and blood vessels is equally positive for vimentin. Monoclonal antibodies to smooth muscle-specific actin only decorates the smooth muscle component present in some of the cavernous lymphatic vessels, whereas in blood vessels of the stroma, this antibody recognizes both pericytes of capillaries and smooth muscle of larger vessels (Fig. 6-3C).

A cellular or hypertrophic type of lymphangioendothelioma has been described.[8, 19] It seems to represent a more active type of cavern-

ous lymphangioma with proliferating endothelium (Fig. 6-8).

CYSTIC LYMPHANGIOMA

It may be difficult to maintain a clear distinction between the cavernous type of lymphangioma and *cystic lymphangiomas,* since mixed types are common.[20, 21] Lymphangiomas containing cysts that are recognizable to the naked eye are usually referred to as being of *cystic type.* Cystic lymphangiomas are often present at birth or develop during the first 2 years of life, the period of greatest lymphatic growth. Rapid increase in size may occur, but in a majority of cases the tumor seems to grow with the

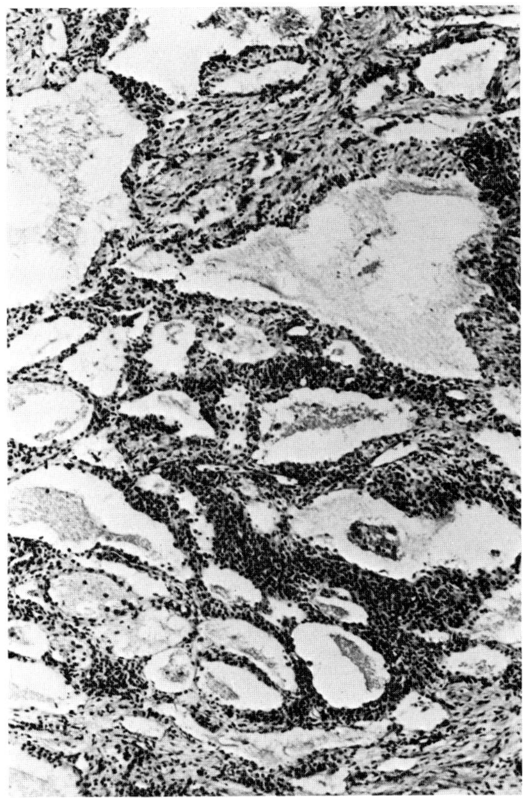

Fig. 6-8. Cavernous lymphangioma with hyperplasia of the endothelium, a so-called lymphangioendothelioma. (H&E, × 180.)

infant and hence only gradually becomes more prominent.[21] The neck region is a predilection site, and here they are most common in the posterior triangle; however, larger masses may extend beyond the sternocleidomastoid muscle into the anterior compartment and often cross the midline. Cystic lymphangiomas in the posterior neck often reach up into the cheek and parotid gland region or down into the mediastinum or axilla. Anterior lymphangiomas tend to involve the floor of the mouth and base of the tongue.[21, 22] When cystic lymphangiomas involve deep structures of the neck or extend into the mediastinum, they may cause alarming symptoms by compressing and stretching the surrounding tissue. On rare occasion, cystic lymphangiomas develop within the retroperitoneum, abdominal cavity, or groin.

The distribution of cystic lymphangioma corresponds to the jugular lymph sac, which normally connects the lymphatic system with the internal jugular vein, and the retroperitoneal cisterna chyli. It has been suggested that cystic lymphangiomas form because the normal lymphaticovenous connections between the lymph sacs and the venous vessels have failed to develop.[23]

Grossly the lesions often appear as multilobular cystic masses in which the larger cystic spaces may reach several centimeters in diameter (Fig. 6-9). Light microscopically the classic cystic hygroma presents as a honeycomb of multiple cisternae lined by a single layer of flattened endothelium. Usually they present a mixture of cystic and cavernous lymph spaces with walls of varying thickness. Larger lymphatic spaces often have a fibrous wall and may present a prominent component of smooth muscle. Characteristically the stroma around the cysts has a loose and sometimes edematous appearance (Fig. 6-10). A prominent feature of the stroma is the presence of inflammatory cells, primarily lymphocytes, some plasma cells and occasionally foci of eosinophils. In certain areas, the lymphocytes form distinct follicular structures with germinal centers. The cisternae appear to be empty or contain a pale-staining thready material, sometimes containing lymphocytes. Lymph thrombus material, containing lymphocytes, may fill some of the lymphatic spaces (Fig. 6-11). In areas with hemorrhage, they may contain a large number of erythrocytes. Coarse papillary fibrous excrescences protruding into the lumen of the vessels may occur (Fig. 6-12). Occasionally, these excrescences contain lymph follicles.

Immunohistochemical staining for factor VIII:RAg helps to identify the abundance of proliferating capillaries within the loose stroma surrounding the cystic spaces (Fig. 6-13A). Staining for smooth muscle-specific actin helps to identify the abundance of proliferating myofibroblasts within the stroma and the smooth muscle component of the lymphatic spaces and blood vessels (Fig. 6-13C & D).

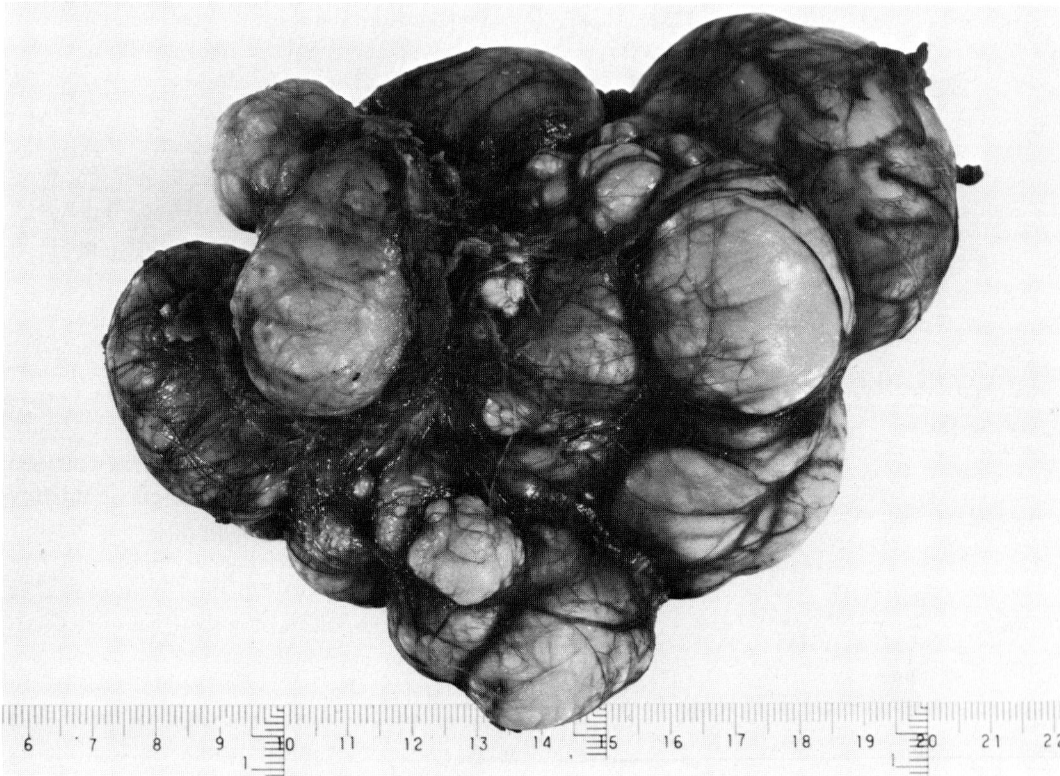

Fig. 6-9. A multicystic lymphangioma of the mesentery of the small intestine in a 20-year-old woman. The cystic spaces contain a thin, milklike fluid.

Intra-abdominal and inguinal cystic mesotheliomas and proliferative mesothelial cysts may be misinterpreted as cystic lymphangiomas. Cytokeratin positivity in such cases is of value in identifying the mesothelial nature of the former lesions (Fig. 6-14).

LYMPHANGIOMATOSIS

When lymphangiomas affect soft tissue and/ or parenchymal organs and bone in a diffuse fashion, the condition is often referred to as *lymphangiomatosis*. At times, these very rare lesions may involve an entire extremity and may cause local gigantism. Most cases occur in children, but they are generally not present at birth, and it seems that a latent period is necessary for the lesion to develop. Light microscopically this type resembles the cavernous lymphangi-

oma. In contrast to patients with lymphangiomatosis restricted to an extremity, patients with widespread lesions involving many visceral organs have a poor prognosis.[24]

LYMPHANGIOMYOMA AND LYMPHANGIOMYOMATOSIS

Lymphangiomyoma is a fairly well-defined lesion. It was first recognized by Enterline and Roberts,[25] who referred to it as *lymphangiopericytoma*. The lesions are usually multiple, and are then referred to as *lymphangiomyomatosis*. Laipply and Sherrick[26] were the first to recognize the association of lymphangiomyomatosis and chylothorax. The lesions characteristically occur within the thoracic cavity and peritoneum and involve lymphatics and lymph nodes. They cause lymph vessel obstruction, leading to chylus effusion into the pleura and abdominal

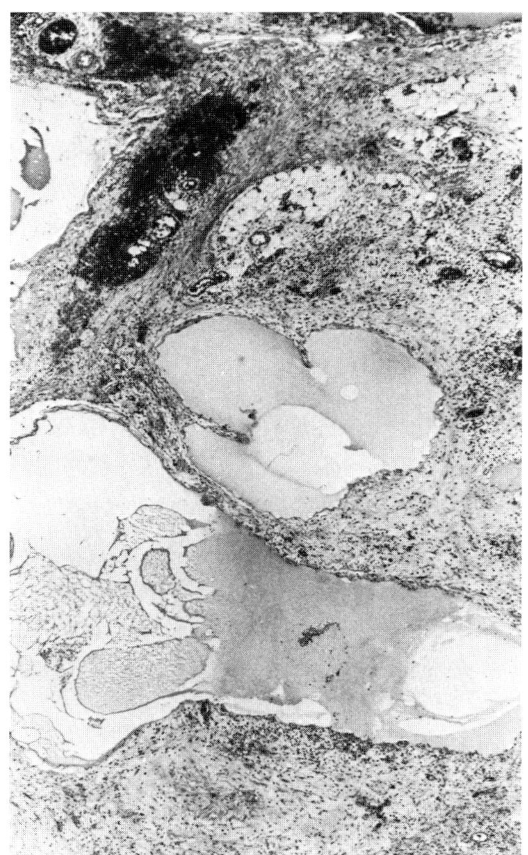

Fig. 6-10. Cystic lymphangioma with a loose, edematous stroma and an abundance of inflammatory cells. (H&E, × 60.)

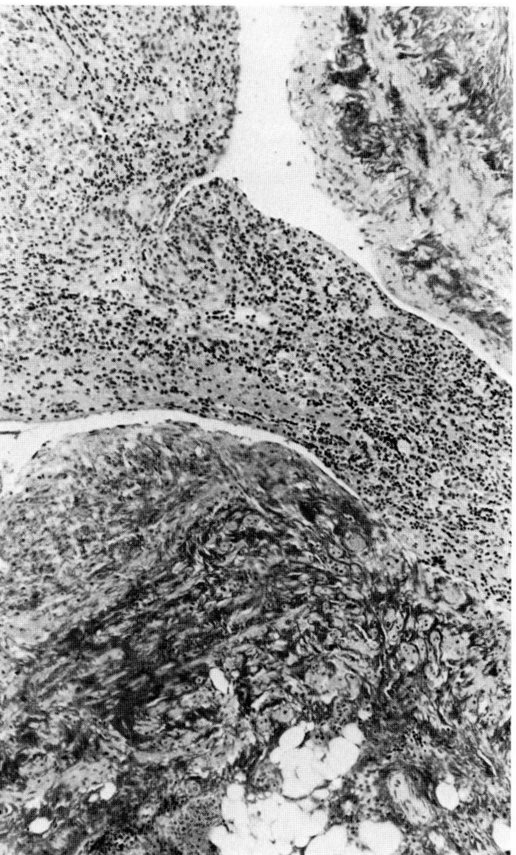

Fig. 6-11. Cystic lymphangioma with a so-called lymph thrombus consisting of coagulated lymph and containing inflammatory cells, predominantly lymphocytes. (H&E, × 180.)

cavity.[27, 28] The lesions are almost exclusively seen in women, the majority occurring during the second to fourth decades of life.

Light microscopically the lesions are characterized by a network of endothelium-lined spaces enclosed within irregularly developed smooth muscle tissue that is composed of short spindle cells without prominent atypia or mitotic activity (Fig. 6-15).[29] The smooth muscle origin of the cellular tissue enclosing the vascular spaces is not always apparent, since the cells may be rather plump and the eosinophilia and picrinophilia are often less prominent than in mature smooth muscle cells (Fig. 6-15B).

The clinical course is highly variable, ranging from a perfectly benign course when the lesions are small and fairly well-circumscribed to a fre-

quently lethal course when the lesions are large and especially when the lungs and mediastinum are involved. The simultaneous occurrence of lymphangiomyoma and renal angiomyolipoma has been reported, and there are observations suggesting a relationship to tuberous sclerosis.[24, 30–33] The relationship between lymphangiomyomatosis and tuberous sclerosis is controversial, however.[34]

LYMPHANGIOSARCOMA

The term *lymphangiosarcoma* has been used to underline the belief that these lesions arise from proliferating lymphatic endothelium, and

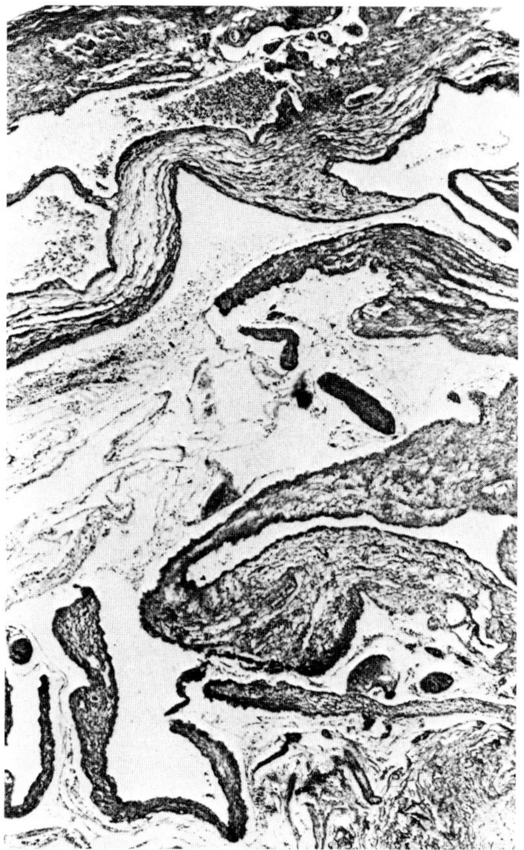

Fig. 6-12. Characteristic cystic lymphangioma with slender papillary processes. (H&E, × 60.)

it has been most widely applied in cases of angiosarcoma occurring in patients with chronic lymphedema. Histologically angiosarcomas originating from blood vessel endothelium cannot be distinguished from those of supposed lymph vessel origin. Therefore, the collective term *angiosarcoma* is today widely used (see Ch. 5).

Lymphangiosarcoma occurring in an arm with chronic lymphedema caused by mastectomy and axillary lymph node resection is referred to as *Stewart-Treves syndrome.* The risk of the development of angiosarcoma in a postmastectomy patient who survives more than 5 years has been estimated at 0.5 percent.[35, 36] The interval between mastectomy and the development of the lymphangiosarcoma may vary considerably, but the median interval is 10 years. It is evident that

chronic lymphedema is an etiologic factor. Lymphangiosarcoma can also develop secondary to congential lymphedema (Milroy's disease) or chronic lymphedema attributable to inflammatory-, surgical-, traumatic-, or radiation-related mechanisms.[36–40] In such instances lymphangiosarcoma may develop in the lower extremities, the inguinal region, scrotum, or penis.[41] Lymphangiosarcoma is virtually nonexistent in childhood,[42] although congenital lymphedema may be a predisposing condition.[43, 44] Angiosarcoma of the skin has been described as arising from lymphangioma circumscriptum in a few cases.[45, 46]

The early stages of a lymphangiosarcoma, arising in a chronic lymphedematous extremity, are often characterized by the occurrence of one or more bruiselike areas and blotchy erythema. These lesions may progress rapidly or over a period of several months, spreading distally, proximally, and circumferentially. Later in the course, multiple red or purple nodules develop and frequently become ulcerated, with signs of hemorrhage and secondary inflammation. Multifocal tumor lesions may involve the whole arm, axilla, and parts of the thoracic wall.

Light microscopically lymphangiosarcomas occurring in chronic lymphedema closely resemble other types of angiosarcoma. Characteristically the lymphangiosarcomas occurring in lymphedematous extremities appear to be multifocal. Abundant ectasic lymph vessels are often present within the surrounding tissues. There may be a continuous spectrum, ranging from areas with ectasic lymph vessels to areas with the appearance of a benign lymphangioma[47] to clearly malignant areas with a solid appearance[36] (Fig. 6-16).

Electron microscopically lymphangiosarcomas are composed of tumor cells that have endothelial features and form solid groups of vascular spaces depending on the degree of vascular differentiation (Fig. 6-17).[48–50] Also, in areas having a solid appearance light microscopically, abortive vascular channels can be recognized at ultrastructural examination (Fig. 6-18).

A clinical picture resembling Stewart-Treves

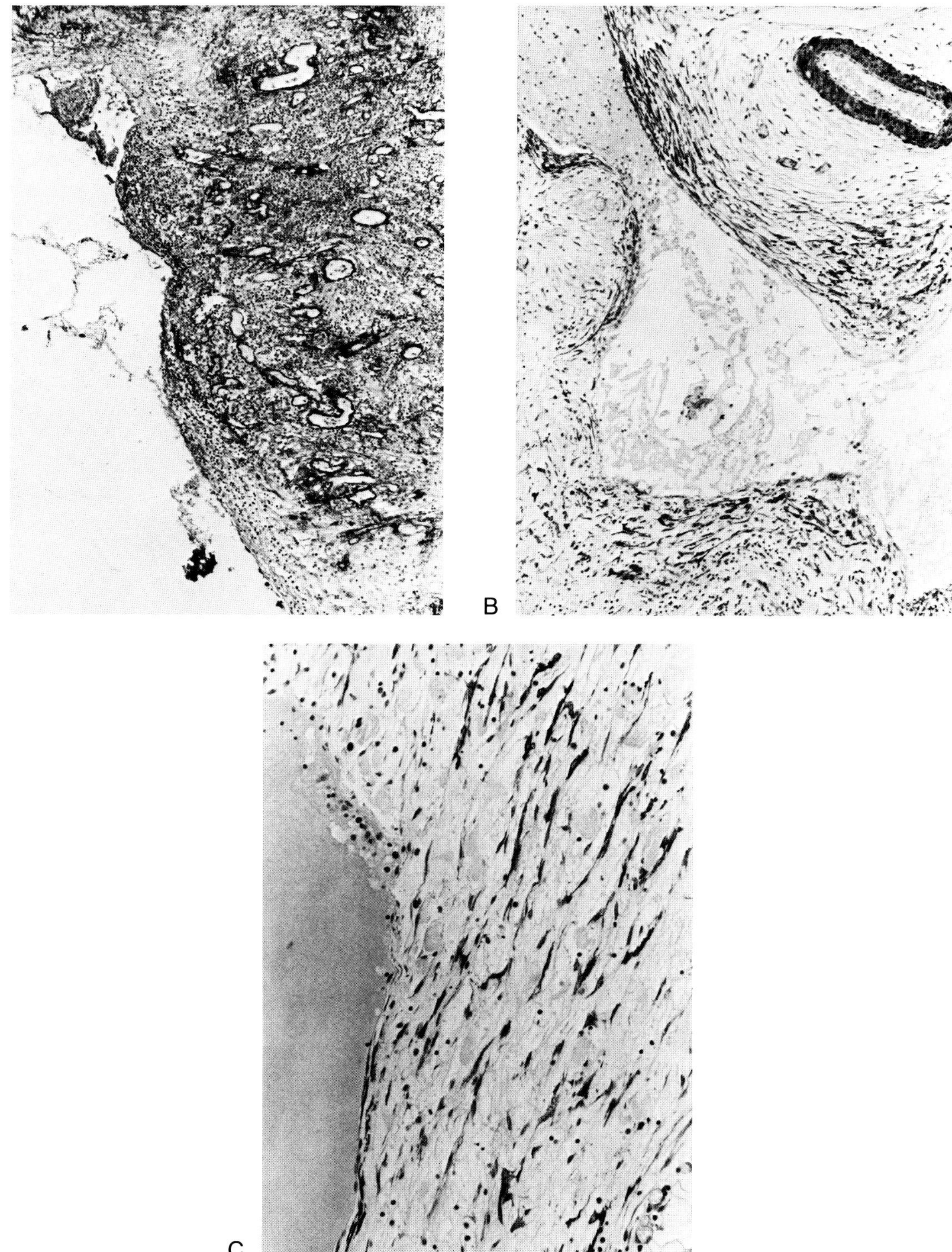

Fig. 6-13. Cystic lymphangioma. (A) Numerous proliferating blood capillaries with the endothelium positively stained for factor VIII:RAg are seen within the loose stroma, which contains numerous inflammatory cells. (B & C) Proliferating myofibroblasts within the stoma, positively stained for smooth muscle-specific actin. In Fig. B there is also positive staining of the smooth muscle of an artery. (Avidin-biotin complex method, Fig. A × 120, Fig. B × 120, Fig. C × 250.)

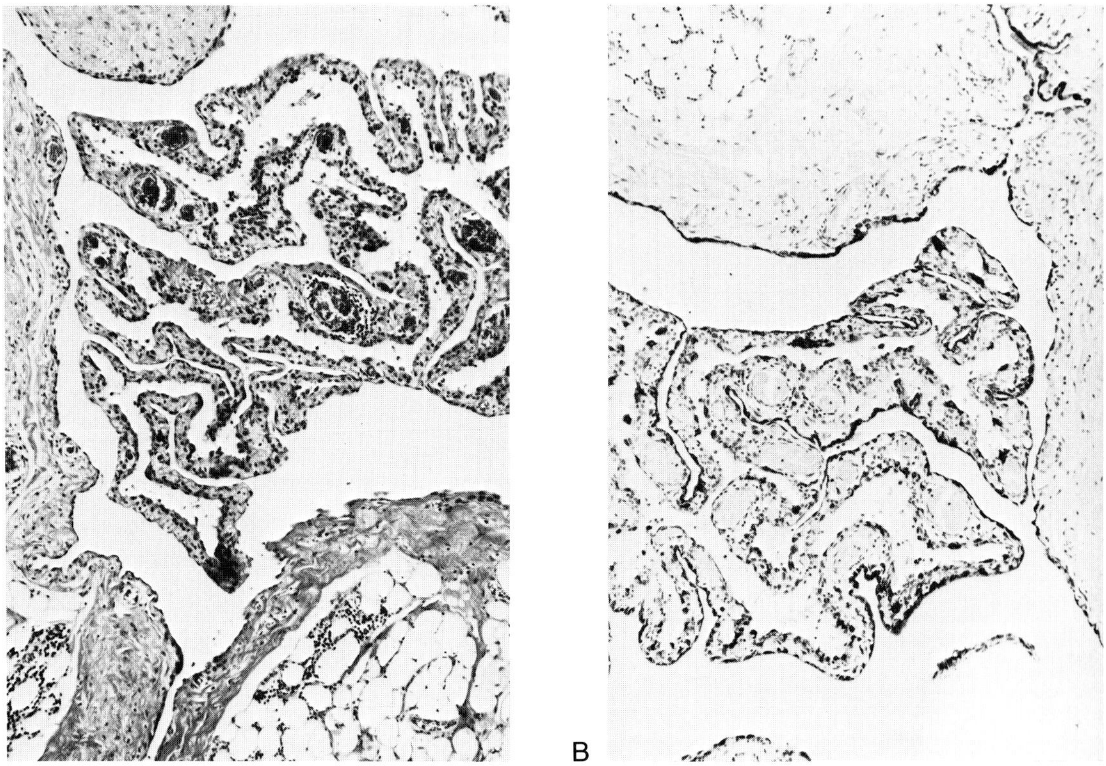

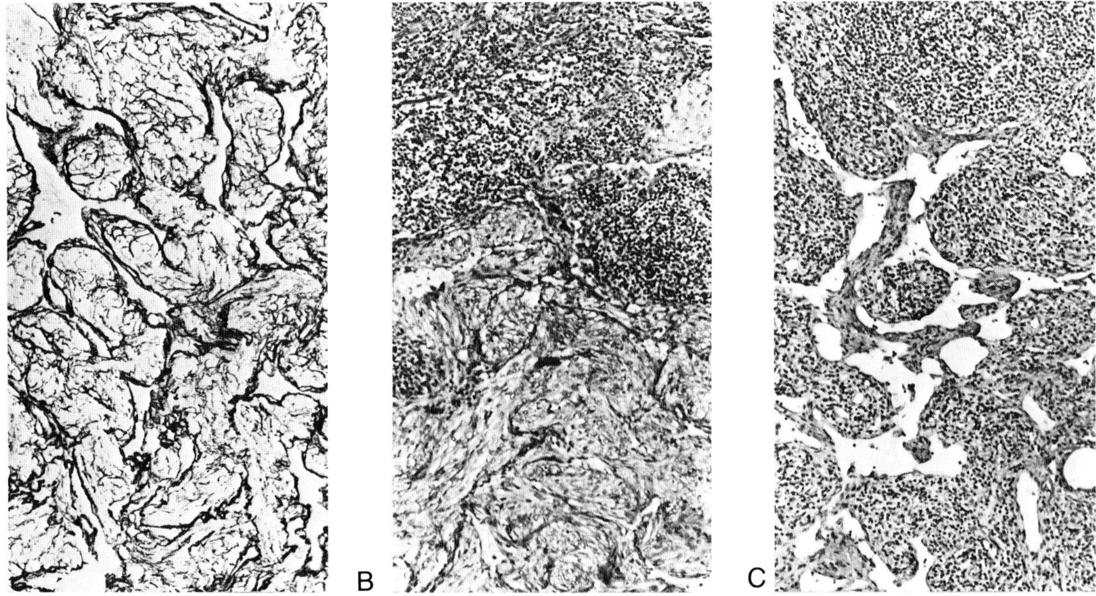

Fig. 6-14. (**A**) An inguinal proliferative mesothelial cyst with characteristic papillary structures giving some resemblance to a cystic lymphangioma. (**B**) Immunohistochemical staining for cytokeratins is positive in the mesothelial cells lining the cyst and papillary structures. This finding distinguishes mesothelial cysts from a lymphangioma. (Avidin-biotin complex method, Figs. A and B × 120.)

Fig. 6-15. (**A & B**) Characteristic lymphangiomyomatosis in a 46-year-old woman, involving inguinal lymphnodes and showing proliferating smooth muscle cells and lymph vessels in a pericytomalike pattern (H&E, × 120). (**C**) Laidlaw reticulin stain, × 120. This case has previously been described by Österborg and co-workers.[29]

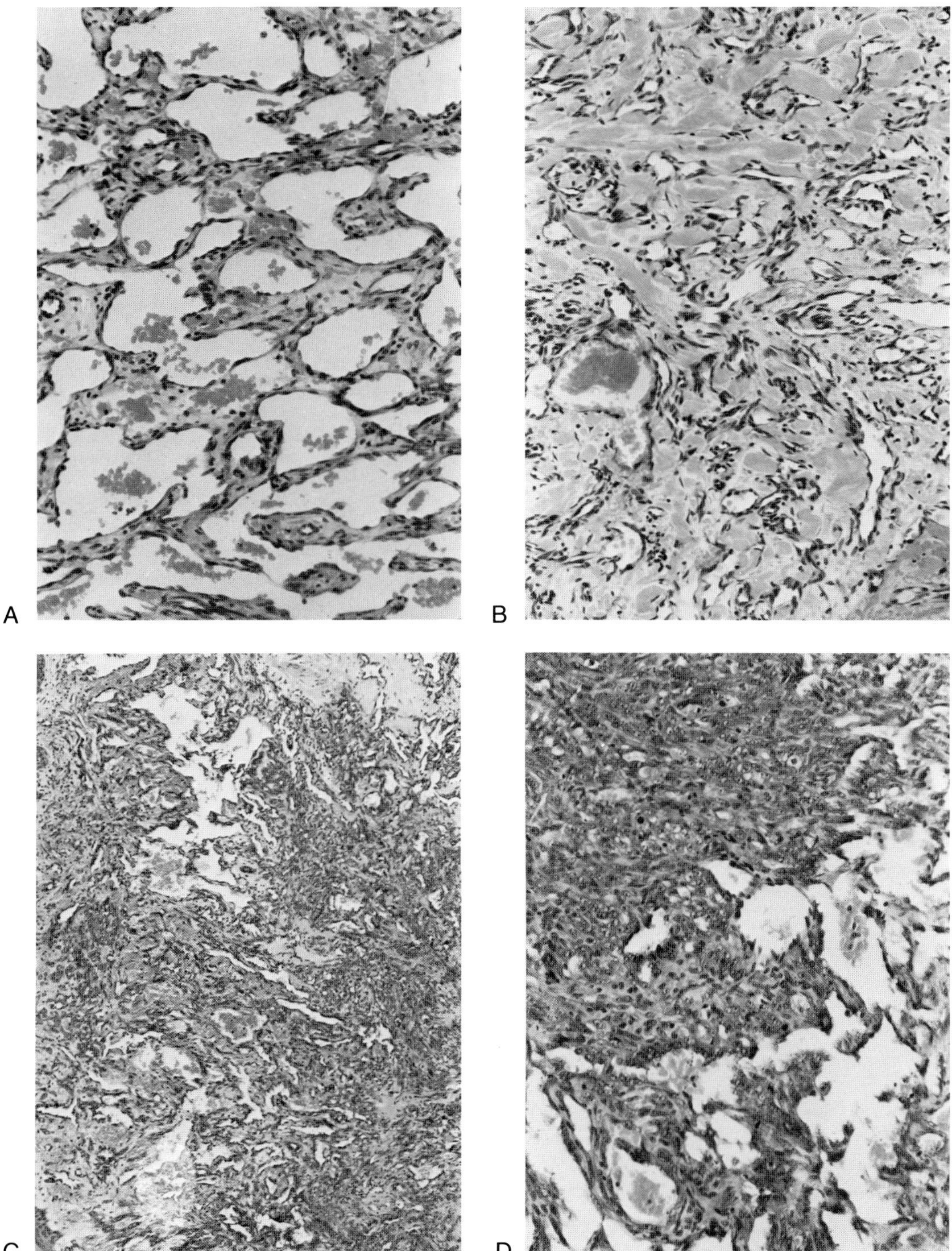

Fig. 6-16. A 53-year-old woman with a lymphangiosarcoma of the left arm and axilla that developed 11 years after surgery and radiotherapy for breast carcinoma. Different areas of the tumor revealed a highly variable degree of cellularity, atypia, and vascular differentiation. Some areas have the appearance of a cavernous lymphangioma with only slight atypia of the endothelial cells (**A**). Whereas others have the appearance of a low-grade lymphangiosarcoma (**B**). Some areas are partly solid, having the appearance of a high-grade lymphangiosarcoma (**C & D**). (H&E, Fig. A × 180, Fig. B × 180, Fig. C × 60, Fig. D × 250.)

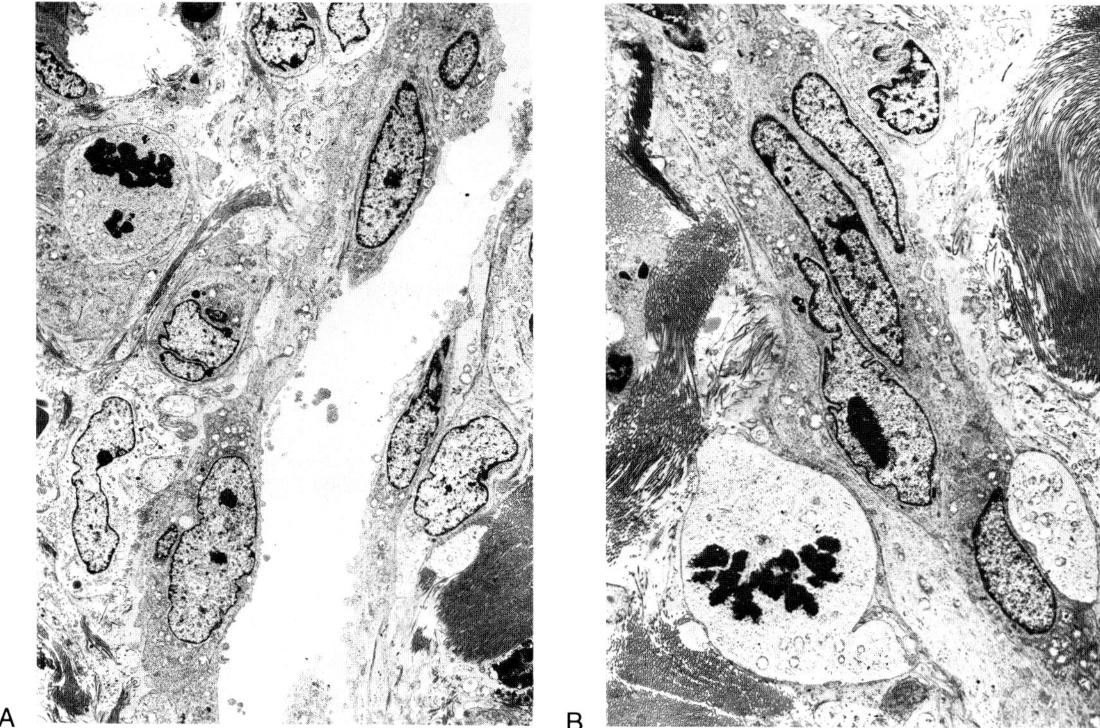

Fig. 6-17. Lymphangiosarcoma, same case as in Fig. 6-16. (**A**) The tumor cells, which have endothelial features, surround a narrow vascular space. (**B**) Solid area composed of spindle-shaped tumor cells surrounded by collagen. A mitotic figure is seen in both Figs. A and B. (Fig. A × 2000, Fig. B × 3,000.)

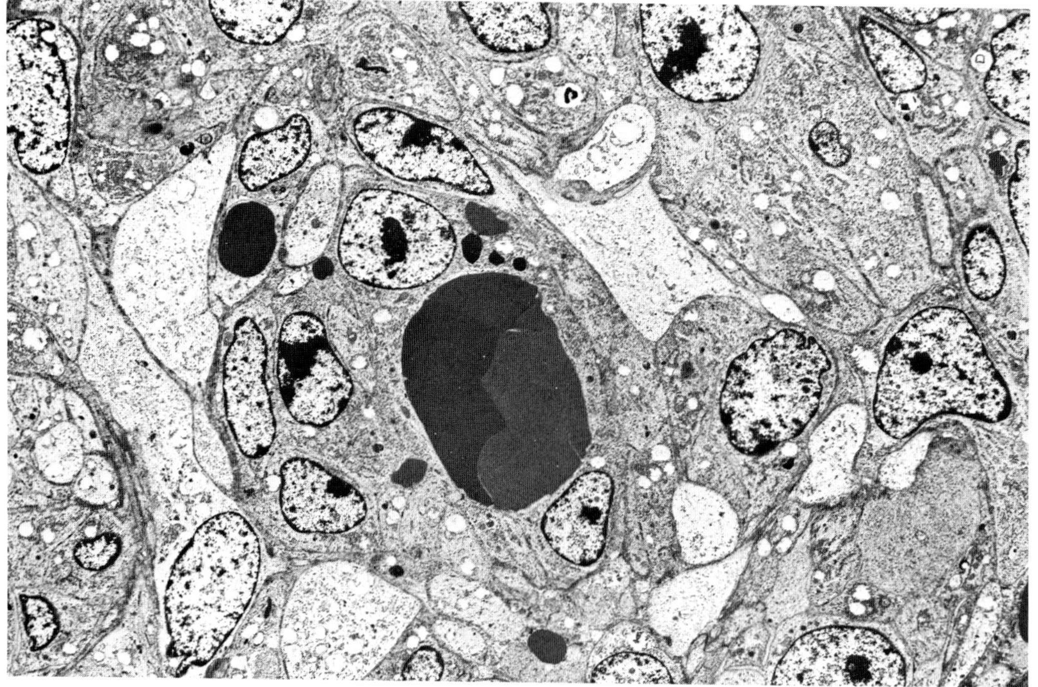

Fig. 6-18. Lymphangiosarcoma, same case as in Figs. 6-16 and 6-17. Solid area consists of tumor cells arranged in nests, one of which shows a paracentric lumen containing erythrocytes, emphasizing the difficulty in clearly distinguishing between lymphangiosarcoma and hemangiosarcoma by electron microscopy. (× 3000.)

syndrome can be caused by cutaneous and lymphatic metastases of a carcinoma, and the term *pseudo-Stewart-Treves syndrome* has been suggested.[51] It is therefore important that the diagnosis of lymphangiosarcoma in a patient presenting with features of the Stewart-Treves syndrome is based on the demonstration of an endothelial and vascular differentiation. For a differential diagnosis between metastatic carcinoma and lymphangiosarcoma, ultrastructural and immunohistochemical analyses are often essential. There are some ultrastructural and immunohistochemical features that distinguish blood vessel capillaries from lymphatic capillaries. However, ultrastructural and immunohistochemical studies are not sufficient to clearly distinguish hemangiosarcomas from lymphangiosarcomas. Angiosarcomas associated with chronic lymphedema generally follow a highly malignant clinical course with a high percentage of metastasis. A mean survival time of 19 months has been observed.[38]

REFERENCES

1. Witte MH, Witte CL: Lymphangiogenesis and lymphologic syndromes. Lymphology 19:21, 1986
2. Levihe C: Primary disorders of the lymphatic vessels—a unified concept. J Pediatr Surg 24:233, 1989
3. Fraley EE, Weiss L: An electron microscopic study of the lymphatic vessels in the penile skin of the rat. Am J Anat 109:95, 1961
4. Leak LV, Burke JF: Fine structure of the lymphatic capillary and the adjoining connective tissue area. Am J Anat 118:785, 1966
5. Barsky SH, Baker A, Siegal GP: Use of anti-basement membrane antibodies to distinguish blood vessel capillaries from lymphatic capillaries. Am J Surg Pathol 7:667, 1983
6. Wegener: Über lymphangiome. Arch Klin Chirurg 20, 1877
7. Taswell HF, Soule EH, Coventry MB: Lymphangiosarcoma in chronic lymphedematous extremities. Report of 13 cases and review of the literature. J Bone Joint Surg 44A:277, 1962
8. Watson WL, McCarthy WD: Blood and lymph vessel tumors; a report of 1,056 cases. Surg Gynecol Obstet 71:569, 1940
9. Flanagan BP, Helwig EB: Cutaneous lymphangioma. Arch Dermatol 113:24, 1977
10. Morris M, Duhring LA, LeLoir H: International Atlas of Rare Skin Diseases. Lewis, London, 1889, p. 1
11. Peachey RDG, Lim C-C, Whimster IW: Lymphangioma of skin, a review of 65 cases. Br J Dermatol 83:519, 1970
12. Whimster IW: The pathology of lymphangioma circumscriptum. Br J Dermatol 94:473, 1976
13. Morson BC, Dawson IMP: Gastrointestinal Pathology. 2nd Ed. Blackwell Scientific Publications, Oxford, 1979, p. 256
14. Prioleau PG, Santa Cruz DJ: Lymphangioma circumscriptum following radical mastectomy and radiation therapy. Cancer 42:1989, 1978
15. Leshin B, Whitaker D, Foucar E: Lymphangioma circumscriptum following mastectomy and radiation therapy. J Am Acad Dermatol 15:1117, 1986
16. Burstein JH: Lymphangioma circumscriptum with congenital unilateral lymphedema. Arch Dermatol 74:689, 1956
17. Abu-Hamad A, Provencher D, Ganjei P: Lymphangioma circumscriptum of the vulva: case report and review of the literature. Obstet Gynecol 73:496, 1989
18. Brown JV, Stenchever MA: Cavernous lymphangioma of the vulva. Obstet Gynecol 73:877, 1989
19. Winkler K: Die Primären Gewäsche des Lymfgefässystems. II. Lymphangioendotheliom. p. 1052. In Henke F, Lubarsch (eds): Handbuch del speziellen patologischen Anatomie und Histologie. II. Herz und Gerfässe. Springer-Verlag, Berlin, 1924
20. Bill AH Jr, Sumner DS: A unified concept of lymphangioma and cystic hygroma. Surg Gynecol Obstet 120:79, 1965
21. Batsakis JG: Tumors of the Head and Neck. Clinical and Pathologic Considerations. 2nd Ed. William & Wilkins, Baltimore/London, 1981, p. 301
22. Goetsch E: Hygroma colli cysticum and hygroma axillare; pathologic and clinical study and report of twelve cases. Arch Surg (Chicago) 36:394, 1938
23. Chervenak FA, Isaacson G, Blakemore KJ: Fetal cystic hygroma: cause and natural history. N Engl J Med 309:822, 1983
24. Enzinger FM, Weiss SS: Tumors of lymph vessels, p. 614. In Soft Tissue Tumors. 2nd Ed. CV Mosby, St. Louis, 1988

25. Enterline HT, Roberts B: Lymphangiopericytoma. Cancer 8:582, 1955
26. Laipply TC, Sherrick JC: Intrathoracic angiomyomatous hyperplasia associated with chronic chylothorax. Lab Invest 7:378, 1958
27. Vadas G, Pare JA, Thurlbeck MW: Pulmonary and lymph node myomatosis: Review of the literature and report of case. Canad Med Assoc J 96:420, 1967
28. Wolff M: Lymphangiomyoma: Clinicopathological study and ultrastructural confirmation of its histogenesis. Cancer 31:988, 1973
29. Österborg A, Christensson B, Silfverswärd C, et al: Lymphangiomyomatosis: immunohistochemical analysis of a case with enlarged inguinal lymph nodes and without pulmonary involvement. Acta Oncol 28:287, 1988
30. Vejlens G: Specific pulmonary alterations in tuberous sclerosis. Acta Pathol Microbiol Scand 18:317, 1941
31. Valensi QJ: Pulmonary lymphangiomyoma, a probable forme fruste of tuberous sclerosis. A case report and review of the literature. Am Rev Respir Dis 108:1411, 1973
32. Monteforte WJ, Kohnen PW: Angiomyolipomas in a case of lymphangiomatosis syndrome: relationships to tuberous sclerosis. Cancer 34:317, 1974
33. Stovin PGI, Lum LC, Flower CDR, et al: The lungs in lymphangiomyomatosis and in tuberous sclerosis. Thorax 30:497, 1975
34. Kreisman H, Robitaille Y, Dionne GP, et al: Lymphangiomyomatosis syndrome with hyperparathyroidism (a case report). Cancer 42:364, 1978
35. Schirger A: Postoperative lymphedema. Etiologic and diagnostic factors. Med Clin North Am 46:1045, 1962
36. Cooper PH: Angiosarcomas of the skin. Semin Diagn Pathol 4:2, 1987
37. Mackenzie DH: Lymphangiosarcoma arising in chronic congenital and idiopathic lymphoedema. J Clin Pathol 24:524, 1971
38. Woodward AH, Ivins JC, Soule EH: Lymphangiosarcoma arising in chronic lymphedematous extremities. Cancer 30:562, 1972
39. Borel Rinkes IHM, de Jongste AB: Lymphangiosarcoma in chronic lymphedema: report of 3 cases and review of the literature. Acta Chir Scand 152:227, 1986
40. Gajraj H, Barker SGE, Burnand KG, Browse NL: Lymphangiosarcoma complicating chronic primary lymphoedema. Br J Surg 74:1180, 1987
41. Lattes R: Tumor of the Soft Tissues. Armed Forces Institute of Pathology, Washington DC, 1982, p. 205
42. Dehner LP: Pediatric Surgical Pathology. 2nd Ed. Williams & Wilkins, Baltimore, 1987, p. 883
43. Banathy LJ: Lymphangiosarcoma arising in a congenitally lymphoedematous arm: case report. Pathology 9:65, 1977
44. Chen KTK, Gilbert EF: Angiosarcoma complicating generalized lymphangiectasia. Arch Pathol Lab Med 103:86, 1979
45. Girard C, Johnson WC, Graham JH: Cutaneous angiosarcoma. Cancer 26:868, 1970
46. King D, Duffy D, Hirose F, et al: Lymphangiosarcoma arising from lymphangioma circumscriptum. Arch Dermatol 115:969, 1979
47. Drachman D, Rosen L, Sharaf D, Weissman A: Postmastectomy low-grade angiosarcoma; an unusual case clinically resembling a lymphangioma circumscriptum. Am J Dermatopathol 10:247, 1988
48. Silverberg SG, Kay S, Koss LG: Postmastectomy lymphangiosarcoma: ultrastructural observations. Cancer 27:100, 1971
49. Yokoyama S, Nakayama I, Tsuji K, et al: Electron microscopic observations of lymphangiosarcoma arising from chronic lymphedema. Acta Pathol Jpn 33:843, 1983
50. Tomita K, Yokogawa A, Oda Y, Terahata S: Lymphangiosarcoma in postmastectomy lymphedema (Stewart Treves syndrome): ultrastructural and immunohistologic characteristics. J Surg Oncol 38:275, 1988
51. Sigal M, Grossin M, Bilet S, et al: Pseudo-syndrome de Stewart-Treves par métastases cutanéolymphatiques d'un carcinome mammaire controlatéral. Ann Dermatol Venereol 114:677, 1987

7

Tumors of Synovial Tissue

Dietmar Schmidt and Dieter Harms

A variety of both benign and malignant lesions are customarily listed under the general heading of tumors of synovial tissue. However, some of these represent only anatomic variants of histogenetically unrelated tumors such as chondroma and hemangioma. Furthermore synovial (osteo)chondromatosis is considered to be a metaplastic or reactive process rather than a true neoplasm. Although their histogenesis still remains controversial, giant cell tumors of the tendon sheath and synovial sarcoma are the most representative tumors traditionally ascribed to synovial tissue.

GIANT CELL TUMOR OF TENDON SHEATH

Giant cell tumor of tendon sheath (GCTTS) is considered to be the prototype of synovial tissue tumors. In the past the term *benign synovioma*[1] was frequently used to designate this tumor. This term is misleading, however, because it connotes a benign form of synovial sarcoma, whereas in its malignant form GCTTS more closely resembles malignant fibrous histiocytoma of giant cell type than synovial sarcoma. Therefore the term GCTTS represents a distinct tumoral entity rather than a benign counterpart of synovial sarcoma.

GCTTS may be classified into localized and diffuse forms. A rare malignant form is also recognized.

LOCALIZED GIANT CELL TUMOR OF TENDON SHEATH

Localized GCTTS is often referred to as *nodular tenosynovitis*[2] as well as *fibrous histiocytoma of synovium.*[3]

Clinical Features

The tumor primarily affects the fingers and arises from the synovium of tendon sheath or the region of the interphalangeal joint. It is most commonly found in those between the fourth and sixth decades of life. There is a slight female preponderance.[1, 3]

Pathologic Findings

The lesions are usually small, circumscribed, and lobulated (Fig. 7-1). As a rule, tumors on the feet are larger and more irregular in shape than those on the hands. Histologically they are characterized by a localized proliferation of rounded cells resembling synoviocytes or histiocytes, accompanied by a variable number of multinucleated giant cells, mononuclear inflammatory cells, siderophages, and foamy macrophages (Fig. 7-2). According to the proportion of these cells and the degree of collagenation, the appearance of this tumor varies greatly, from highly cellular to more hyalinized and hypocel-

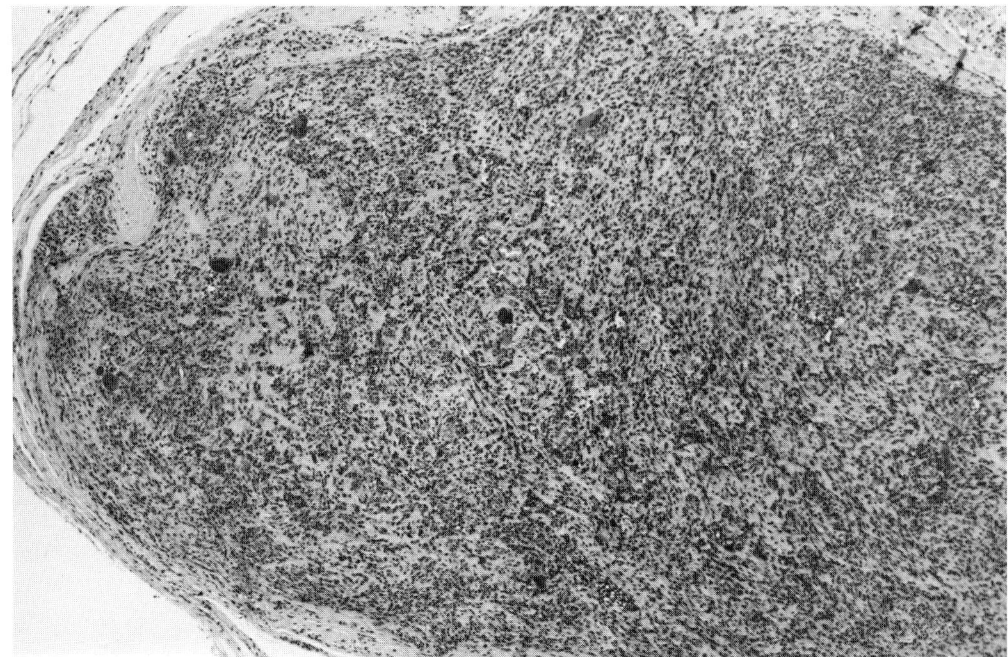

Fig. 7-1. Localized giant cell tumor of tendon sheath showing typical low-power histomorphologic findings. A collagenous "capsule" appears to penetrate into the tumor. (H&E, × 60.)

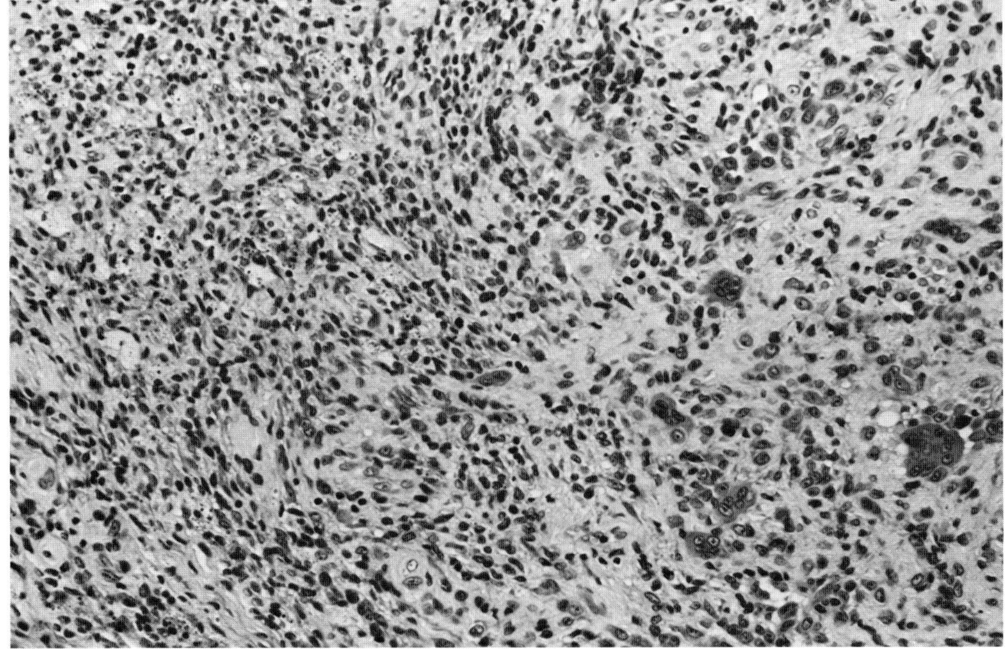

Fig. 7-2. High-power view demonstrating various fibrohistiocytic cells, including siderophages, foamy macrophages, and multinucleated giant cells, which are intermingled with mononuclear inflammatory cells. (H&E, × 250.)

lular forms. In less than 2 percent of cases, the tumor grows into small vascular spaces: although worrisome, this feature does not indicate malignancy.

Prognosis

Surgical excision is curative in the majority of patients, although a local recurrence has been reported in approximately 20 percent of cases.[4]

DIFFUSE GIANT CELL TUMOR OF TENDON SHEATH

Unlike the localized variant, diffuse GCTTS usually occurs in large, weight-bearing, joints (i.e., the knee and ankle), and in most cases it represents an extra-articular extension of pigmented villonodular synovitis. Therefore, the term *diffuse GCTTS* is often used to refer to a poorly circumscribed mass of similar histology occurring in soft tissues with or without apparent joint involvement.[4]

Clinical Features

This variant is relatively uncommon compared with the localized form and tends to affect younger persons.

Pathologic Findings

In comparison with the localized form, which is usually "encapsulated," diffuse GCTTS shows an infiltrative growth pattern with indistinct borders. The lesion is highly cellular, with fewer giant cells than the localized form (Figs. 7-3 and 7-4). Prominent cleftlike or pseudoglandular spaces are frequently observed.

Differential Diagnosis

Because of its intense cellularity, coupled with the clinical impression of a destructive mass, a more cautious approach to diagnosis is required in the assessment of this benign tumor.

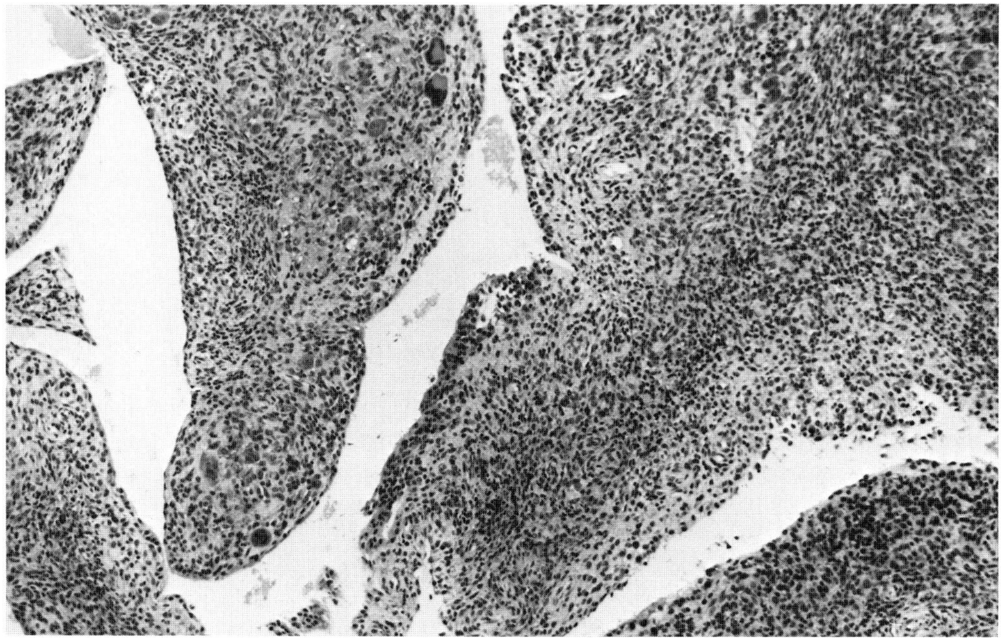

Fig. 7-3. Intra-articular form of diffuse giant cell tumor of tendon sheath exhibiting villous projections reminiscent of pigmented villonodular synovitis. (H&E, × 125.)

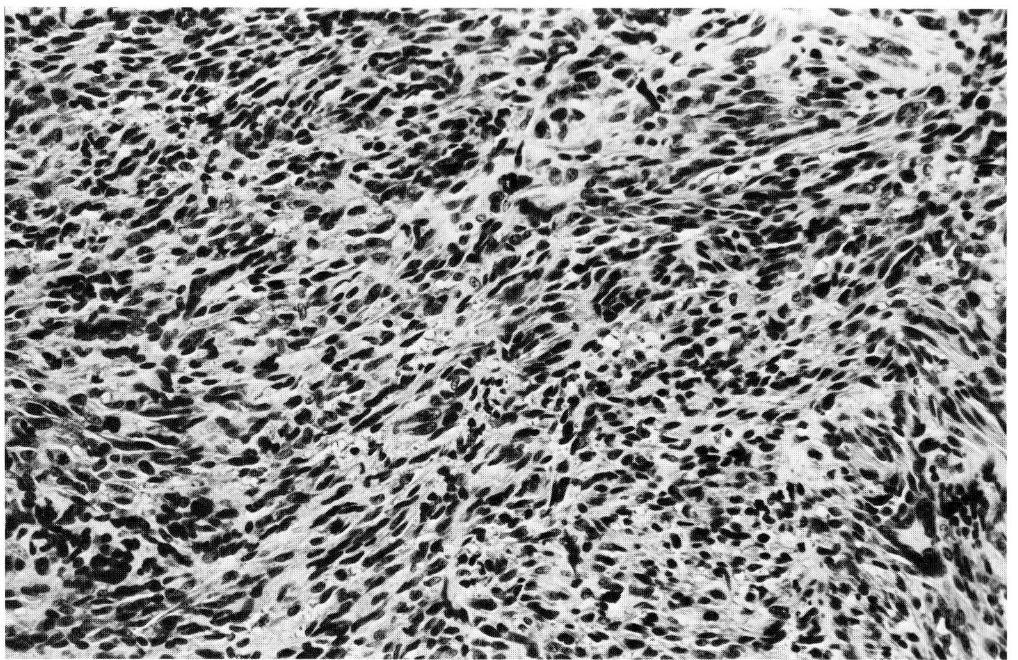

Fig. 7-4. Extra-articular portion of the same tumor shown in Fig. 7-3. Note the rounded synoviocytelike cells admixed with more spindle-shaped cells, siderophages, xanthoma cells, and multinucleated giant cells. (H&E, × 250.)

Prognosis

About 50 percent of patients develop local recurrence.

Malignant Giant Cell Tumor of Tendon Sheath

A heterogeneous group of sarcomas that contain giant cells and arise in the vicinity of a tendon has been referred to as *malignant GCTTS*. This group includes clear cell sarcoma,[5] fibrosarcoma, epithelioid sarcoma,[6] and malignant fibrous histiocytoma. The designation of malignant GCTTS, however, should be reserved for lesions in which benign GCTTS co-exists with obvious malignant areas or when the initial lesion was a typical benign GCTTS and the subsequent recurrence appeared malignant, often with a histologic similarity to malignant fibrous histiocytoma of giant cell type (Figs. 7-5 and 7-6). These tumors are very rare and are characterized by their local aggressiveness. Metastases are reported to occur following repeated recurrences over a period of many years.[7]

SYNOVIAL SARCOMA

Since the first adequate description of synovial sarcoma by Lejars and Rubens-Duval[8] in 1910, innumerable reports on this type of malignant soft tissue tumor have been published that discuss its histogenetic relationship and clinicopathologic features. It has become evident that synovial sarcoma is not derived from synovial cells, but merely assumes a light-microscopic appearance in some cases that is reminiscent of synovial lining tissue. Its origin is now presumed to be a multipotent mesenchymal stem cell that is capable of differentiation into cells with epithelial and mesenchymal features. Among the soft tissue malignancies of all age groups it ranks fourth after malignant fibrous histiocytoma, liposarcoma, and rhabdomyo-

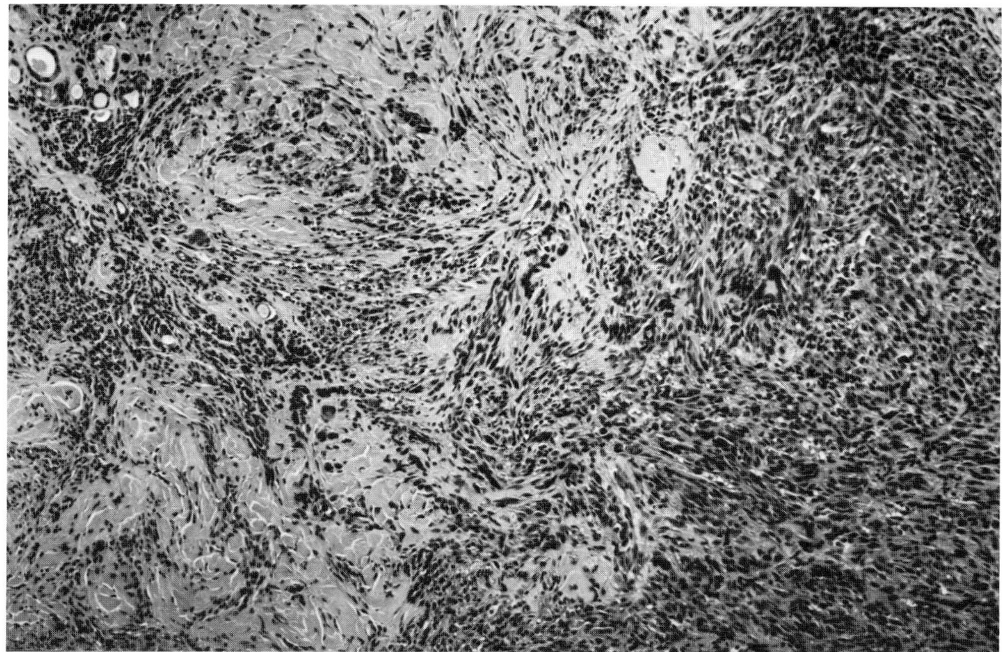

Fig. 7-5. Recurrent atypical GCTTS that produced lung metastasis in a 62-year-old man. A typical GCTTS had been removed from his finger 2 years previously. Note the infiltrative growth pattern and entrapped sweat glands. (H&E, × 125.)

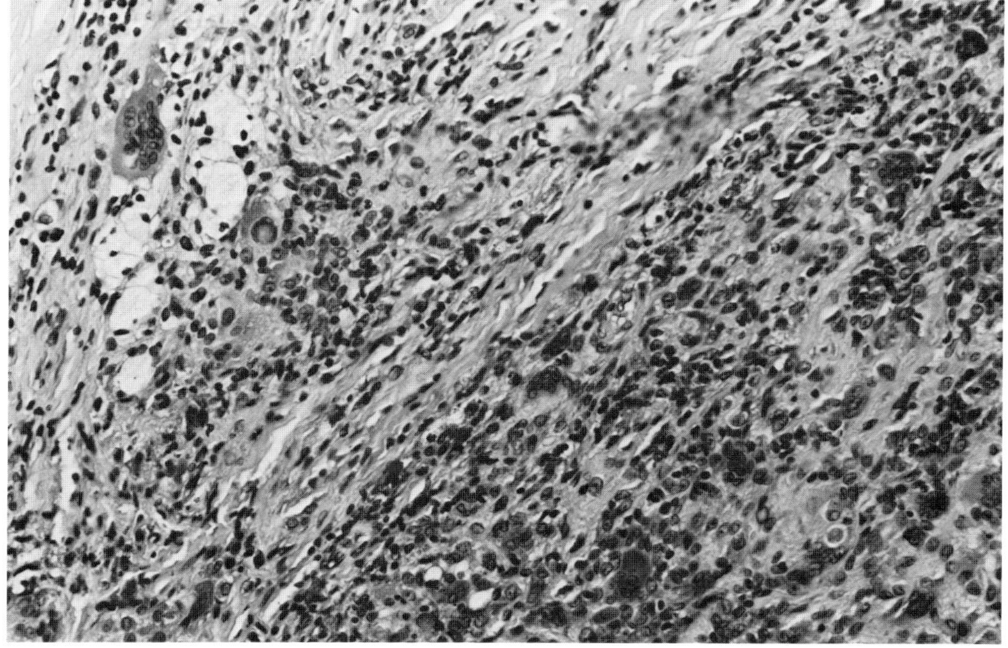

Fig. 7-6. High-power view of the same tumor shown in Fig. 7-5. Note the vague storiform pattern mimicking malignant fibrous histiocytoma. (H&E, × 250.)

Table 7-1. The Most Frequently Occurring Soft Tissue Sarcomas in the Kiel Pediatric Tumor Registry (1965–1989)

Type	No.	%
Rhabdomyosarcoma	480	43.2
PNET	179	16.1
Synovial sarcoma	79	7.1
Malignant schwannoma	66	5.9
Leiomyosarcoma	56	5.1
Extraskeletal Ewing's sarcoma	53	4.8
MFH	26	2.3
Fibrosarcoma	23	2.0
Liposarcoma	21	1.9
Other	129	11.6
Total	1,112	100%

PNET, primitive peripheral neuroectodermal tumor; MFH, malignant fibrous histiocytoma.

sarcoma.[4] In children and adolescents synovial sarcoma is the third most frequent tumor after rhabdomyosarcoma and primitive peripheral neuroectodermal tumor (Table 7-1). The incidence among all malignant tumors of somatic soft tissues varies between 5.6 percent[9] and 10 percent.[10]

Clinical Features

The main clinical features of synovial sarcoma are summarized in Table 7-2.

The tumor usually presents as a palpable deep-

Table 7-2. The Main Clinical Features of Synovial Sarcoma

Symptoms:	Tender or nontender, deep-seated mass, pain in about 25% of cases
Age:	Predominantly adolescents and young adults (range 0–72 yrs)
Sex:	Males affected more often than females
Localization:	Limbs, abdominal wall, head and neck

seated mass or swelling that may or may not be tender and causes pain in about 25 percent of cases. The duration of symptoms before diagnosis varies between 2 and 4 years. However, it may take as long as 20 years before a patient seeks medical advice. In a number of cases, the patient becomes aware of a mass only following a trauma. Rarely synovial sarcoma causes numbness, radiating pain, and paresthesia owing to secondary involvement of nerves. Although it may occur in newborns[11] and in patients as old as 72 years,[10] the vast majority of patients are between 15 and 50 years of age (the reported mean age is between 30 years[12] and 35 years[13]). Based on our own experience, however, the mean age is 15.6 years, with a range from 14 months to 43 years. Ninety-two percent of patients are less than 20 years old at the time of diagnosis. Most reports indicate a male predominance (2.1:1), whereas our experience coincides with that of Moberger et al.,[14] who found no apparent sex preference. The most frequent sites of occurrence are the extremities (95 percent), notably the vicinity of the knee and the distal thigh. Less frequently synovial sarcoma is found in the abdominal wall and in the trunk, including the retroperitoneum.[15] Unusual sites of occurrence are the head and neck area, with possible origin in the base of the tongue,[16] pharynx,[17] and the orofacial region.[18]

Pathologic Findings

On macroscopic examination a multilobular pseudoencapsulated neoplasm with a yellow to grayish white cut surface is often found. Areas of hemorrhage and pseudocyst formation may be present (Fig. 7-7).

Histomorphologically three basic cell types can be distinguished (Table 7-3). The first and most prevalent cell type is a spindle-shaped fibroblastlike cell with an elongated nucleus possessing a dense chromatin pattern. These cells are usually arranged in sheets and bundles, but, unlike fibrosarcoma, they do not display a herringbone pattern. The second cell type is a cuboidal or tall columnar cell with epithelial differen-

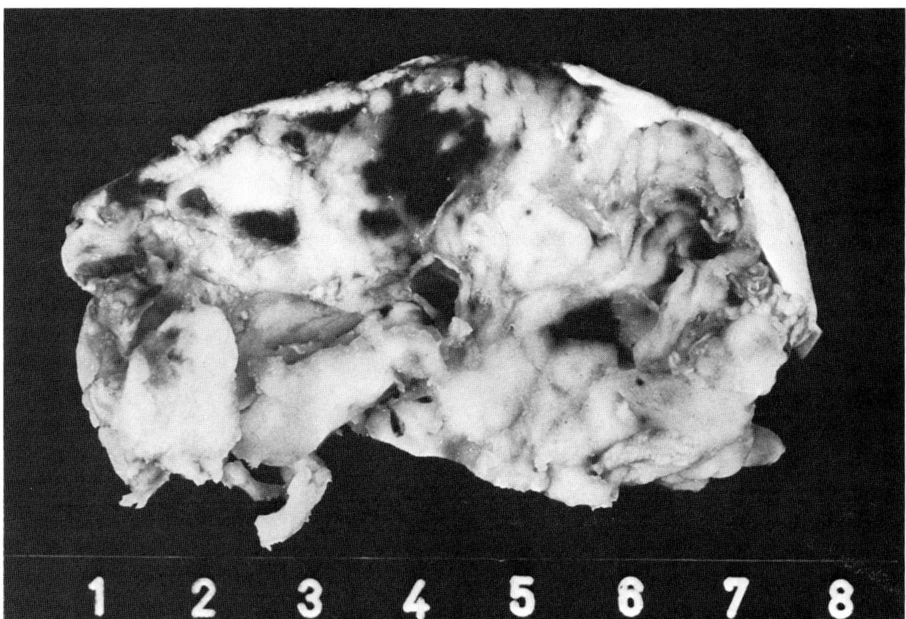

Fig. 7-7. Gross appearance of synovial sarcoma located in the foot of a 33-year-old man. On the cut surface areas of hemorrhage and pseudocystic spaces may be seen.

tiation that lines cleftlike spaces or glandular structures (Fig. 7-8). The third cell type corresponds to a polygonal cell that is often found in solid groups of varying size (Fig. 7-9) distributed between the spindle-shaped cells. This latter type of cell is considered to represent a transitional stage between the spindle-shaped fibroblastlike cells and the epithelial cells. The proportion of each cell type may vary, to a large extent, from tumor to tumor and within individual tumor specimens, resulting in different growth patterns. This variability is reflected in the definitions of various subtypes of synovial

Table 7-3. Summary of Microscopic Findings in Synovial Sarcoma

Histology:	Three cell types: fibroblastlike spindle cell, polygonal cell (epithelioid), epithelial cell
Ultrastructure:	Microvilli, filopodia, basal lamina, desmosomes
Immunohistochemistry:	Fibroblastlike spindle cell (vimentin +), epithelioid cell (vimentin +, cytokeratin +), epithelial cell (cytokeratin +)

sarcoma and the relative frequency of each tumor subtype. Traditionally the tumor is divided into two broad categories, namely biphasic (Fig. 7-10) and monophasic synovial sarcoma. The latter can be either monophasic-fibrous, consisting predominantly of spindle cells (Fig. 7-11), or monophasic-epithelial, which is difficult to distinguish from adenocarcinoma, except for the presence of a subtle spindle cell component. No sharp delineation has been drawn between the monophasic-fibrous form with a few polygonal, epithelioid cells and the biphasic tumors with large, solid nests of epithelioid cells but lacking epithelial-lined spaces (Fig. 7-12). The distinction between the cells with early epithelial differentiation and the fibroblastlike cells is usually enhanced by the reticulin pattern: the solid groups of epithelioid cells are almost devoid of reticulin fibers, whereas a large number of fibers can be found between the fibroblastlike cells.

The presence of a hemangiopericytomalike pattern (Fig. 7-13) and focal areas of hyalinization with an osteoidlike appearance (Fig. 7-14) are other characteristic findings that aid in the

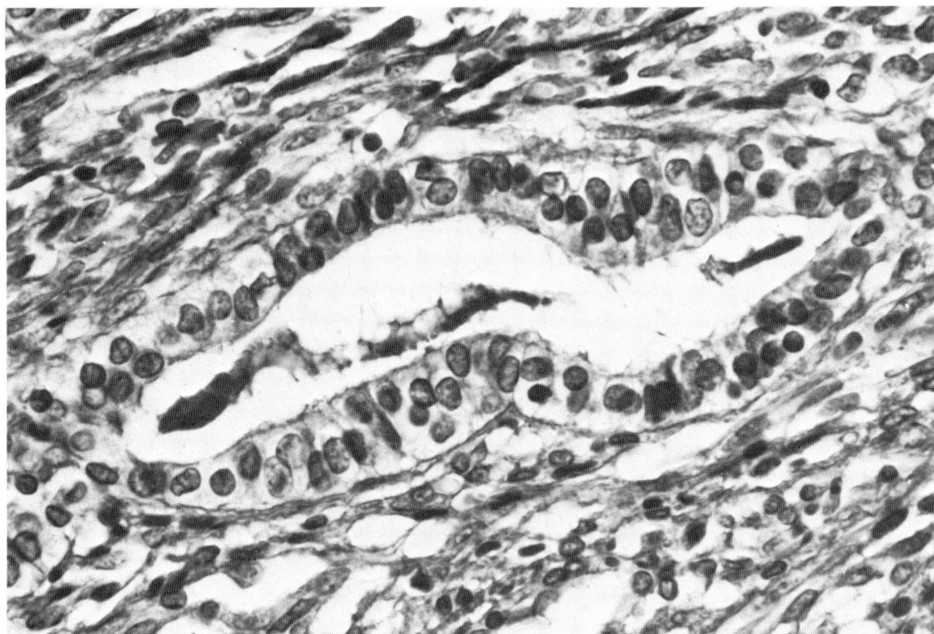

Fig. 7-8. Biphasic synovial sarcoma showing a cleftlike space lined with columnar epithelial cells and a PAS-positive substance in the lumen. (PAS. × 560.)

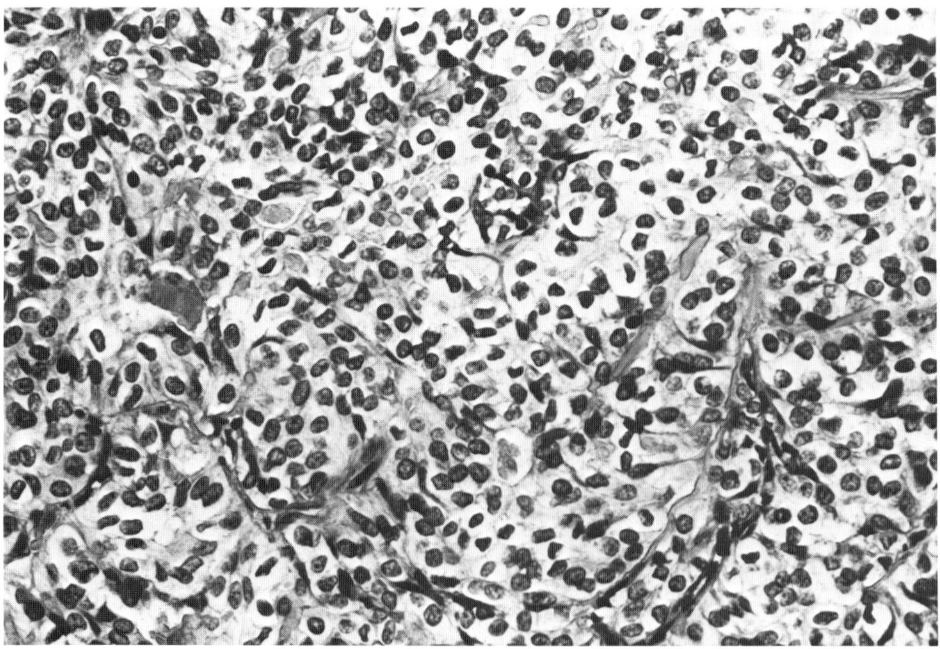

Fig. 7-9. Biphasic synovial sarcoma showing an area of epitheloid cells without gland formation. (H&E, × 350.)

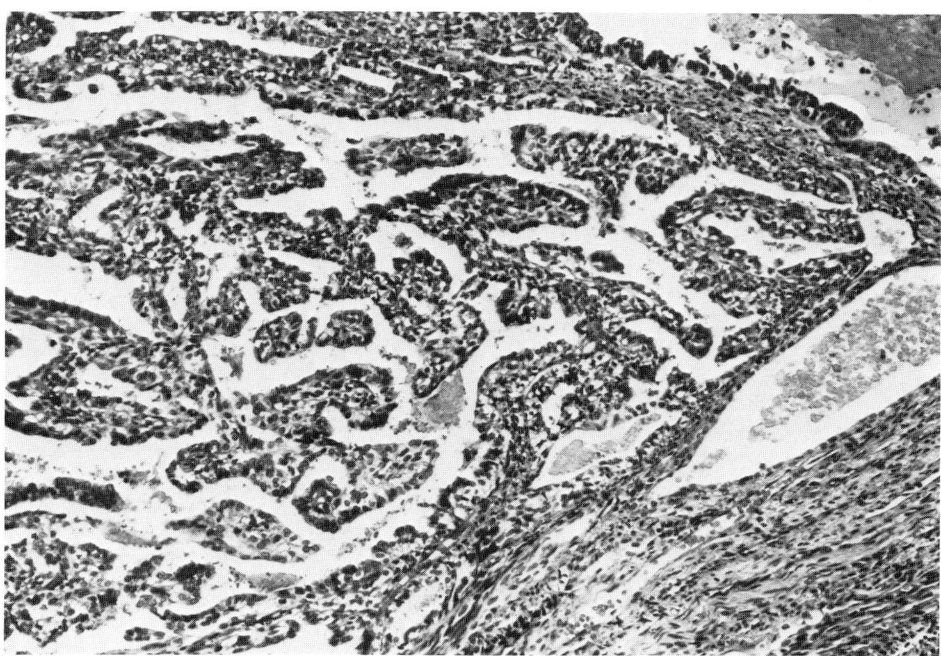

Fig. 7-10 Biphasic synovial sarcoma showing a glandular component with papillary fronds protruding into the lumen. (H&E, × 350.)

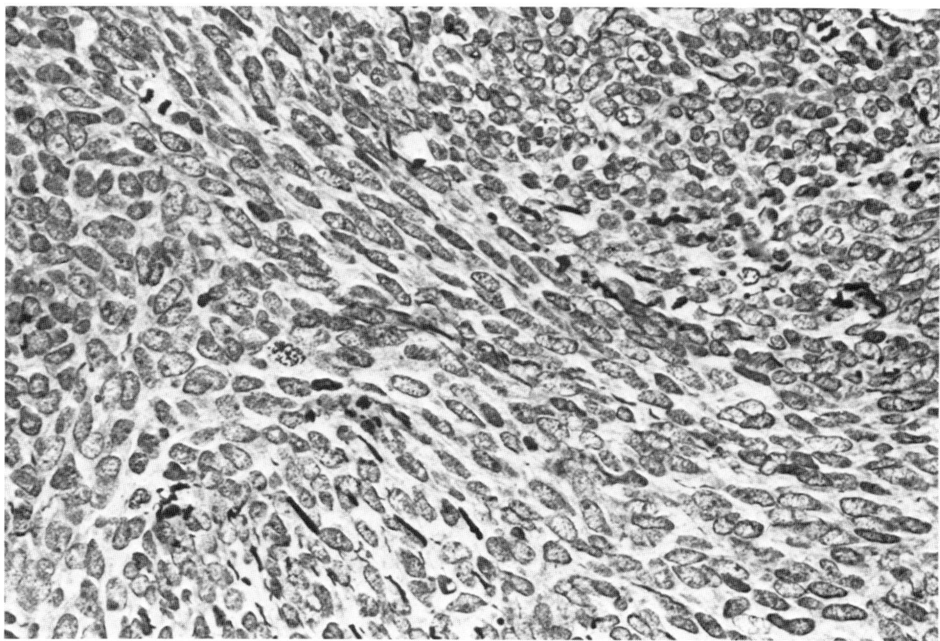

Fig. 7-11. Monophasic fibrous synovial sarcoma. Most cells are spindle-shaped. In the left half the cells have plump nuclei. Few reticulin fibers are present between the cells. (Reticulin silver stain, × 350.)

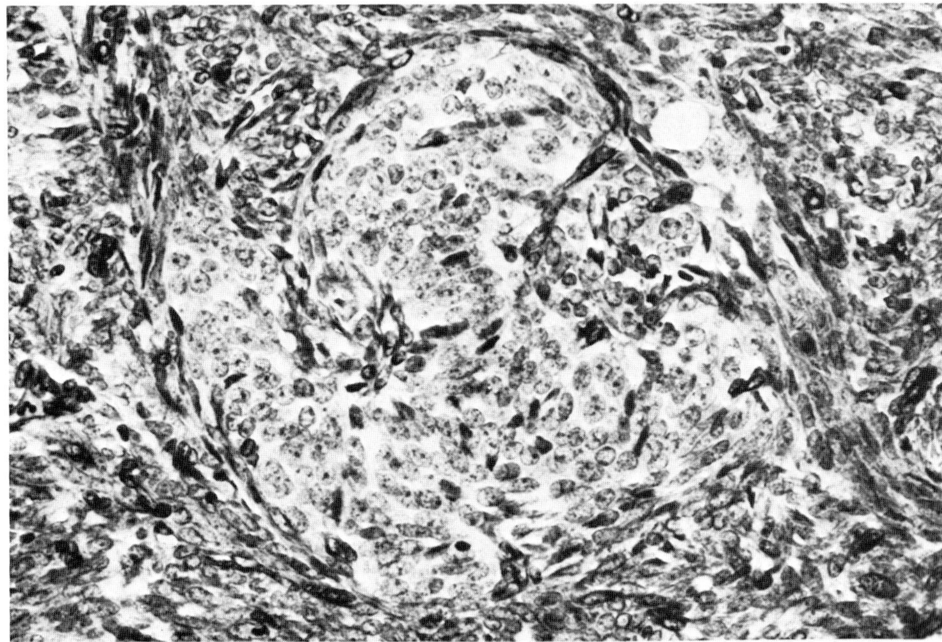

Fig. 7-12. Biphasic synovial sarcoma. A solid cluster of epithelioid cells is surrounded by spindle-shaped cells. The histologic appearance is accentuated by vimentin positivity in the spindle cells. (Monoclonal antibody V9, APAAP method, × 350.)

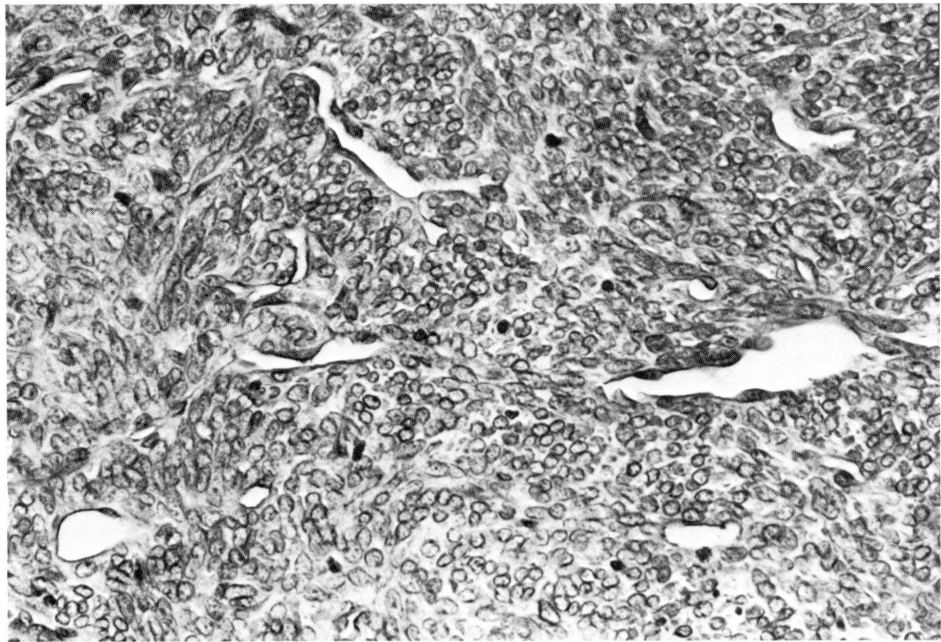

Fig. 7-13. Monophasic fibrous synovial sarcoma showing a hemangiopericytomalike pattern. (H&E, × 350.)

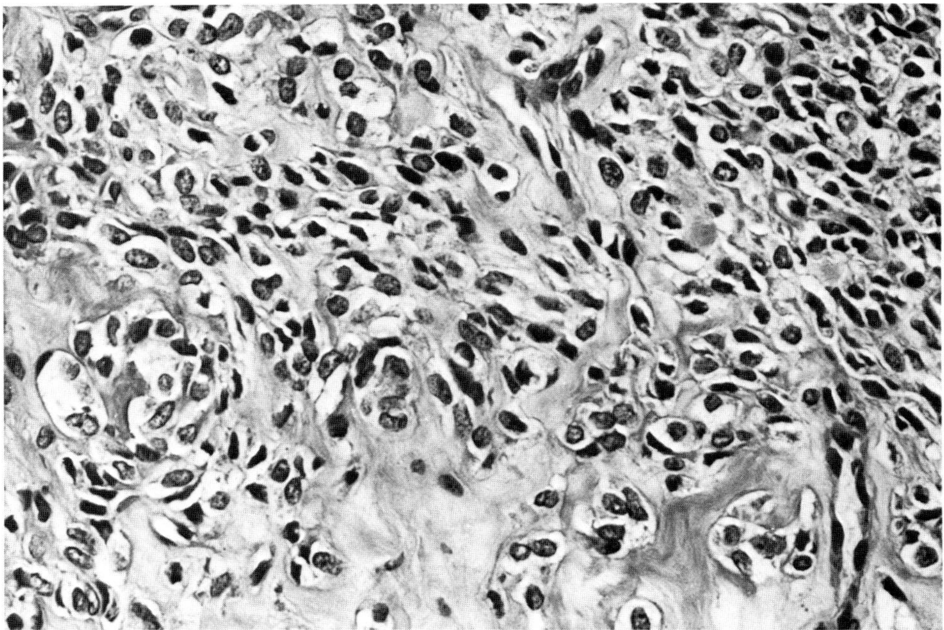

Fig. 7-14. Biphasic synovial sarcoma showing an area with hyalinization. (PAS. × 350.)

distinction from other spindle cell soft tissue sarcomas.

The histopathologic appearance of metastatic lesions is generally similar to that of the primary tumors, although morphologic changes do occur. Usually a biphasic synovial sarcoma assumes a monomorphic spindle cell pattern in the metastasis. In a case of monophasic fibrous synovial sarcoma with two local recurrences, a biphasic form has been described in the first recurrence, whereas the second recurrence consisted of a tumor with predominant glandular differentiation.[19]

Ultrastructural Findings

As suggested by conventional light microscopy there is no significant difference between the spindle cell component of biphasic synovial sarcoma and the monophasic fibrous synovial sarcoma.[19] Moreover, there is no essential difference between the cytoplasmic constituents of the spindle and epithelioid cells.[20] A constant finding is the presence of microvilli on the surface of the glandular lining cells. Interdigitating cell processes and filopodia can be detected along the lateral borders and between the spindle cells. Amorphous moderately electron-dense material is present on the surface of the epithelial cells and between the spindle cells.[21] Both cell types are connected by specialized junctions in the form of desmosomes or macula adhaerens-type junctions (Table 7-3). Although a continuous basal lamina surrounds the glandular spaces (Fig. 7-15), basal lamina formation is incomplete in the spindle cell areas. Collagen fibers are usually sparse. Cytoplasmic filaments include microfilaments, intermediate filaments, and interestingly, in some cases of biphasic synovial sarcoma, tonofilaments.[22, 23]

Immunohistochemical Findings

In accordance with the cytologic composition as defined by conventional light microscopy three types of cells can be distinguished by immunohistochemical means employing antisera against intermediate filament proteins (Table

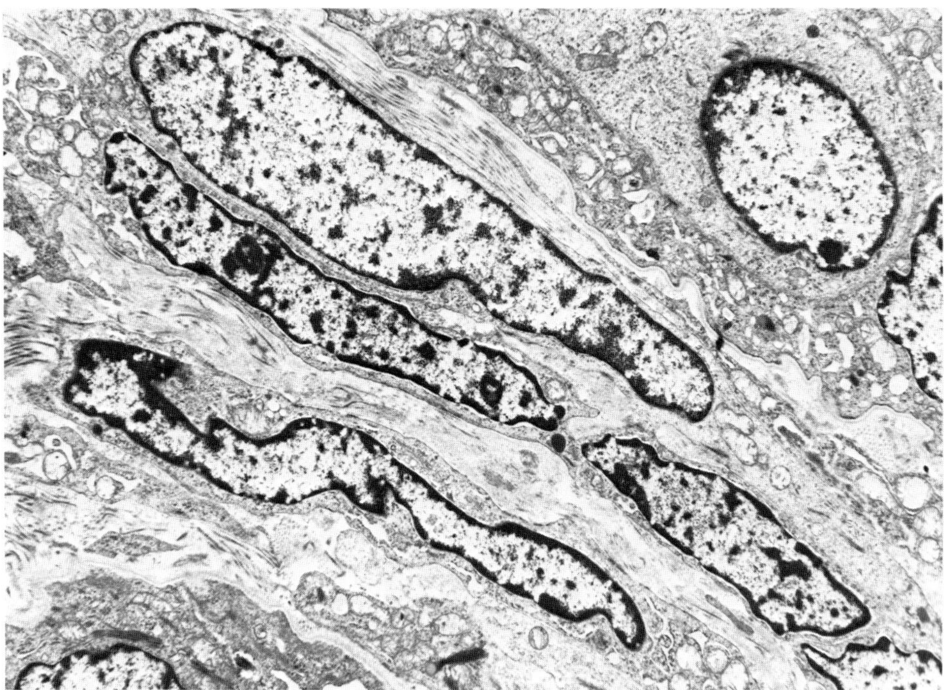

Fig. 7-15. Electron micrograph of biphasic synovial sarcoma. Two clusters of epithelioid cells are surrounded by a distinct basal lamina. A few collagen fibers are present between the spindle cells. (Uranyl acetate and lead citrate, × 6000.)

7-3). Most of the fibroblastlike cells contain vimentin only (Fig. 7-16), whereas the epithelial cells lining the cleftlike spaces and the glandular structures express cytokeratins, but lack vimentin. In the cytoplasm of the transitional polygonal cells vimentin and cytokeratins are expressed. Cytokeratins are also detected in a minor portion of the spindle cells (Fig. 7-17), indicating very early epithelial differentiation not detectable by conventional light microscopy. Essentially similar findings have been obtained for epithelial membrane antigen (EMA), which, interestingly, is found in the spindle cells in a diffuse manner and is located in the epithelial-like cells at the cell membrane.[24] Various other antisera have also been employed, but none of them was as useful in the distinction of the cellular composition of synovial sarcoma as those against intermediate filaments and EMA. These stains include reactants for *Ulex europaeus* agglutinin I (UEA I), human milkfat globulin 2 (HMFG$_2$), Leu 7 (HNK1), carcinoem-

bryonic antigen (CEA), actin, desmin, and protein S-100.[25, 26] The latter has usually been claimed to be absent in synovial sarcoma,[23, 27] however, we found protein S-100-positive cells in both biphasic and monophasic tumors in about 30 percent of the cases (Fig. 7-18). Moreover, Leu 7 may be positive in synovial sarcoma, making the differentiation from malignant schwannoma, notably the glandular subtype, difficult.

Histochemical Findings

Various histochemical stains have been applied, lending further support to the concept of there being two distinct components in synovial sarcomas. Pisa et al.[28] found that the epithelial-like cells contain alkaline and acid phosphatase, ATPase, and nonspecific esterase, whereas these enzymes were absent in the spindle cells. Periodic acid-Schiff (PAS)-positive glycopro-

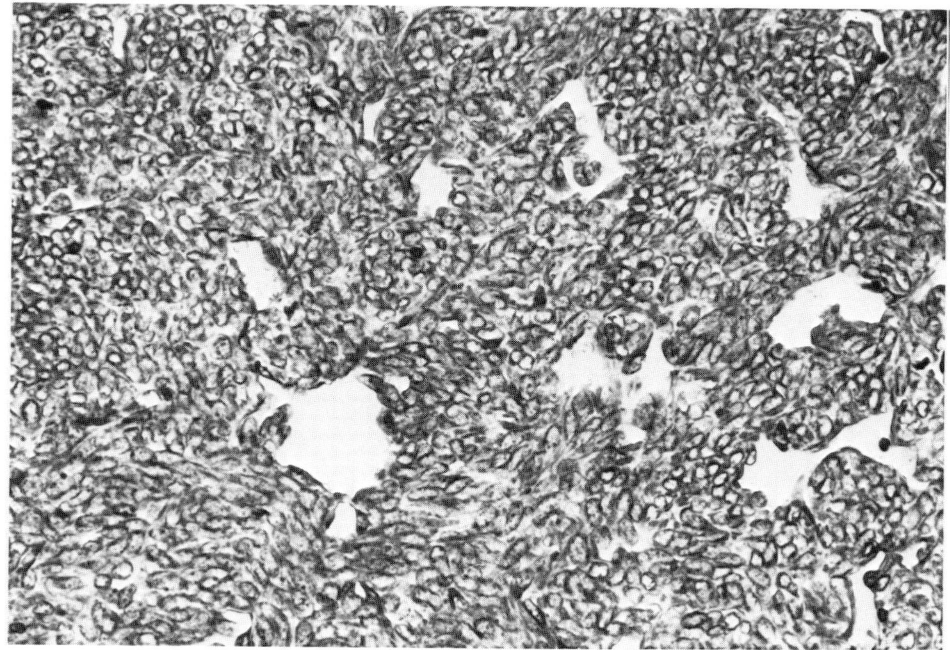

Fig. 7-16. Monophasic fibrous synovial sarcoma. Fibroblastlike cells contain vimentin. (Monoclonal antibody V9, APAAP method, × 350.)

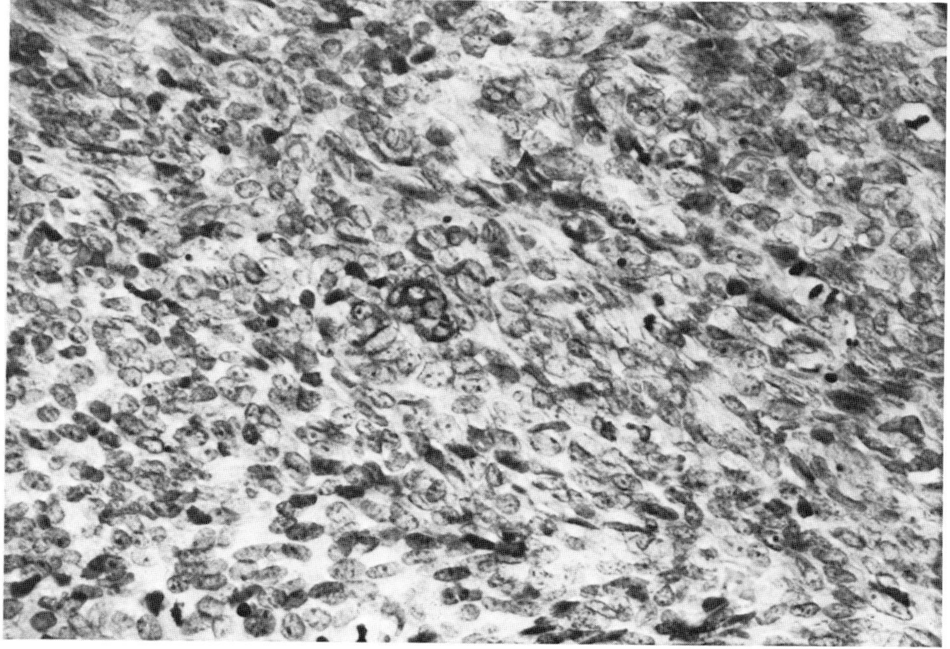

Fig. 7-17. Monophasic fibrous synovial sarcoma. Cytokeratin positivity in small groups of cells indicates early epithelial differentiation. (Monoclonal antibody AE1, APAAP method, × 350.)

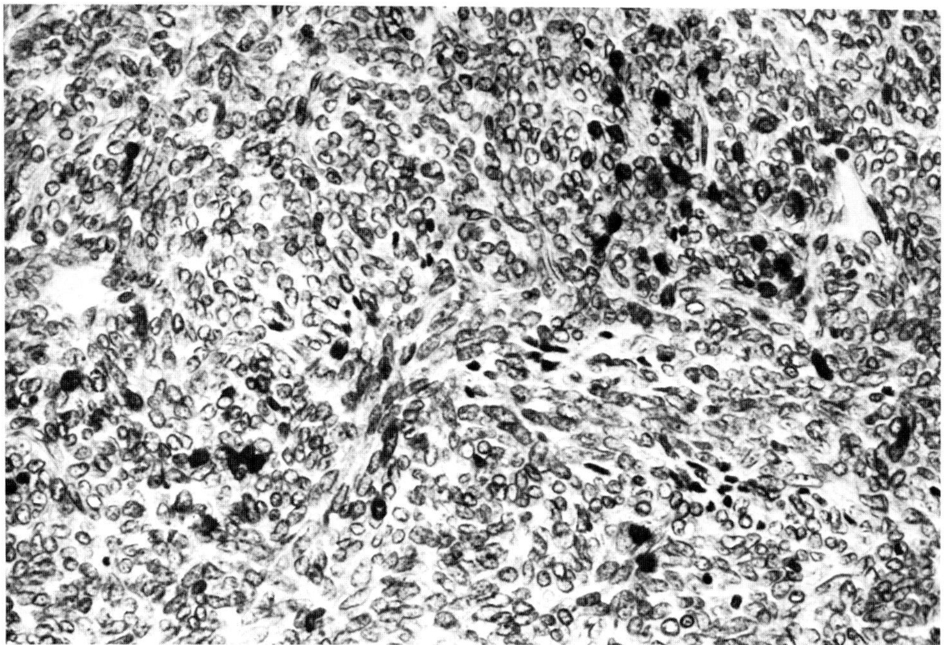

Fig. 7-18. Monophasic fibrous synovial sarcoma. Some of nuclei are S-100 protein positive. (Polyclonal antibody, APAAP method, × 350.)

teins with various amonts of sialic acid were described by Nakamura et al.[29] in the epithelioid regions in addition to hyaluronic acid and chondroitin sulfate. In the spindle cell areas sialic acid was absent, but hyaluronic acid, chondroitin sulfate, and heparitin sulfate were detected. The luminal content of the glandular structures is PAS positive, but the mucinous material in the interstitial space of the spindle cell areas is PAS negative. Both substances, however, stain positively with Alcian blue.

Cytogenetic Findings

As in other types of malignant tumors a common translocation has been discovered in synovial sarcoma. This consists of a translocation between a chromosome X and the autosome 18,t (X;18) (p11; q11).[30–32] In cases of spindle cell sarcoma with uncertain diagnosis this could be a useful diagnostic tool in establishing the differential diagnosis from other soft tissue sarcomas. It is especially helpful, since it is expressed in the mono- and biphasic forms.

Prognosis

Among other factors, the clinical course is highly dependent on treatment strategies. In the past treatment consisted of local excision (local recurrence rates were as high as 70 percent, sometimes with multiple recurrences), followed by radiotherapy. Chemotherapy has been recently introduced in to the treatment. However, the question is still unresolved whether modern treatment plans will significantly improve survival rates. Earlier reports have shown that survival is frequently determined by the occurrence of late metastases and late recurrences, which may even develop after 20 years.[33] Most frequently metastases occur in the lung (up to 90 percent), followed by lymph nodes (approximately 20 percent) and bone, and more rarely in the skin[33] and the brain.[34]

Prognostic Factors

Better survival has been associated with young age,[35] female sex,[12] distal localization,[36] and tumor size less than 5 cm.[37]

Contradictory results have been reported when histologic features are correlated with prognosis. Those reports that claim there is a relationship between histology and prognosis have found a better survival in biphasic synovial sarcoma, especially in tumors with a high proportion of glandular structures and low mitotic rates.[38] An additional favorable prognostic factor is the presence of extensive calcification. In these cases the 5-year survival rate may be as high as 82 percent.[39]

REFERENCES

1. Wright CJE: Benign giant cell synovioma. Br J Surg 38:257, 1951
2. Jaffe HL, Lichtenstein L, Sutro CJ: Pigmented villonodular synovitis, bursitis, and tenosynovitis: a discussion of the bursal equivalents of the tenosynovial lesion commonly denoted as xanthoma, xanthogranuloma, giant cell tumor or myeloplaxoma of the tendon sheath, with some consideration of this tendon sheath lesion itself. Arch Pathol 31:731, 1941
3. Jones FE, Soule EH, Coventry MB: Fibrous xanthoma of the synovium (giant-cell tumor of the tendon sheath, pigmented nodular synovitis). A study of one hundred and eighteen cases. J Bone Joint Surg 51A:76, 1969
4. Enzinger FM, Weiss SW: Soft Tissue Tumors. 2nd Ed. CV Mosby, St. Louis, 1988
5. Kahn LB: Malignant giant cell tumor of the tendon sheaths. Ultrastructural study and review of the literature. Arch Pathol 95:203, 1973
6. Bliss BO, Reed RJ: Large cell sarcomas of the tendon sheath. Malignant giant cell tumor of the tendon sheath. Am J Clin Pathol 49:776, 1968
7. Carsten PHB, Howell RS: Malignant giant cell tumor of the tendon sheaths. Virchows Arch [A] 382:237, 1979
8. Lejars F, Rubens-Duval H: Les sarcomes primitive des synoviales articulaires. Rev Chir 41:751, 1910
9. Enjoji M, Hashimoto H: Diagnosis of soft tissue sarcomas. Pathol Res Pract 178:215, 1984
10. Cadman NL, Soule EH, Kelly PJ: Synovial sarcoma. An analysis of 134 tumors. Cancer 5:613, 1965
11. Evans RW, Thomas GE, Walker NM: A congenital malignant synovial tumor of bone. J Bone Joint Surg 42B:742, 1960
12. Wright PA, Sim FH, Soule EH, Taylor WF: Synovial sarcoma. J Bone Joint Surg 64A:112, 1982
13. Geiler G: Gelenktumoren. p. 647. In Doerr W, Seifert G (eds): Pathologie der Gelenke und Weichteiltumoren. Springer-Verlag, Heidelberg, 1984
14. Moberger G, Nilsonne U, Friberg Jr S: Synovial sarcoma. Histologic features and prognosis. Acta Orthop Scand Suppl 111:3, 1968
15. Shmookler BM: Retroperitoneal synovial sarcoma. A report of four cases. Am J Clin Pathol 77:686, 1982
16. Holtz F, Magielski JE: Synovial sarcomas of the tongue base. The seventh reported case. Arch Otolaryngol 111:271, 1985
17. Choux R, Jaquemier J, Chrestian MA, et al: Synovialo-sarcoma pharyngé. Etude ultrastructurale d'un cas. Bull Cancer 65:3, 1978
18. Shmookler BM, Enzinger FM, Brannon RB: Orofacial synovial sarcomas: a clinical pathologic study of 11 new cases and a review of the literature. Cancer 50:269, 1982
19. Fisher C: Synovial sarcoma: ultrastructural and immunohistochemical features of epithelial differentiation in monophasic and biphasic tumors. Hum Pathol 17:996, 1986
20. Katenkamp D, Stiller D: Synovial sarcoma of the abdominal wall. Light microscopic, histochemical and electron microscopic investigations. Virchows Arch [A] 388:349, 1980
21. Lombardi L, Rilke F: Ultrastructural similarities and differences of synovial sarcoma, epithelioid sarcoma, and clear cell sarcoma of the tendons and aponeuroses. Ultrastruct Pathol 6:209, 1984
22. Klein W, Huth F: The ultrastructure of malignant synovioma. Beitr Pathol 153:194, 1974
23. Abenoza P, Manivel JC, Swanson PE, Wick MR: Synovial sarcoma: Ultrastructural study and immunohistochemical analysis by a combined peroxidase-antiperoxidase/avidin-biotin-peroxidase complex procedure. Hum Pathol 17:1107, 1986

24. Miettinen M, Virtanen I: Synovial sarcoma—a misnomer. Am J Pathol 117:18, 1984
25. Borisch B, Harms D: Untersuchungen mit *Ulex europaeus* Agglutinin I (UEA I) an Normalgeweben sowie Synovialsarkomen, Mesotheliomen und Karzinomen. Pathologe 6:260, 1985
26. Corson JM, Weiss LM, Banks-Schlegel SP, Pinkus GS: Keratin proteins and carcinoembryonic antigen in synovial sarcomas: an immunohistochemical study of 24 cases. Hum Pathol 15:615, 1984
27. Salisbury JR, Isaacson PG: Synovial sarcoma: an immunohistochemical study. J Pathol 147:49, 1985
28. Pisa R, Bonetti F, Chilosi M, et al: Synovial sarcoma. Enzyme histochemistry of a typical case. Virchows Arch [A] 398:67, 1982
29. Nakamura F, Nakata K, Hata S, et al: Histochemical characterization of mucosubstances in synovial sarcoma. Am J Surg Pathol 8:429, 1984
30. Limon J, Dal Cin P, Sandberg AA: Translocations involving the X chromosome in solid tumors: Presentation of two sarcomas with t (X,18) (q13, p11). Cancer Genet Cytogenet 23:87, 1986
31. Turc-Carel C, Dal Cin P, Limon J, et al: Letter to the editor. Translocation X;18 in synovial sarcomas. Cancer Genet Cytogenet 23:93, 1986
32. Noguera R, Lopez-Gines C, Gil R, et al: Translocation X;18 in a synovial sarcoma: a new case. Cancer Genet Cytogenet 33:311, 1988
33. Cameron HU, Kostuik JP: A long-term follow-up of synovial sarcoma. J Bone Joint Surg 56B:513, 1974
34. Lee SM, Hajdu SI, Exelby PR: Synovial sarcoma in children. Surg Gynecol Obstet 138:701, 1974
35. Buck P, Mickelson MR, Bonfiglio M: Synovial sarcoma: a review of 33 cases. Clin Orthop 156:211, 1981
36. Treuner J, Suder J, Gerein V, et al: Behandlungsergebnisse der nichtrhabdomyosarkomatösen Weichteilmalignome im Rahmen der CWS-81-Studie. Klin Pädiatr 199:209, 1987
37. Hajdu SI, Shin MH, Fortner JG: Tenosynovial sarcoma. A clinico-pathological study of 136 cases. Cancer 39:1201, 1977
38. Cagle LA, Mirra JM, Storm FK: Histologic features relating to prognosis in synovial sarcoma. Cancer 59:1810, 1987
39. Varela-Duran J, Enzinger FM: Calcifying synovial sarcomas. Cancer 50:345, 1982

8

Mesothelial Tumors and Tumorlike Lesions

Dieter Harms and Dietmar Schmidt

Mesothelial tumors and tumorlike mesothelial lesions may present with various histologic patterns. Consequently it may be difficult to identify and classify these lesions. Moreover, it can be extremely difficult to distinguish between mesothelial and nonmesothelial tumors. In the differential diagnosis many other soft tissue tumors as well as epithelial tumors and even tumorlike conditions have to be taken into consideration.

The development of new immunohistochemical techniques has made diagnosis more precise, and as a result the proportion of unclassifiable cases has decreased considerably. This is also true for mesothelial tumors.

DIFFUSE MALIGNANT MESOTHELIOMA

Diffuse malignant mesothelioma (DMM) is the most important mesothelial tumor. Its annual incidence in North America in 1972 was estimated at 2.8 per million males and 0.8 per million females aged 15 years and over.[1] About 70 percent of the cases develop in the pleura, whereas 20 to 25 percent arise in the peritoneum. Occurrence in other primary locations (e.g., the pericardium) is rare.[2] Most tumors appear in adult patients, and many tumors are associated with asbestos exposure.[2–4] However, DMM does develop without previous exposure to asbestos, and may even occur in early childhood.[5–7] Macroscopically pleural mesothelioma usually presents with many tumor nodules in the parietal and visceral pleura. In general, the nodules in the parietal pleura are larger and/or more numerous than those in the visceral pleura. As the tumor progresses, it forms large masses, often encoating the lung and extending to the pericardium. Peritoneal diffuse malignant mesothelioma usually presents with multiple nodules, mimicking macro- and micronodular peritoneal carcinosis, and is often associated with formation of scarlike plaques.

Microscopically epithelial, sarcomatous (fibrous), and biphasic (mixed epithelial/sarcomatous) subtypes are distinguished.[2, 4, 8–10] Desmoplastic mesothelioma is a variant of sarcomatous mesothelioma.

Epithelial mesothelioma is the most common subtype of mesothelioma, accounting for about 50 percent of all DMM; about 25 to 30 percent of the cases are biphasic, whereas slightly more than 20 percent of the cases are sarcomatous. In sarcomatous mesotheliomas the desmoplastic variant is less common than the frankly sarcomatous tumor.[11] Epithelial mesotheliomas are relatively more frequent in females than in males. Adams and coworkers[11] reported that 76 percent of mesotheliomas in females were epithelial, whereas only 37 percent of tumors occurring in males were purely epithelial.

Generally, the prognosis of DMM is poor, and ultimately almost every patient will die. Nevertheless, there are differences in median survival period and 2-year survival rates between the various subtypes. Thus, 2-year survival probability is 32 percent in epithelial, 8 percent in mixed, and 5 percent in sarcomatous subtype.[11]

195

Epithelial Mesothelioma

Epithelial mesothelioma usually displays tubulopapillary structures, but may also show a glandular or diffuse pattern. The tumor cells are usually medium-sized and cuboidal, but sometimes are flattened or cylindrical, and possess an eosinophilic cytoplasm that is sometimes vacuolated, thus mimicking signet ring cells. The cell membrane is distinct. The nuclei are predominantly centrally located and contain a moderately prominent nucleolus. In spite of variable cell size, the nuclear:cytoplasmic ratio is comparatively constant (low to moderate).

Immunohistochemically the epithelioid tumor cells contain low- and high-molecular-weight cytokeratins (Table 8-1 and Fig. 8-1). The reactions against carcinoembryonic antigen (CEA) and LeuM1 are usually negative, in contrast to many adenocarcinomas, including adenocarcinoma of the lung.

Sarcomatous Mesothelioma

Sarcomatous mesothelioma (Fig. 8-2) is composed of plump to spindle-shaped fibroblastlike cells with considerable nuclear atypia. The cells are often arranged in bundles. A storiform pattern or irregular cell arrangement can occur. Many reticulin and collagen fibers are found between the cells, both with and without hyalinization.

The tumor cells are strongly positive for vimentin. Co-expression of cytokeratin may occur, indicating "early" epithelial differentiation. Cases with a significant number of cytokeratin- and vimentin-positive cells have been called *transitional mesotheliomas.*[4]

In differential diagnosis sarcomatous mesothelioma must be distinguished from fibrosarcoma, malignant fibrous histiocytoma, leiomyosarcoma, malignant schwannoma, and other malignant, predominantly spindle cell soft tissue tumors. In many cases, detailed information

Table 8-1. Differential Diagnosis between Adenocarcinoma and Malignant Epithelial Mesothelioma by Conventional Light Microscopy, Histochemistry, Immunohistochemistry and Electron Microscopy.[a]

	Adenocarcinoma	Malignant Epithelial Mesothelioma[b]
Predominant cell type	Columnar	Cuboidal (flat)
Mucicarmine	+	0
Diastase-PAS	+	0
Hyaluronic acid	0	+
Low-molecular-weight cytokeratins	+	+
High-molecular-weight cytokeratins	0	+
Carcinoembryonic antigen (CEA)	+	0[c]
LeuM1	+	0
Microvilli	Few, short, stubby	Many, long, slender
Desmosomes	Small	Large
Tonofilaments	Variable	Frequent

[a] Note that none of the single criteria is axiomatic (diagnostic or exclusive).
[b] Including epithelial components of biphasic mesothelioma.
[c] Some weakly positive cells may occur.

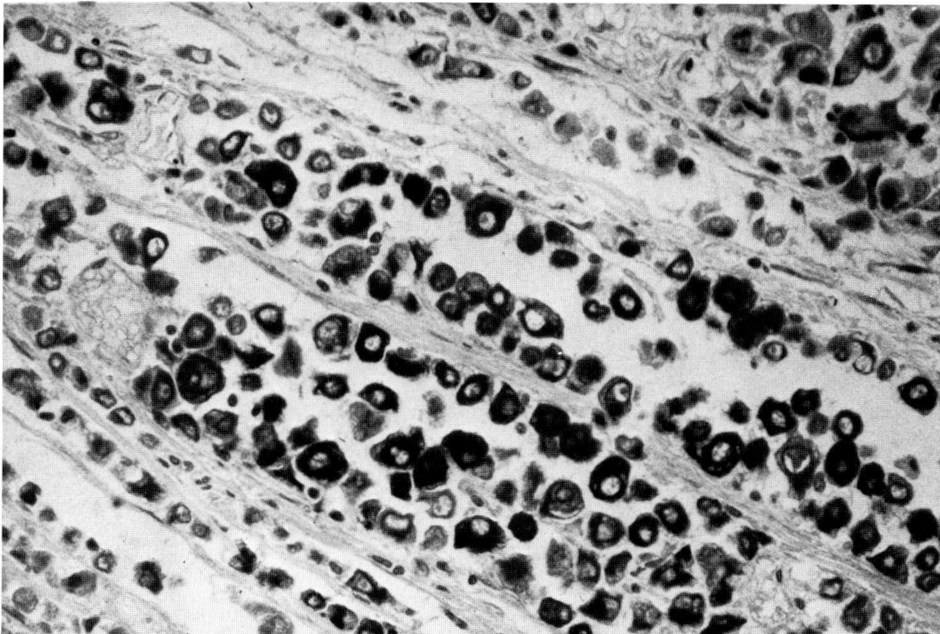

Fig. 8-1. Diffuse malignant mesothelioma, epithelial subtype, with prominent tubular pattern. The spaces are lined by moderately atypical epithelioid tumor cells, which reacted strongly with an antibody against cytokeratin. (Monoclonal antibody KL1, APAAP method, × 280.)

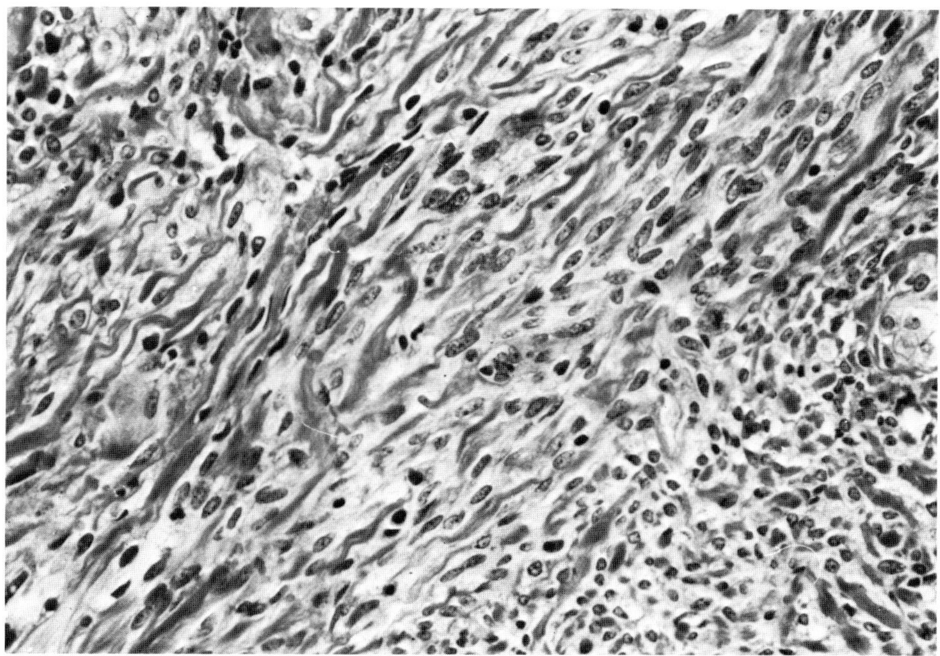

Fig. 8-2. Diffuse malignant mesothelioma, sarcomatoid subtype, presenting as a spindle cell tumor with some hyalinization. (H&E, × 280.)

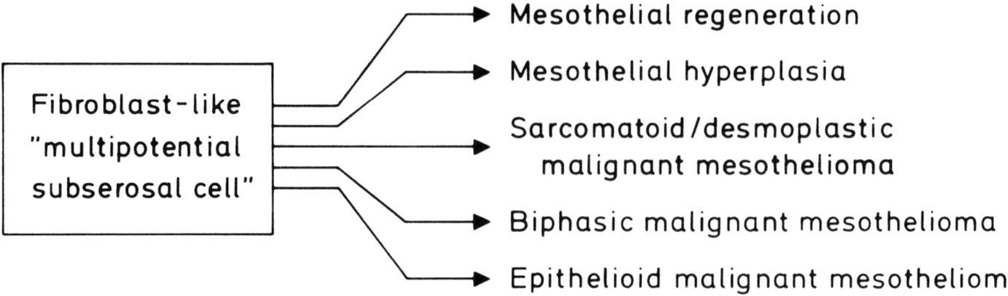

Fig. 8-3. A fibroblastlike "multipotential subserosal cell" is considered to be the precursor cell of different reactive and neoplastic mesothelial lesions.[12]

concerning tumor location as well as additional immunohistochemical stains are necessary for the diagnosis and differential diagnosis of sarcomatous mesotheliomas.

DESMOPLASTIC MESOTHELIOMA

Desmoplastic mesothelioma is a highly collagenous variant of sarcomatous mesothelioma. In contrast to the typical sarcomatous mesothelioma, it is hypocellular, and the individual tumor cells look quite bland. Areas of necrosis, absence of inflammatory infiltrates, and invasion of adjacent structures are useful criteria in the differential diagnosis with reactive fibroblastic lesions. In old scars the collagenous fibers tend to be arranged in a more parallel fashion. Despite the bland histology, the prognosis of desmoplastic mesothelioma is as poor as that of conventional sarcomatous mesothelioma.[11]

BIPHASIC MESOTHELIOMA

Biphasic (mixed epithelial/sarcomatous) mesothelioma is a combination of epithelial and sarcomatous mesothelioma. It may be interpreted, like biphasic synovial sarcoma, as a carcinosarcomatous tumor showing both atypical epithelial and sarcomatous elements. The quantitative proportion of the tumor components can vary considerably, not only from tumor to tumor, but also between different areas of the same tumor. If one considers epithelial and sarcomatous mesothelioma to be the extremes of a continuous spectrum, biphasic mesothelioma is located quantitatively between these extremes.

The precursor cell of diffuse malignant mesothelioma is thought to be a subserosal fibroblastlike cell, the so-called multipotential subserosal cell.[4, 12] This fibroblastlike cell is considered to be the stem cell of mesothelial regeneration, common mesothelial hyperplasia, and the various subtypes of malignant mesothelioma (Fig. 8-3). The multipotential subserosal fibroblastlike cell contains vimentin, low-molecular-weight cytokeratins, actin, and desmin. With increasing epithelial differentiation the cells develop high-molecular-weight cytokeratins, whereas the expression of vimentin, actin and desmin is lost (Table 8-2).

Table 8-2. Expression of Immunohistochemical Markers during Differentiation of Mesothelial Cells

	Vimentin	Actin	Desmin	Cytokeratin
Conventional fibroblast	+	0	0	0
Subserosal fibroblastlike cell	+	+	+	+
Mesothelial cell	0	0	0[a]	+

[a] Exceptionally, epithelioid mesothelial cells express desmin.

WELL-DIFFERENTIATED (LOCALIZED) PAPILLARY MESOTHELIOMA

Well-differentiated papillary mesothelioma is a predominantly benign tumor that occurs mostly in the peritoneum of women (median age 40 years). Adjuvant therapy is not necessary, except in the rare cases with tumor progression.[13]

The tumor presents either with multiple nodes with a diameter up to 2 cm or more, or as a solitary mass. Microscopically the arborescent tumor shows a well-developed papillary pattern (Fig. 8-4), with papillary structures lined by a single layer of cuboidal epithelial cells without nuclear atypia and mitotic activity. The epithelium may be vacuolated at the base of the cells. The fibrous stroma can be edematous or sclerotic. Occasionally a tubulopapillary pattern can be seen. In such cases diffuse malignant mesothelioma and well-differentiated serous papillary carcinomas of the peritoneum or the ovary must be excluded.[14, 15]

MULTICYSTIC PERITONEAL MESOTHELIOMA

Like well-differentiated papillary mesothelioma, multicystic peritoneal mesothelioma occurs predominantly in middle-aged women.[2, 9, 16, 17] It is usually a large tumor, consisting of multiple thin-walled cysts that are separated by narrow bands of fibrous tissue. The lumina of the cystic spaces are lined by a layer of flat to cuboidal cells with mostly regular nuclei and without mitotic activity. In most cases the lining cells react with anticytokeratin antibodies. Important variations from the common histologic appearance are squamous metaplasia and adenomatoid changes, which occur in a significant number of cases.[17]

In differential diagnosis, mesothelial pseudocysts and cystic lymphangiomas must be considered, the former mostly presenting as a solitary cyst and the latter reacting with endothelial markers such as BMA 120 and antibodies against factor VIII-associated antigen.

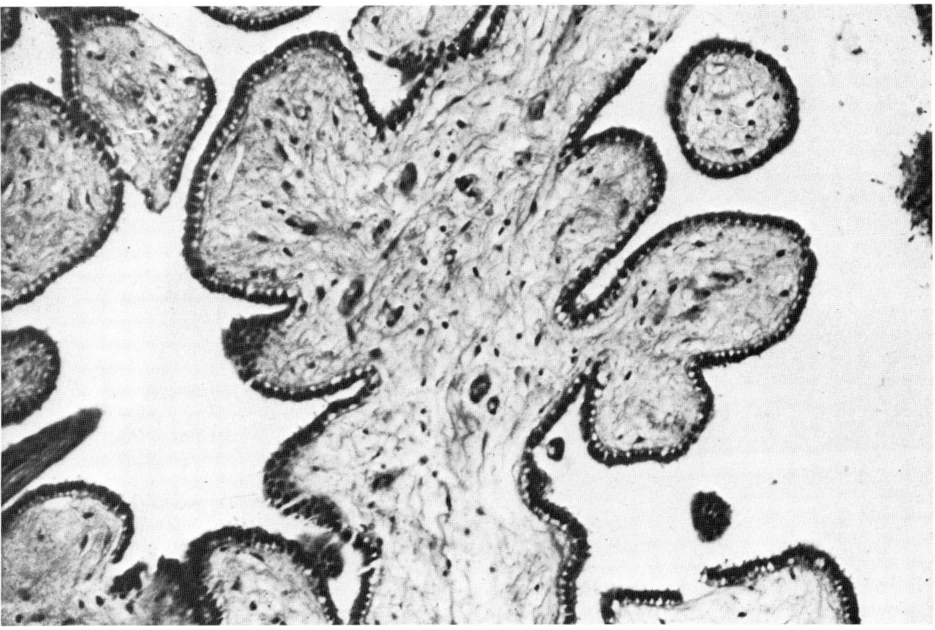

Fig. 8-4. Localized papillary epithelial mesothelioma of the peritoneum showing a monolayer of cuboidal cells at the surface. No cellular atypia. (H&E, × 140.)

ADENOMATOID TUMOR

Adenomatoid tumor is usually a small and incidentally detected tumor that occurs almost exclusively in the genital tract. Microscopically tubulocanalicular or glandular structures are present; these are surrounded by a stroma that often contains smooth muscle fibers. The tumor cells are flat to cuboidal, frequently with distinct vacuolization of the eosinophilic cytoplasm. It has now been proved by electron microscopy and immunohistochemistry that adenomatoid tumor is a mesothelial/epithelial tumor.[18–22] The tumor cells express cytokeratins and epithelial membrane antigen.

The most important entity to be considered in differential diagnosis is embryonal rhabdomyosarcoma. In the paratesticular location, embryonal rhabdomyosarcoma frequently shows cytoplasmic vacuolization (and cytokeratin expression may also occur). The signs that are diagnostic for rhabdomyosarcoma are nuclear atypia, mitotic activity, and, most importantly, expression of desmin, muscle actin, and myoglobin.

LOCALIZED FIBROUS MESOTHELIOMA

Localized fibrous mesothelioma, a rare and often pedunculated tumor, usually originates from the visceral pleura, shows no sex predilection, and is not associated with asbestos exposure. Microscopically it is composed mainly of irregularly arranged, vimentin-positive spindle cells surrounded by abundant reticulin and collagen fibers. The vascular pattern resembles hemangiopericytoma. Localized fibrous mesothelioma is a tumor that obviously develops from subserosal fibroblasts. There is no evidence of true epithelial differentiation, but some cytokeratin-positive spindle cells may be seen.

MESOTHELIAL HYPERPLASIA

Mesothelial hyperplasia is very common. It develops from irritation of the serosal layers as a result of chronic infection, radiation therapy, foreign body granulomas, or primary or metastatic tumors.[3, 4, 10, 12] The hyperplastic

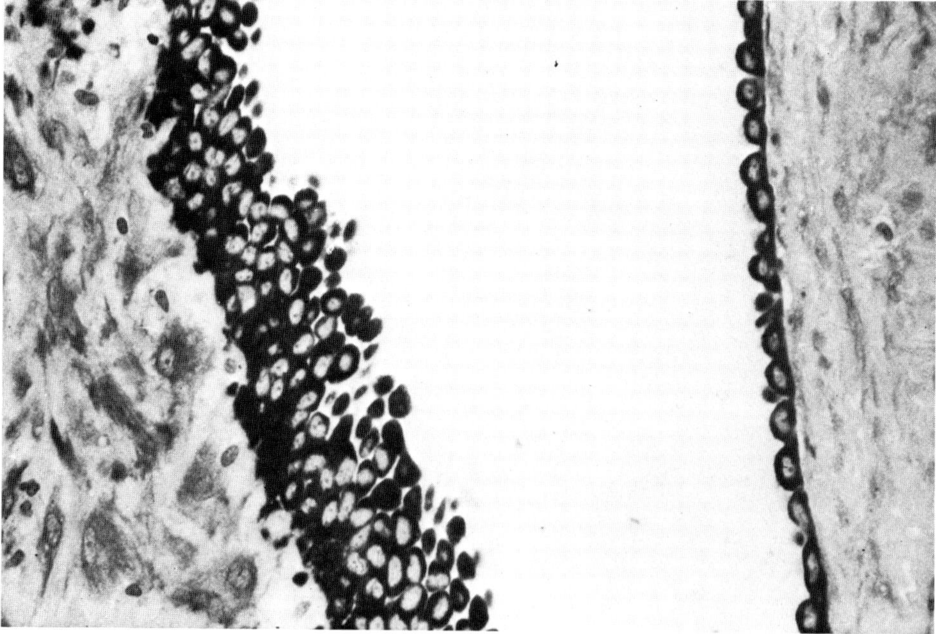

Fig. 8-5. Reactive mesothelial hyperplasia (left) attributable to chronic inflammation of the large omentum. Multilayered cytokeratin-positive mesothelial cells with some loss of cell cohesion. (Monoclonal antibody KL1, APAAP method, × 280.)

mesothelium may be multilayered (Fig. 8-5) or present with a papillary, tubular (Fig. 8-6), or combined tubular-papillary or nodular (Fig. 8-7) pattern. Some nuclear atypia and pseudoinvasion may occur, but mitotic activity is generally absent or low.

In *conventional mesothelial hyperplasia* the flat to cuboidal mesothelial cells react strongly with antibodies against cytokeratins (Figs. 8-5 and 8-6). The adjacent fibrous tissue frequently contains spindle-shaped, fibroblastlike cells that are arranged parallel to the surface. The elongated fibroblastlike cells show co-expression of vimentin and cytokeratin. In contrast to conventional fibroblasts, these subserosal fibroblastlike cells show additional expression of actin and desmin (Table 8-2). Possibly they are "stem cells" of the mesothelium,[3, 4, 12, 23] and represent a transitional stage between conventional vimentin-positive fibroblasts and cytokeratin-positive mesothelial cells. With further epithelial differentiation, the expression of vimentin, actin, and desmin decreases, whereas that of cytokeratin rises.

NODULAR MESOTHELIAL HYPERPLASIA

A rare yet characteristic variant of mesothelial hyperplasia, nodular mesothelial hyperplasia, was described by Rosai and Dehner[24] and later discussed by Harms.[25] It is often found in inguinal hernial sacs of young children and may simulate an undifferentiated malignant tumor. The diagnostic clue is a simple mesothelial hyperplasia adjacent to the main nodular lesion. The nodules (Fig. 8-7) are composed of round cells with eosinophilic and sometimes vacuolated cytoplasm. Mitotic activity can occur, leading to the incorrect diagnosis of a malignant tumor.

In contrast to conventional mesothelial hyperplasia, cells in nodular mesothelial hyperplasia react strongly with antibodies against vimentin and monocytes/macrophages. In our laboratory we use the monoclonal antibody Ki-M1P, which was raised against supernatants of detergent-soluble fraction of human lymph node tissue[26] and can be used on paraffin sections. Moreover the cells of nodular mesothelial hyperplasia do not express cytokeratins. Thus, nodular me-

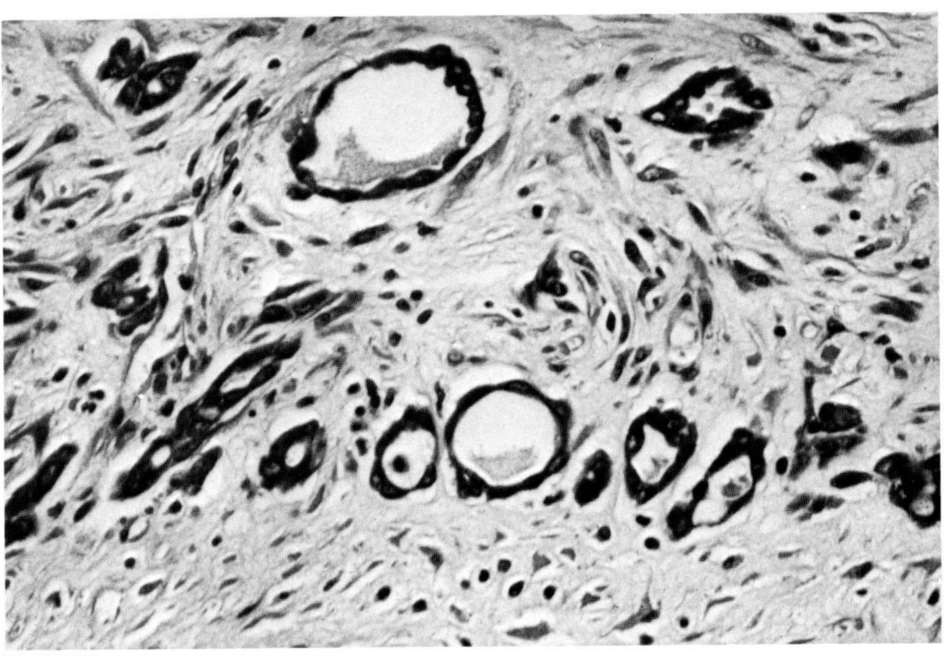

Fig. 8-6. Mesothelial hyperplasia in a peritoneal scar showing cytokeratin-positive tubules arranged in a parallel manner. (Monoclonal antibody KL1, APAAP method, × 280.)

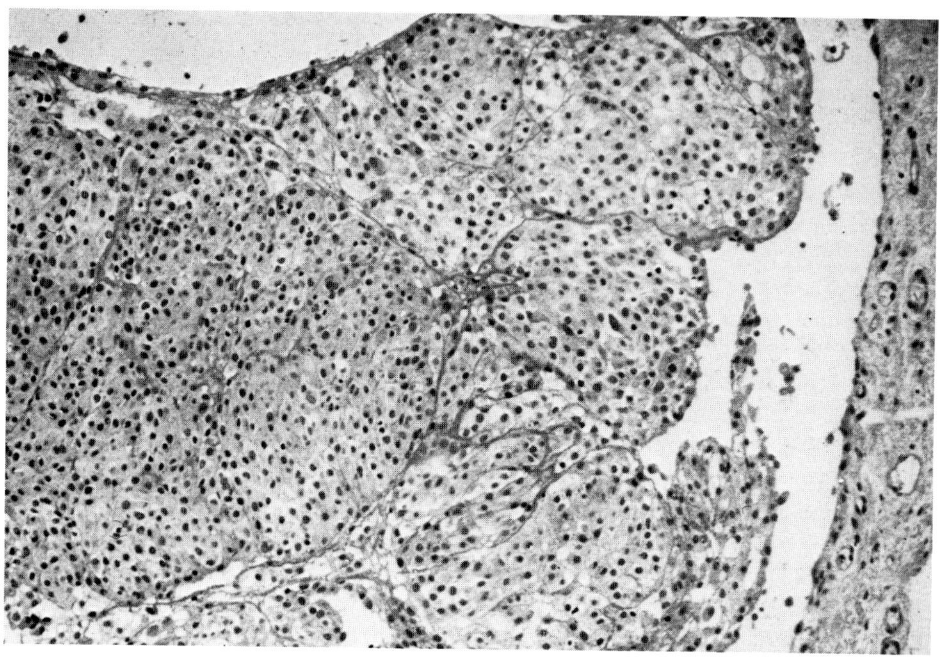

Fig. 8-7. Nodular mesothelial hyperplasia in an inguinal hernia sac of a 5-month-old boy. Solid nodule beneath a thin mesothelial-lined membrane. (H&E, × 140.) (From Harms,[25] with permission.)

sothelial hyperplasia is basically of macrophage and not of mesothelial origin.

In conclusion, at least two different cell types may contribute to mesothelial regeneration and hyperplasia: subserosal fibroblastlike cells in "conventional" mesothelial hyperplasia, and peritoneal macrophages[27] in nodular mesothelial hyperplasia.

REFERENCES

1. McDonald AD, McDonald JC: Malignant mesothelioma in North America. Cancer 46:1650, 1980

2. McCaughey WTE, Kannerstein M, Churg J: Tumors and pseudotumors of the serous membrane. In Atlas of tumor pathology. 2nd series. Fasc. 20. Armed Forces Institute of Pathology, Washington, DC, 1985

3. Craighead JE: Current pathogenetic concepts of diffuse malignant mesothelioma. Hum Pathol 18:544, 1987

4. Hammar SP, Bolen JW: Pleural neoplasms. p. 937. In Dail DH, Hammar SP (eds): Pulmonary Pathology. Springer-Verlag, New York, 1988

5. Kauffman SL, Stout AP: Mesothelioma in children. Cancer 17: 539, 1964

6. Grundy GW, Miller RW: Malignant mesothelioma in childhood. Report of 13 cases. Cancer 30:1216, 1972

7. Nishioka H, Furusho K, Yasunaga T, et al: Congenital malignant mesothelioma. A case report and electron-microscopic study. Eur J Pediatr 147:428, 1988

8. Adams VI, Unni KK: Diffuse malignant mesothelioma of pleura: diagnostic criteria based on an autopsy study. Am J Clin Pathol 82:15, 1984

9. Enzinger FM, Weiss SW: Soft Tissue Tumors. 2nd ed. CV Mosby, St. Louis, 1988

10. Battifora H: The pleura. p. 829. In Sternberg SS (ed): Diagnostic Surgical Pathology. Raven Press, New York, 1989

11. Adams VI, Unni KK, Muhm JR, et al: Diffuse malignant mesothelioma of pleura. Diagnosis and survival in 92 cases. Cancer 58:1540, 1986

12. Bolen JW, Hammar SP, McNutt MA: Reactive and neoplastic serosal tissue. A light-microscopic, ultrastructural, and immunocytochemical study. Am J Surg Pathol 10:34, 1986

13. Daya D, McCaughey WTE: Well-differentiated papillary mesothelioma of the peritoneum. A clinicopathologic study of 22 cases. Cancer 65:292, 1990

14. Foyle A, Al-Jabi M, McCaughey WTE: Papillary peritoneal tumors in women. Am J Surg Pathol 5:241, 1981

15. Bell DA, Weinstock MA, Scully RE: Peritoneal implants of ovarian serous borderline tumors. Histologic features and prognosis. Cancer 62:2212, 1988

16. Katsube Y, Mukai K, Silverberg SG: Cystic mesothelioma of the peritoneum. A report of five cases and review of the literature. Cancer 50:1615, 1982

17. Weiss SW, Tavassoli FA: Multicystic mesothelioma: an analysis of pathologic findings and biologic behavior in 37 cases. Am J Surg Pathol 12:737, 1988

18. Mackay B, Bennington JL, Skogland RW: The adenomatoid tumor: fine structural evidence for a mesothelial origin. Cancer 27:109, 1971

19. Ferenczy A, Fenoglio J, Richart RM: Observations on benign mesothelioma of the genital tract (adenomatoid tumor). A comparative ultrastructural study. Cancer 30:244, 1972

20. Salazar H, Kanbour A, Burgess F: Ultrastructure and observations on the histogenesis of mesotheliomas. "Adenomatoid tumors" of the female genital tract. Cancer 29:141, 1972

21. Said JW, Nash G, Lee M: Immunoperoxidase localization of keratin proteins, carcinoembryonic antigen and factor VIII in adenomatoid tumors. Evidence for a mesothelial derivation. Hum Pathol 13:1106, 1982

22. Stephenson TJ, Mills PM: Adenomatoid tumors: an immunohistochemical and ultrastructural appraisal of their histogenesis. J Pathol 148:327, 1986

23. Raftery AT: Regeneration of parietal and visceral peritoneum: an electron microscopical study. J Anat 115:375, 1973

24. Rosai J, Dehner LP: Nodular mesothelial hyperplasia in hernia sacs. A benign reactive condition simulating a neoplastic process. Cancer 35:165, 1975

25. Harms D: Diagnostic pitfalls in solid childhood tumors. Pathol Res Pract 182:183, 1987

26. Radzun HJ, Hansmann ML, Heidebrecht HJ, et al: Detection of a monocyte/macrophage-restricted differentiation antigen in routinely processed paraffin-embedded tissue by monoclonal antibody Ki-M1P. Lab. Invest, submitted for publication.

27. Ryan GB, Grobéty J, Majno G: Mesothelial injury and recovery. Am J Pathol 71:93, 1973

9

Tumors and Tumorlike Conditions of the Peripheral Nerve

James M. Woodruff

For the purposes of this discussion, the term *peripheral nerves* includes not only the derivatives of the spinal nerves but also the extradural portions of the cranial nerves, excluding the optic nerve. The conditions discussed include both non-neoplastic cystic and hyperplastic lesions as well as true neoplasms (tumors). In order to understand the differences between these lesions and the somewhat varied terminology applied to them, a short review of the normal histology of the peripheral nerve is necessary.

NORMAL ANATOMY OF THE PERIPHERAL NERVE

In the simplest terms, the peripheral nerve consists of groups of axonal processes emanating from centrally or peripherally situated neurons, and their investing supportive sheath (Fig. 9-1). The cell of this sheath of greatest interest to the pathologist, and one that is presumed to play a prominent role in tumor formation is the Schwann cell. The Schwann cell is the supportive cell in closest proximity to the axon. Beginning at the point where oligodendrogliocytes cease lining the axonal processes emanating from the brain or spinal cord, Schwann cells line up to form a continuous periaxonal coat. Fine structural studies (Fig. 9-2) show that individual Schwann cells encircle an axon or axons, and where the encircling processes meet, they overlap like crossed fingers. The channel formed where the processes cross is called a *mesaxon*

(Fig. 9-2). Schwann cells are interconnected by rare cell junctions, and each is lined externally by a continuous basal lamina. Schwann cells, like oligodendrogliocytes, may form myelin.

The Schwann cell coat represents the innermost aspect of the endoneurium, which in addition to Schwann cells consists of fibroblasts, collagen fibers, and small blood vessels. External to the endoneurium is the middle layer of the peripheral nerve sheath, the perineurium (Fig. 9-2). The perineurium is a sleeve or a few sleeves of circumferentially arranged flattened cells interconnected by tight cell junctions. The perineurial sleeves are separated from the endoneurium and the epineurium by boundary basement membrane (Fig. 9-2). Each perineurial sleeve is one cell thick, and basement membrane is also present between sleeves.[1] A feature of perineurial cells not found in Schwann cells is the presence of numerous pinocytotic vesicles. The epineurium is made up of connective tissue that externally coats the nerve.

Knowledge of the histogenesis of the cells of the peripheral nerve sheath is crucial to an understanding of the types of tumors arising from it. Schwann cells are derived from the neural crest,[2,3] and there is good evidence that perineurial cells are modified fibroblasts[4] and therefore are derived from the mesenchyme. The observations that Schwann cells immunostain for S-100 protein[5] but not for epithelial membrane antigen (EMA),[6] whereas perineurial cells stain for EMA but not for S-100 protein,

205

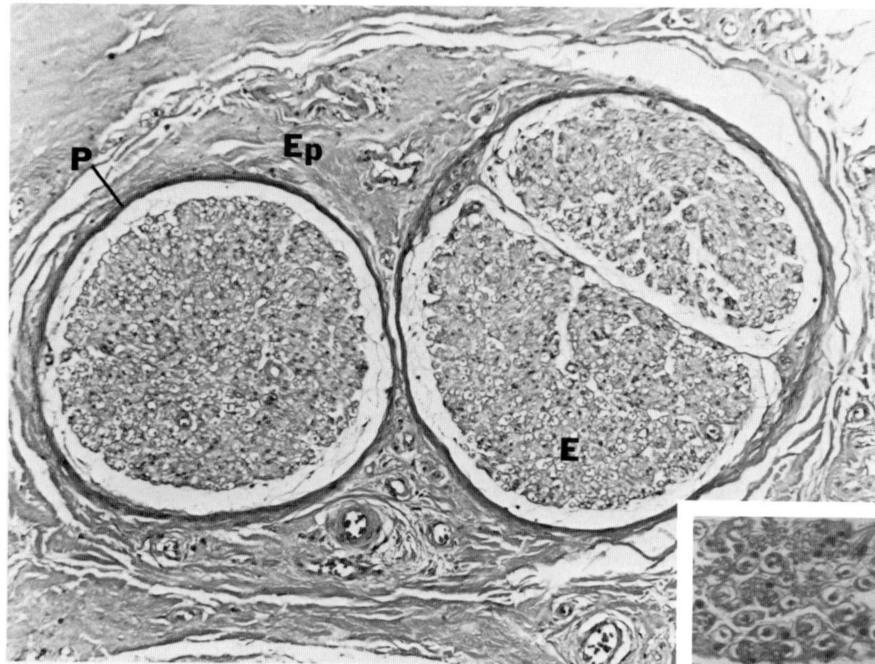

Fig. 9-1. A peripheral nerve and its supportive sheath: endoneurium (*E*), perineurium (*P*), and epineurium (*EP*). (Inset) Endoneurium at higher-power magnification shows dotlike axons and encircling thin rim of Schwann cell cytoplasm.

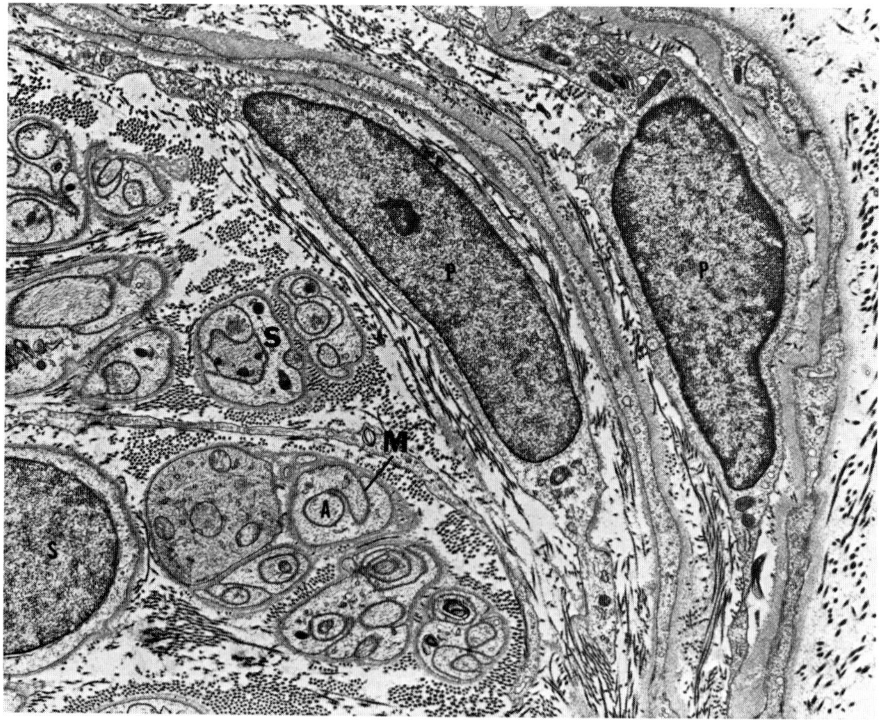

Fig. 9-2. Fine structure of peripheral nerve: axons (*A*), Schwann cells (*S*), mesaxon (*M*), perineurial cells (*P*). (× 8,000). (From Erlandson and Woodruff,[31] with permission.)

are reflections of this histogenetic difference. Axons stain by antisera to neurofilament.

TUMORLIKE LESIONS OF THE PERIPHERAL NERVE

Tumorlike lesions of the peripheral nerve include lesions ranging from cystic and fibrotic changes of the nerve that may be traumatically induced, to pseudo and true neuromas. True neuromas are, in effect, hyperplastic nerves in which the number of axons and Schwann cell tracts is approximately equal.

Nerve Cyst (Ganglion; Mucinous Ganglion Cyst)

Endoneurial or perineurial mucin-filled cysts[7–9] have been reported to cause nerve compression, with resulting tenderness, radiating pain, and weakness. The perineal nerve is the favored site of origin, and the lesion is often found close to a joint. The cyst wall is fibrous and devoid of an epithelial lining. These cysts should be distinguished from cysts external to the peripheral nerve.

Plantar Neuroma (Morton's Neuroma; Interdigital Neuritis)

The plantar neuroma, a painful lesion that afflicts women who wear ill-fitting footwear, is a fibrosing process affecting the endoneurium, perineurium, and epineurium of the interdigital plantar nerves.[10, 11] The nerve most commonly involved lies between the third and fourth metatarsals. There is associated axonal and myelin degeneration. Clues to look for in diagnosing a plantar neuroma are a lamellar fibrosis of the perineurium and fibrosed and hyalinized small blood vessels.[12]

Fibrolipomatous Hamartoma of the Nerve

Pain, numbness, compression neuropathy, and carpal tunnel syndrome result from a fibrolipomatous hamartoma affecting the ulnar nerve.

Silverman and Enzinger[13] found that of 26 patients with this disorder, 10 either had the lesion at birth or had developed it in the first 2 years of life. Twenty-seven percent of the patients had an associated macrodactyly. Microscopically fibrolipomatous tissue expands the epineurium, separates nerve bundles, and causes both a perineurial and an endoneurial fibrosis.

Neuromuscular Choristoma (Neuromuscular Hamartoma)

First described by Louhimo and Rapola in 1972,[14] neuromuscular choristoma is a rare lesion primarily involving the root of a limb (brachial plexus and sciatic nerve) of infants. Males and females are equally affected. Despite an intimate involvement of nerves, nerve dysfunction was noted initially in only one of six cases.[14–16] The reported lesions have ranged in size from 1 to 5 cm. Neuromuscular choristomas are benign and may regress with time; since two patients developed palsy and paralysis after total surgical resections, it has been recommended that total excisions not be attempted. Histologically neuromuscular choristomas are multinodular and exhibit an intermingling of nerves and mature striated muscle fibers (Fig. 9-3). Fibrous sheaths subdivide the tumor. The likely explanation for this unusual combination of tissues is a developmental abnormality in which mesenchyme destined to form striated muscle becomes trapped within the developing nerve sheath.

Amputation Neuroma

Amputation neuroma, the most common form of true neuroma, represents an attempted but failed regeneration of a peripheral nerve after its disruption or transection. The lesion is usually painful on palpation. After disruption of the nerve the Schwann cells of the proximal stump proliferate in an attempt to bridge the gap between the two parts of the nerve. If unsuccessful, the Schwann cells may grow aimlessly, within fibrous tissue, giving the growth the ap-

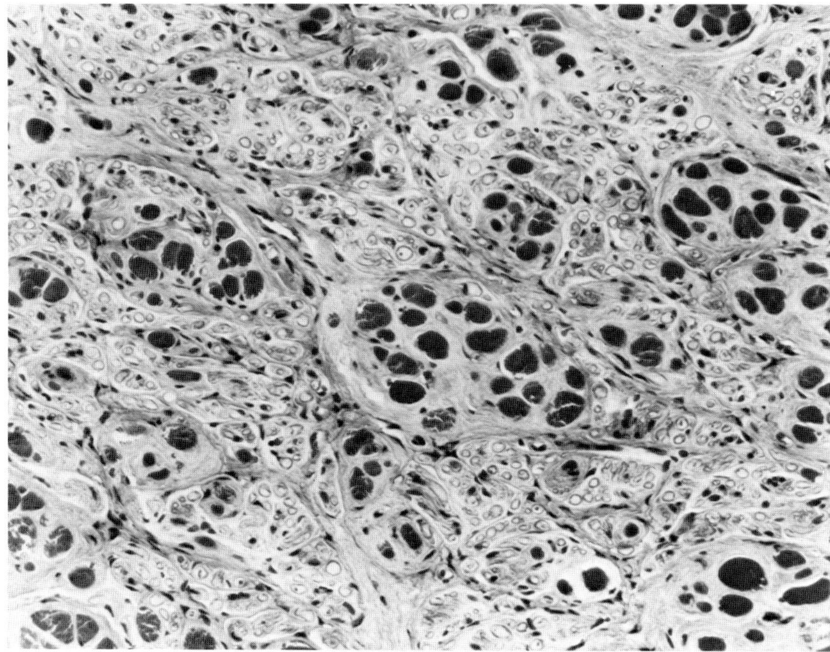

Fig. 9-3. Neuromuscular choristoma. (Case courtesy of R. Bonneau, M.D. and R. Brochu, M.D.)

pearance of a jumble of fascicles, each of which may simulate an individual nerve.[12] An amputation neuroma may be distinguished from a peripheral nerve neoplasm by the presence of axons within most of the Schwann cell fascicles.

MUCOSAL NEUROMA (NEUROMA OF MEN TYPE IIB)

A second type of true neuroma was described by Williams and Pollock in 1966.[17] Not allied to von Recklinghausen's neurofibromatosis (type I NF), mucosal neuroma involves the lips, tongue, oral mucosa, eyelids, cornea, and intestinal tract of patients with type IIB multiple endocrine neoplasia (MEN). MEN type IIB is closely related to MEN type IIA and differs from it in that patients with type IIB have mucosal neuromas. Like MEN type I, both disorders are genetically transmissible and familial. Both MEN types IIA and B are characterized by adrenal hyperplasia and pheochromocytoma, C-cell hyperplasia and medullary carcinoma of the thyroid, and parathyroid hyperplasia.[18]

Young individuals of both sexes develop the syndrome, and they are at great risk of an early death from metastatic thyroid medullary carcinoma unless treated by the second decade of life with a total thyroidectomy. Patients then should be closely followed for the development of a pheochromocytoma,[19] which is bilateral in over 60 percent of patients.

Histologically mucosal neuromas affecting the lips, tongue, and oral mucosa consist of numerous separate, tortuous nerve bundles (Fig. 9-4). Intestinal lesions appear as thick linear bands of hyperplastic nerves that involve myenteric plexuses and are associated with an increased number of ganglionic neurons.[20] The intestinal lesions are referred to as *ganglioneuromatosis*, and they may cause intestinal obstruction.

This is one peripheral nerve disorder in which the pathologist can play a key role in saving lives. He may be the first to recognize the neuromas that herald this disorder, and his findings are often easily confirmed by examination of the lip and tongue of the patient (Fig. 9-5). The clinician can then be alerted to the need to examine siblings of the affected individual.

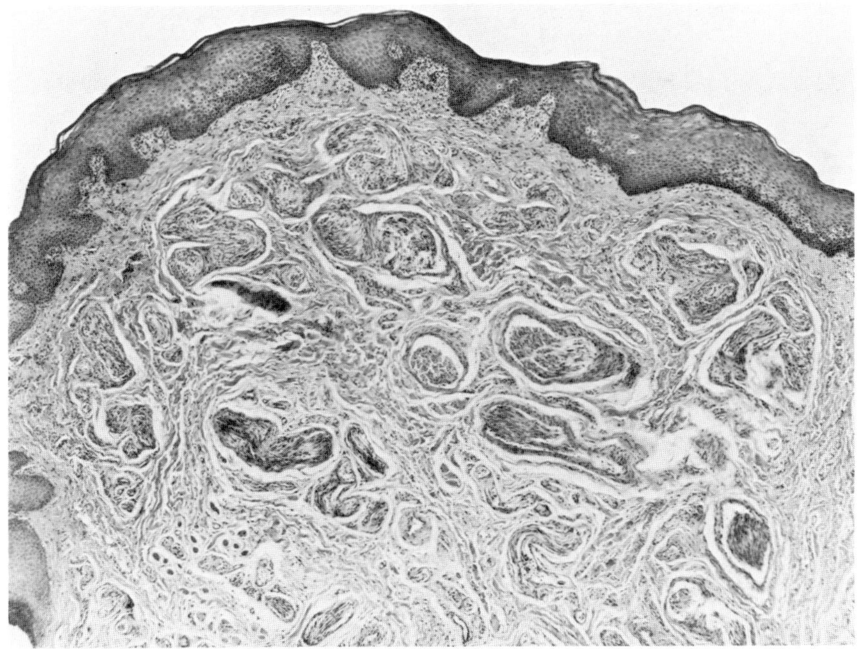

Fig. 9-4. Lingual mucosal neuroma in patient with MEN type IIB.

PALISADED, ENCAPSULATED CUTANEOUS NEUROMA

Described in 1972 by Reed et al.,[21] palisaded, encapsulated cutaneous neuroma (PEN), the third form of true neuroma, characteristically presents as a solitary dermal lesion near a mucocutaneous junction on the face of men and women in the middle decades of life. There usually is a history of a slowly and progressively enlarging, nontender, firm lesion. Microscopically the neuroma is typically sausage shaped with a bulbous expansion forming the main mass (Fig. 9-6). The lesion consists of compact fasi-

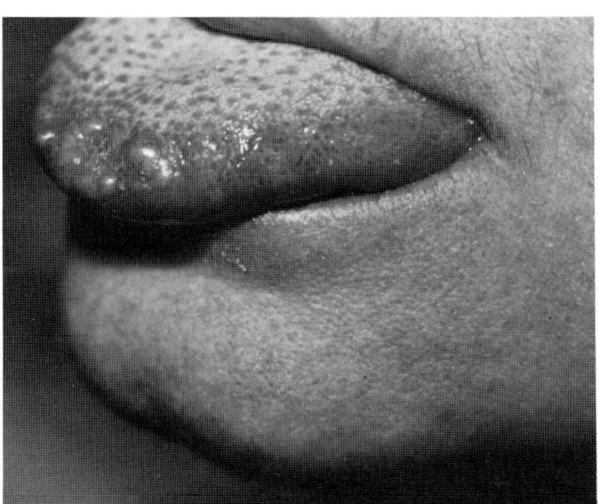

Fig. 9-5. Clinical appearance of lingual mucosal neuroma in a patient with MEN type IIB.

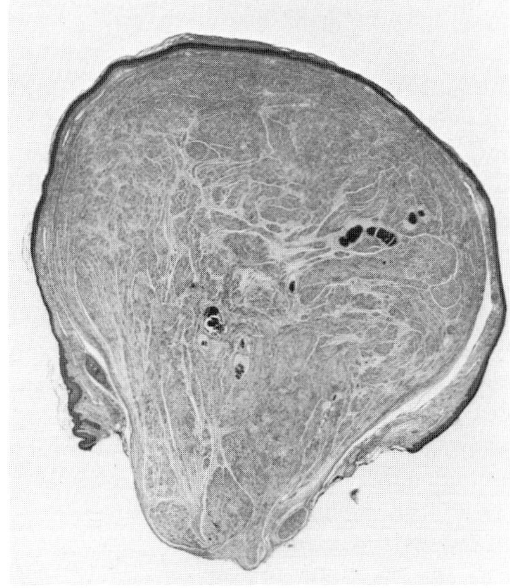

Fig. 9-6. Bulbous PEN of skin. (Case courtesy of A. B. Ackerman, M.D.)

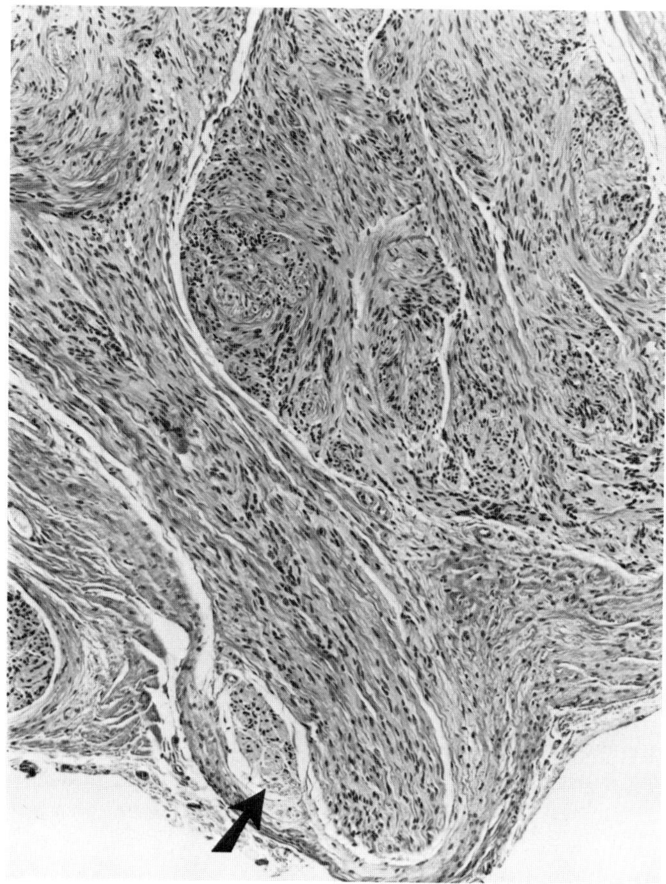

Fig. 9-7. Higher-power magnification of base of the PEN seen in Figure 9-6. Compact fascicles of Schwann cells. Normal nerve (arrow).

cles of Schwann cells (Fig. 9-7) that enwrap axons (Fig. 9-8). Continuity with a peripheral nerve may be seen. The fascicles of Schwann cells may be arranged in subtle palisades. The three lesions most closely resembling PEN are the amputation neuroma, schwannoma, and leiomyoma. Unlike the amputation neuroma, the Schwann cell fascicles of this neuroma are not subdivided by fibrous tissue. A schwannoma will be devoid of intratumoral axons, as will a leiomyoma.

sists of hyperplastic pacinian corpuscles and can take several forms. It can be grapelike and attached to a digital nerve by a fine filament, it can line a stretch of a digital nerve, or it can take the form of a single large corpuscle or multiple corpuscles just beneath the epineurium of a digital nerve.[23] Most of each corpuscle consists of lamellae of perineurial cells (they express epithelial membrane antigen) that surround an axon and its coating Schwann cell.[24, 25]

PACINIAN NEUROMA

Included in the differential diagnosis of finger pain, pacinian neuromas are most often found on the digits.[22] At least half of the cases have a history of antecedent trauma. The lesion con-

LOCALIZED HYPERTROPHIC NEUROPATHY (INTRANEURAL NEUROFIBROMA; ONION BULB PERINEURIAL CELL HYPERPLASIA)

Responsible for muscle weakness and atrophy, but for minimal sensory symptoms, localized hypertrophic neuropathy (LHN) affects pa-

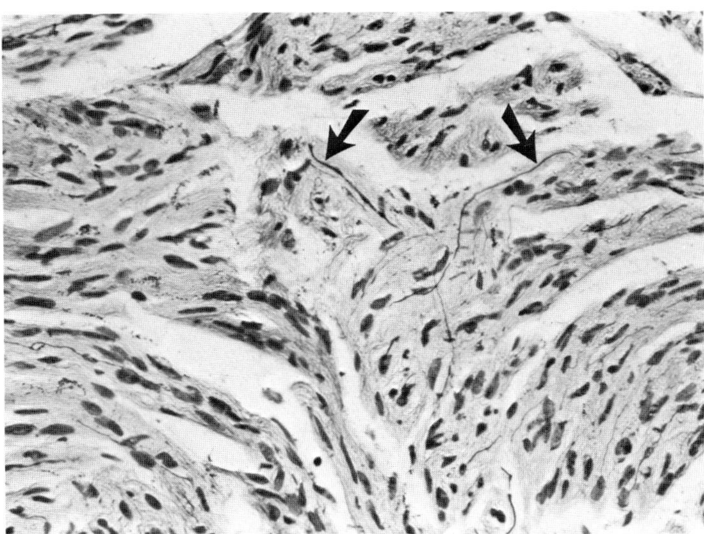

Fig. 9-8. Axonal component (arrows) of a PEN. (Bodian stain.) (Case courtesy of R. J. Reed, M.D.)

tients ranging in age from 10 to 40 years (mean age for 14 cases in the literature is 23 years). LHN arises in males slightly more often than in females. The posterior interosseous is the nerve most often involved. The affected nerve shows a localized cylindrical enlargement, usually measuring no more than a few centimeters in length. Three examples between 10 and 14 cm long have been reported.[26]

Microscopically cross sections of the affected nerve present sheets of onion bulblike structures[26–28] (Fig. 9-9). Ultrastructurally, each "onion bulb" consists of a central axon or axons with their Schwann cell coat, enveloped in turn by layers of cells with long, curved attentuated cell processes[26, 28] (Fig. 9-10). The processes of the enveloping cells possess pinocytotic vesicles,[26] are lined in part by basal

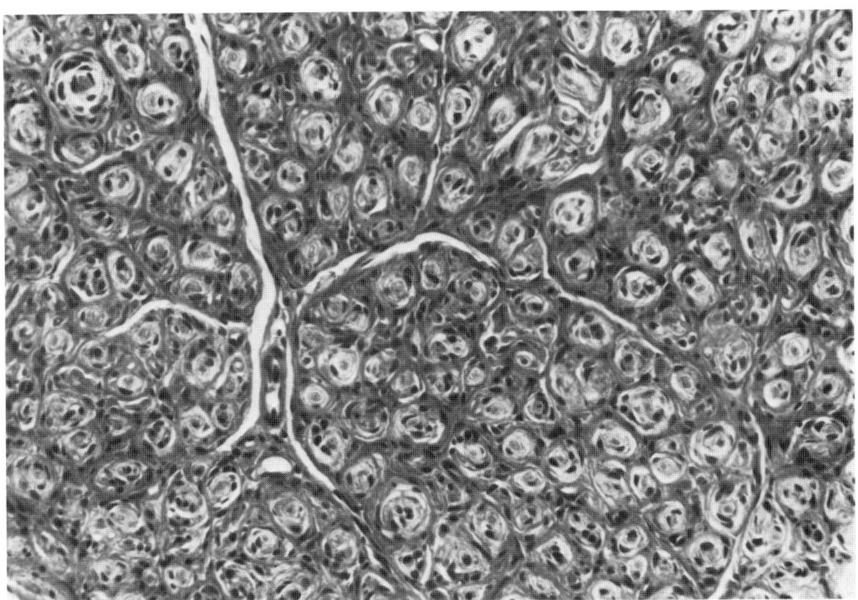

Fig. 9-9. LHN on cross section has the appearance of sheets of onion bulbs. (Case courtesy of B. W. Scheithauer, M.D.)

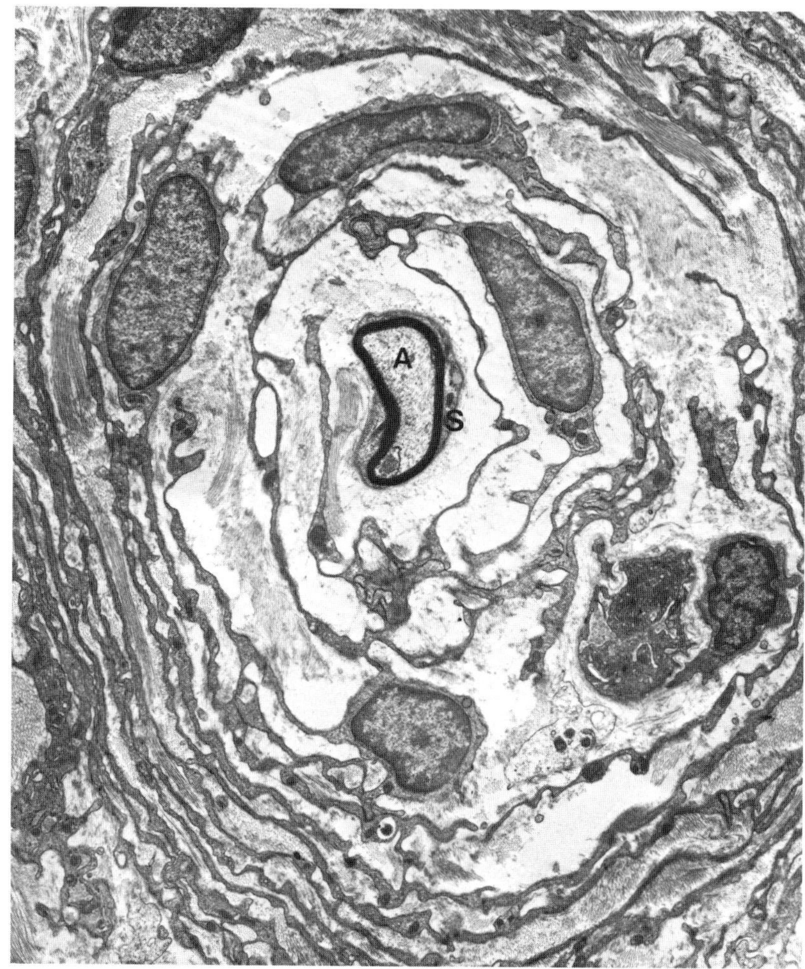

Fig. 9-10. Proliferative cells forming the "onion bulbs" of LHN have the fine structural and immunohistochemical characteristics of perineurial cells. Axon (*A*), Schwann cell (*S*). (Case courtesy of B. W. Scheithauer, M.D.)

lamina,[26, 28] and express epithelial membrane antigen but not S-100 protein.[24] The cells therefore qualify as perineurial cells.

No example of LHN has been reported to undergo malignant transformation, and although the lesion has been variously classified as a neurofibroma[27] or perineurioma,[26, 28] the preservation of a constant spatial relationship between axons and various elements of the nerve sheath in the face of a proliferative process is more in keeping with a hyperplastic than a neoplastic lesion.

NEOPLASTIC TUMORS OF THE PERIPHERAL NERVE

Peripheral nerve tumors (PNT) are among the most varied of all soft tissue tumors, a circumstance brought about by several factors. First, there are several cell types in the peripheral nerve sheath from which tumors may theoretically arise. Second, axonal processes are a component of at least one type of PNT. Third, at least one cellular component of the peripheral nerve sheath, which from all available evidence is probably the Schwann cell, when neoplastic, exhibits a remarkable plasticity of phenotypic expression. Fourth, some malignant melanomas have a growth affinity for the peripheral nerve sheath and may present as primary PNT. This section surveys the varieties of PNT and points out some of the problems faced by pathologists in the evaluation of these tumors.

One major problem results from a long-standing lack of knowledge of the specific cell of origin of most types of PNT. This lack of knowledge is reflected in the use of two forms of the same term, *nerve sheath tumor* (neurilemoma[29] and neurothekeoma[30]), for two quite different PNT. As with soft tissue tumors in general, the most consistently meaningful criterion available for classifying PNT is their cellular differentiation, not their presumed cytogenesis. Such information is best attained by fine structural and immunohistochemical studies.

Schwannomas, for example, consist of a group of mostly benign tumors whose cells on fine structure resemble differentiated Schwann cells either very closely (the classic schwannoma[31] or neurilemoma, and the cellular schwannoma[31, 32]) or closely enough to warrant a designation of schwannoma (melanotic schwannoma[33]). All three tumors also express S-100 protein, but not EMA, thus satisfying the immunohistochemical requirements for Schwann cells. Another tumor, the granular cell tumor, frequently displays some Schwann cell traits,[34] but not enough to warrant a designation of schwannoma, and although most granular cell tumors express S-100 protein, some do not.

Using this approach, it has been shown that the neurofibroma differs significantly from the schwannoma. On fine structure the neurofibroma is hamartomalike, being composed of multiple cell types that include Schwann cells coating axons or wrapped around collagen fibers, unwrapped cells having Schwann cell characteristics, a perineurial-like cell that is usually the predominant cell, and rare fibroblasts.[31] Neurofibromas express S-100 protein, but generally to a lesser extent than schwannomas. Like schwannomas, they do not express epithelial

membrane antigen.[24] Using this approach, relatively specific definitions of the schwannomas and neurofibroma can be drawn, and it is clear that electron microscopy plays a key role in the formulation of these definitions.

MAIN TYPES OF PERIPHERAL NERVE TUMORS

The main types of peripheral nerve tumors or neoplasms are the schwannomas, neurofibroma, and malignant peripheral nerve sheath tumor.

Schwannoma

Classic Schwannoma (Neurilemoma). The classic schwannoma is a widely distributed tumor presenting most often in the middle decade of life and affecting women more often than men. Included in its distribution are intracranial nerves (most often the acoustic nerve); spinal nerves; small and medium-sized nerves of the face, neck, intercostal region; flexor surfaces of extremities (including hands but rarely feet); infrequently nerves of the skin and trunk; and rarely nerves of the lung and heart. A few intracerebral examples have also been reported. The classic schwannoma is a solitary lesion and is unrelated to von Recklinghausen's neurofibromatosis (NF-I).[29] However, schwannomas may be multiple,[35] and bilateral acoustic schwannomas are a recognized feature of type II NF. NF-II is not associated with many peripheral neurofibromas and café au lait spots.[36] The disorder characterized by many schwannomas is designated *schwannomatosis* or *neurilemomatosis*.[35] Classic schwannomas are slowly growing tumors and almost never undergo malignant change.[29, 37]

Grossly the tumors are globoid and encapsulated, and on cut section vary from light tan with hemorrhagic and yellow areas, to a darker tan with cysts and hemorrhages. No necrosis is grossly evident, and frequently no nerve is identified. If very hemorrhagic, a classic schwannoma may be mistaken grossly for a paraganglioma, or thought to be focally necrotic. Classic schwannoma of the acoustic nerve may grow into the cerebellopontine angle, deforming the brain stem and cerebellum.[38] The largest examples of this tumor arise in the posterior mediastinum and pelvis, and may exceed 10 cm in greatest dimension. Uncommonly the tumor may be plexiform.[39–41]

The histology of the classic schwannoma is well known: an encapsulated mass of interlacing spindle cells that pushes the intact nerve from which it arose to one side;[9, 12] alternating loose (Antoni B) and more dense (Antoni A) areas; palisaded nuclei and Verocay bodies; thick-walled, hyalinized blood vessels and hemorrhage; and clusters of foamy histiocytes. Rare examples have foci of calcification. Although Antoni A and B areas are not exclusively found in the classic schwannoma, true Verocay bodies are. Verocay bodies (Fig. 9-11) are formed by roughly parallel columns of palisaded nuclei

that are separated by an anucleated lightly fibrillar eosinophilic tissue: on ultrastructure, the eosinophilic tissue consists of closely packed alternating layers of cytoplasmic processes and thickened basal lamina.[31]

The histology of the classic schwannoma can be mimicked by palisaded examples of both benign and malignant smooth muscle tumors, and by the recently defined palisaded myofibroblastoma of inguinal lymph nodes (PMILN).[42, 43] Palisading in smooth muscle tumors tends to be more exaggerated than that in the classic schwannoma, and the eosinophilic tissue in the center of their Verocaylike bodies is coarsely, not finely, fibrillar. The eosinophilic bodies in the PMILN (Fig. 9-12) are amianthoid collagen[43] rather than cell processes and basal lamina material and, as pointed out by Weiss et al.,[42] earlier misinterpretations of the PMILN as a classic schwannoma led to the erroneous conclusion on the one hand that a classic schwannoma had metastasized to a lymph

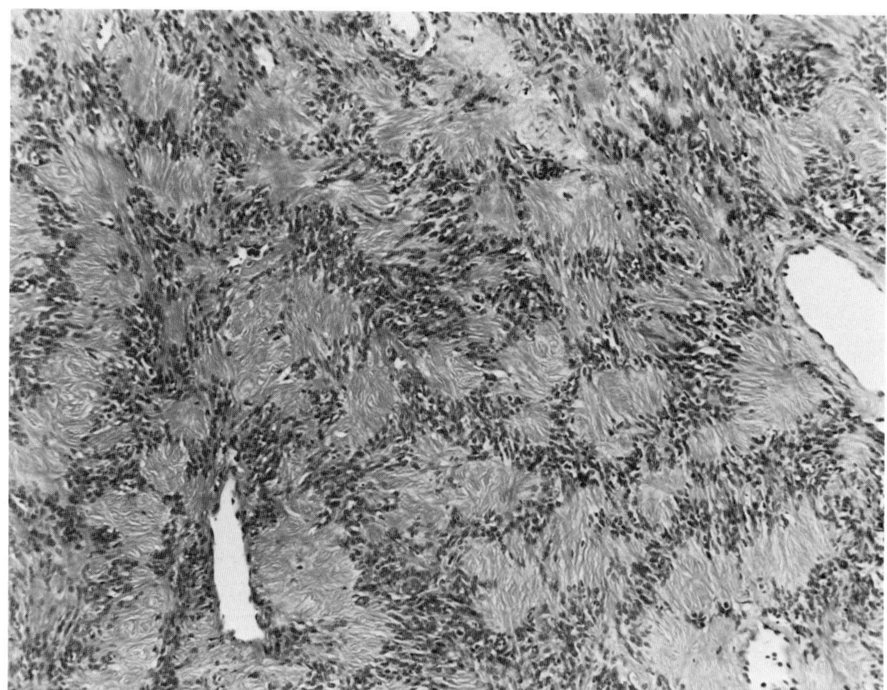

Fig. 9-11. Verocay bodies of a classic schwannoma. Like the inconstant open hand in David's paintings, Verocay bodies are not always found in schwannomas. (From Woodruff et al.,[12] with permission.)

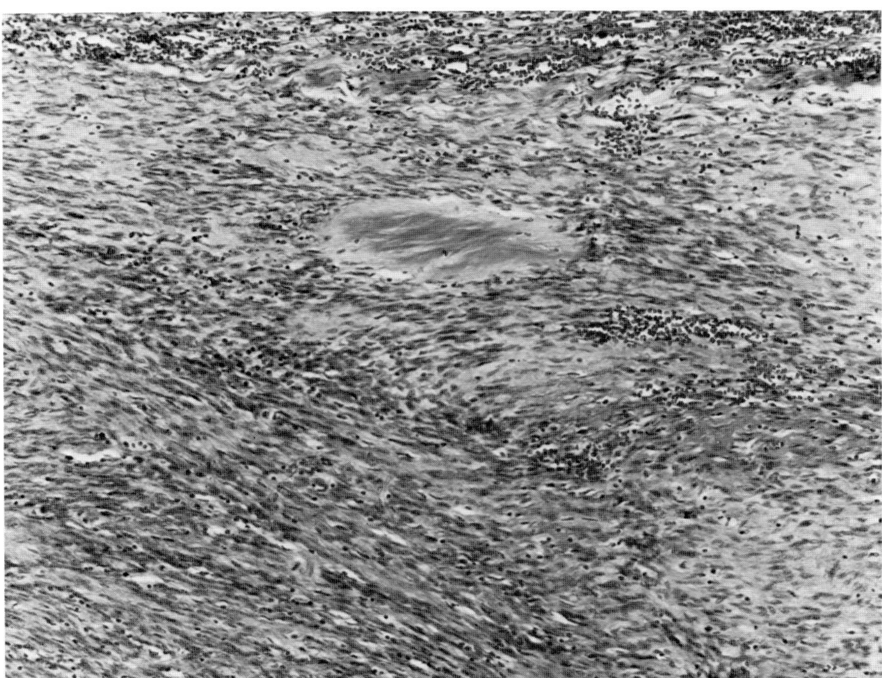

Fig. 9-12. Patch of amianthoid collagen fibers in a palisaded myofibroblastoma of an inguinal lymph node simulates a Verocay body. (Case courtesy of N. S. McNutt, M.D.)

node,[44] and on the other hand that some classic schwannomas arise in lymph nodes.[45] It cannot be overemphasized that classic schwannomas almost never undergo malignant change, and in this writer's experience, with extremely rare exceptions, the presence of hyperchromatic nuclei and mitotic figures carries no prognostic import. Also, this writer has never seen a classic schwannoma involving a lymph node.

Cellular Schwannoma (Cellular Neurilemoma). Sharing many features with the classic schwannoma, cellular schwannoma, described in detail by Woodruff et al.[32] in 1981, and subsequently confirmed as a distinctive lesion by Fletcher et al.,[46] is not uncommonly mistaken for a sarcoma or fibrous histiocytoma. In a recent and as yet unpublished study of 57 such cases, my colleague, Dr. Warren White, and I found a mean age of 44 years and a 63 percent female predominance for this neoplasm. The tumor most commonly occurs in the posterior mediastinum and pelvis, but may also arise on the extremities, including the fingers. They

also involve cranial nerves. An attached nerve was identified clinically in 36 percent of our cases. The most common presenting complaints were a palpable mass and neurologic problems, including pain, paresthesias, and weakness. Examples arising from spinal nerves may erode bone, giving the impression of a malignant tumor. Some cases had been present for years (15 years in one case) before resection. Most of the tumors were completely surgically excised, but some were incompletely removed. Twenty-eight percent of the cases in our study had been diagnosed as malignant, yet follow-up (available for 36 patients and greater than 5 years for 20 patients) revealed re-excisions for local recurrences in three cases, but no metastases or deaths attributable to tumor.

Grossly the tumors are ovoid and encapsulated, and range in size from 1.0 to 19.5 cm. The cut surfaces are usually solid, firm, and tan, with occasional white and yellow patches. Focal hemorrhages are occasionally noted, but there is no gross evidence of necrosis. Rare examples are plexiform, and some of these are in cutaneous sites.

Microscopy reveals a more cellular neoplasm than the classic schwannoma. Interlacing fascicles of spindle cells lacking Verocay bodies predominate in every tumor (Fig. 9-13). This represents Antoni A tissue. Its fascicles may simulate the growth pattern of a smooth muscle tumor, are often focally arranged in a storiform pattern, and may form whorls. Collections of lipid-laden histiocytes and focal fibrosis may be seen.

Frequent findings are a lymphocytic infiltration that is commonly perivascular but may also occur as a dense patchy infiltration and hyalinized blood vessels. The little Antoni B tissue present sometimes has neurofibromatous features and may contain pools of mucin. Moderate hyperchromasia, nuclear pleomorphism, and mitotic activity (up to eight mitotic figures in a single high-power field in one case) are not uncommon, but have no prognostic significance. Nor does focal microscopic necrosis. We have seen focal microscopic necrosis in four cases, and it was represented by a circumscribed necrosis, not the geographic type of necrosis seen in malignant PNST. Major hurdles for the pathologist examining this lesion are a recognition of its neural nature and an appreciation that it is not a sarcoma.

Melanotic Schwannoma. Since the early 1970s there has been an increasing awareness of a melanin-containing and probably melanin-producing (premelanosomes have been found in some cases), usually benign tumor consisting of cells that otherwise have the histologic and ultrastructural features of Schwann cells. This unusual combination of cytocharacteristics is explained as a melanocytic differentiation by a cell (the Schwann cell) sharing a common lineage (neural crest) with the melanocyte. This common lineage theory will prove useful when explaining the unusual histology of some other PNT.

In a literature review of 34 such cases,[47] there was a slight female predominance (19 females and 15 males), an age range of 10 to 84 years, and a mean age of 38 years. The most frequent

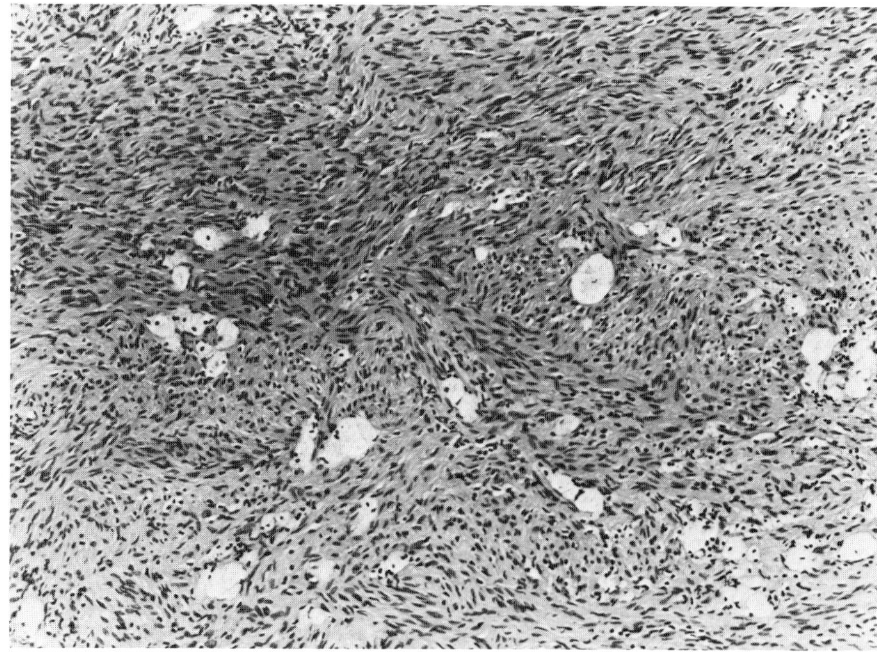

Fig. 9-13. Cellular schwannoma with closely packed interlacing spindle cells and scattered lipid-laden histiocytes.

locations of the tumors were spinal nerve roots and soft tissues, although a few involved the stomach, heart, and acoustic nerve. While the vast majority of the tumors had an indolent growth and were cured by surgical resection, six cases recurred, and a few patients died because of their tumor. Two patients with very similar neoplasms arising from sympathetic ganglia died with metastatic tumor.[48] The tumors typically are encapsulated or circumscribed, with pigmented spindle and epithelioid cells arranged in fascicles and sheets. Nuclear palisading and mitotic figures are not uncommonly found. In addition to the common expression of S-100 protein, one melanotic schwannoma was reported to be positive for HMB-45.

The melanotic schwannoma has been reported to be a component of the familial[49] complex of cardiac and cutaneous myxomas, spotty pigmentation (lentigines and blue nevi), pigmented nodular adenocortical disease with endocrine overactivity, and large cell calcifying Sertoli cell tumors of the testis. This complex was described in 1985 by Carney and his co-workers.[50] Carney has just completed an exhaustive review of 40 psammomatous melanotic schwannomas (PMS) (Fig. 9-14) in 31 patients (aged 10 to 63 years) and found that 55 percent of the patients had the above complex.[51] Many of these cases had been reported before as simply melanomatous schwannomas. The mean age for patients with PMS and the complex was 22 years, a full decade earlier than for patients with ordinary melanotic schwannomas. Multiple tumors were found in 19 percent of patients with PMS. The most common sites for the tumors were the posterior spinal nerve roots and alimentary tract (64 percent of those in the alimentary tract were in the stomach), a different distribution from nonpigmented schwannomas. Two-thirds of the tumors caused symptoms. Most of the tumors were successfully treated by surgical excision, but a few recurred locally, and four patients died with metastatic PSM.

Neurofibroma

In all aspects, neurofibroma is a different tumor from the schwannomas. Clinically it as-

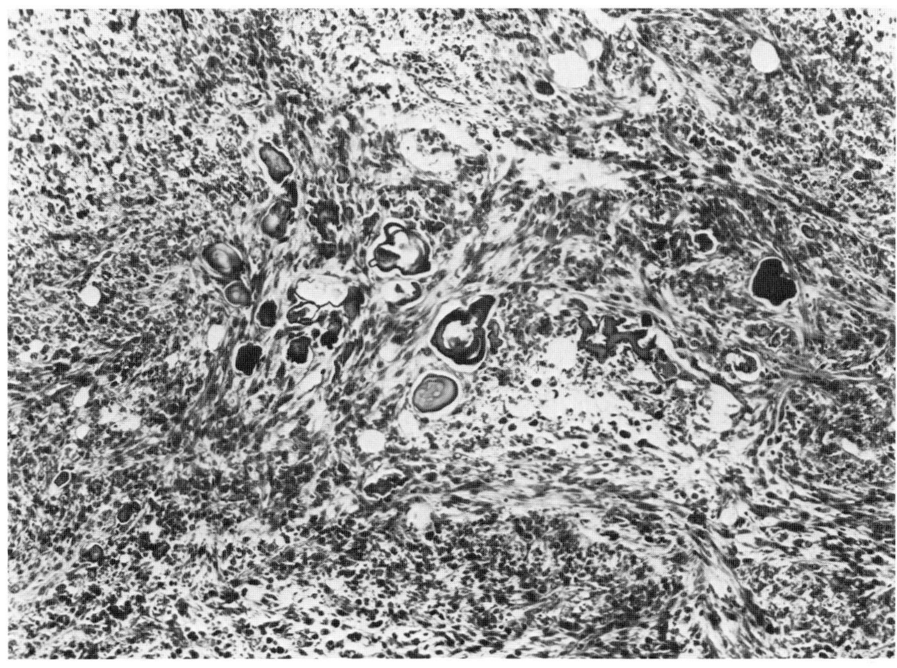

Fig. 9-14. Melanotic schwannoma with psammoma bodies. (Case courtesy of J. A. Carney, M.D.)

sumes at least four forms: (1) discrete cutaneous lesions that are usually sessile but are occasionally polypoid[9, 12] and, in a given patient, are more often solitary than multiple; (2) solitary fusiform enlargements of medium-sized and large nerves[9, 12]; (3) fusiform and globoid enlargements of a plexus of nerves or a series of such enlargements along the course of a single nerve, sometimes imparting a ropy appearance (plexiform neurofibroma)[12]; (4) a diffuse, nondiscrete involvement of the skin, subcutaneous tissues, and soft tissues that may cause a localized gigantism[9, 12] or massive enlargement of a part of the body referred to as *elephantiasis.*[9] Virtually any peripheral nerve may be involved by a neurofibroma, including intestinal nerves. Cranial nerve involvement is very uncommon.

Multiple neurofibromas, plexiform neurofibromas, and diffuse neurofibromas that cause a localized gigantism or elephantiasis are all hallmarks of NF-I. There is a wide age distribution for neurofibromas. Neurofibromas may cause pain, and extremely rarely, deaths may result from compression of vital structures by a plexiform neurofibroma or, more often, as a result of a neurofibroma undergoing malignant transformation.

Grossly neurofibromas are gray-tan, almost translucent, and firm to gelatinous. Those involving medium-sized and large nerves are usually fusiform. An individual tumor can be mistaken grossly for lipoma, a hyperplastic lymph node, dermatofibroma, or dermatofibrosarcoma protuberans.

Histologically neurofibromas vary considerably. The most typical finding is roughly parallel collagen bundles of varying thickness, between and beside which are widely scattered round, ovoid, and more elongated wrinkled nuclei (Fig. 9-15). These nuclei stain darkly. The cells have thin, attenuated bi- and tripolar cell processes that generally are not visable with routinely stained material. The collagen fiber formation often imparts a shredded carrot appearance to the lesion.[12] Accompanying the collagen fibers is a mucinous matrix that may pool. A component of many neurofibromas, best seen in specimens stained for neurofilament, is scattered ax-

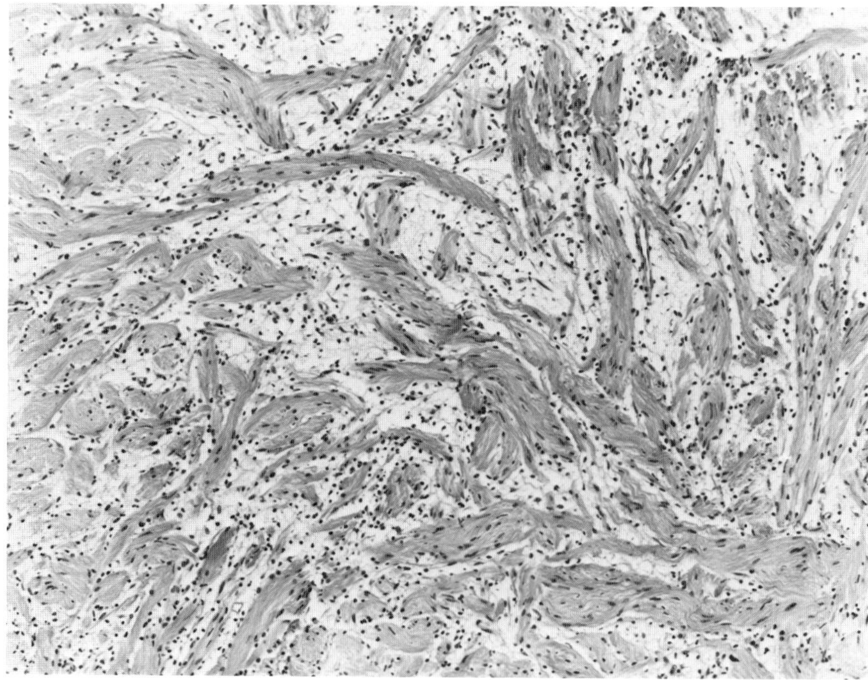

Fig. 9-15. Scattered collagen bundles often give neurofibromas the histologic appearance of shredded carrots.

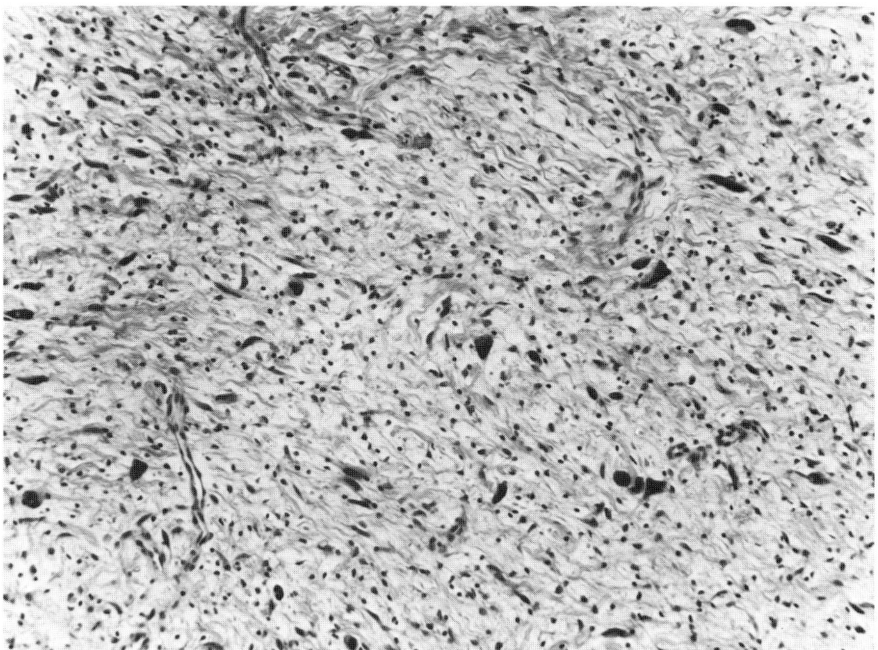

Fig. 9-16. Atypical neurofibroma with scattered, enlarged, pleomorphic, hyperchromatic nuclei.

ons; fine structure shows them to be coated by Schwann cells. The neurofibroma has an insinuative growth that separates axons and often expands the nerve into a fusiform mass encased by its epineurium.[9, 12] At other times the tumor will breach the epineurium and infiltrate soft tissues, a behavior that can be misinterpreted by the inexperienced as aggressive or malignant behavior. Other less common histologic findings are Wagner-Meissner-like corpuscles,[52] structures resembling pacinian corpuscles,[53] epithelial glands,[54] and melanin-containing tumor cells. Atypical neurofibromas[12] (Fig. 9-16) have scattered, enlarged, pleomorphic, hyperchromatic nuclei, but no one has shown that they have a prognosis that is different from other neurofibromas.

Malignant Peripheral Nerve Sheath Tumor; Malignant Schwannoma

This writer prefers the term *malignant peripheral nerve sheath tumor* (malignant PNST) for primary malignant tumors of the peripheral nerve. The often-used term *malignant schwannoma* implies that all malignant PNST arise from the Schwann cell, and does not provide for the possibility that some examples may originate from fibroblasts or perineurial cells of the peripheral nerve sheath.[55] A majority of malignant PNST arise from neurofibromas or in patients with NF-I,[56] but a second, sizeable group of tumors arise directly from the nerve sheath (de novo malignant PNST). Many of the de novo tumors develop in nerves that were in a portal of radiation given most often for Hodgkin's disease, mammary carcinoma, or carcinoma of the uterine cervix and endometrium.[57] Postradiation cases account for 6 to 11 percent of all malignant PNST.[57–59] The classic schwannoma (neurilemoma) almost never undergoes malignant change, so the term *malignant neurilemoma* is of little use. There have, however, been several examples of malignant melanotic schwannoma. Malignant PNST may also arise from ganglioneuromas and ganglioneuroblastomas[60] (the supportive tissues of both tumors is the Schwann cell).

There is a wide range of criteria for the diagnosis of malignant PNST that includes (1) a demonstrated origin from a nerve[9, 12]; (2) origin from a benign PNT or from a ganglioneuroma or ganglioneuroblastoma[60]; (3) existence of a soft tissue sarcoma in a patient with NF-I, if the tumor has the histology typical of a majority of the malignant PNST shown arising from nerves[56, 61]; (4) existence of a soft tissue sarcoma in a patient without NF-I, but displaying a histology similar to that in criterion 3, and, in addition, expressing S-100 protein[5] or Leu-7 antigen[62, 63] (an exception is the malignant Triton tumor). The expression of myelin basic protein is not included as a criterion for the diagnosis of malignant PNST because it has recently been questioned whether malignant PNST express myelin basic protein.[64]

Some pathologists base a diagnosis of malignant PNST strictly on a histology they believe to be consistent with this tumor type. Although this approach may be valid for treatment purposes, published data of this nature should be clearly segregated from the data based on more rigid criteria.[65, 66] Electron microscopy may also be used in diagnosing malignant PNST. Fine structural findings of cells with processes lined by basement membrane substance may be seen in several soft tissue tumors, but its presence may serve as supportive evidence for a diagnosis of malignant PNST. Unfortunately, over 50 percent of the malignant PNST are ultrastructurally undifferentiated.[31]

Malignant PNST afflict females more often than males.[58] This is true whether the patients have NF-I or not. The tumors rarely present before the second decade of life and not in infancy. In patients with NF-I the mean age for presentation is in the late 20s and early 30s, a decade earlier than for the de novo tumors. The tumors often involve larger nerves than those involved by schwannomas, and although widely distributed, they have a proclivity for nerves of the brachial and lumbar plexuses, and sciatic and spinal nerves. The sciatic nerve is the most commonly affected nerve. Malignant PNST are extremely rarely multifocal. The lifetime risk for a malignant PNST developing in a patient with NF-I is about 2 percent.[67]

Pain, dysesthesia, and a mass are the most common presenting complaints. Malignant PNST are highly malignant tumors that often recur locally after surgical resection. A majority eventually metastasize distantly, most often to the lung. Regional lymph node metastasis is rare. In a recent study of 43 malignant PNST of the lower extremity we found an overall survival rate of 57 percent at 24 months, and 39 percent at 60 months.[61] The median survival from diagnosis was 35 months. In one study of 120 patients, the survival rate at 5 years was 34 percent and that at 10 years was 23 percent. We found that patients with tumors less than 10 cm in size did significantly better than those with larger tumors. Several groups report a poorer prognosis for patients with NF-I than for those without NF-I.

Grossly, malignant PNST are spherical, ovoid (Fig. 9-17), fusiform, or sausage shaped. If involving a large nerve, they are often eccentric. We found an average size of 12 cm, but have seen examples as small as 3.4 cm. The cut surfaces are firm, tan-yellow, and in over half of the cases, focally necrotic. Some cases are partly mucoid or gelatinous.

The microscopic appearance of malignant PNST is the most varied of any soft tissue tumor. The most common histology is that of tightly packed, hyperchromatic spindle cells that are usually smaller than smooth muscle cells and are arranged in interlacing and woven fascicles (Fig. 9-18). The nuclei may be wrinkled, especially if there was a pre-existing neurofibroma, and the cytoplasm is devoid of the longitudinal cytoplasmic fibrils seen in leiomyosarcomas. Mitotic figures are virtually always found and, in a majority of the tumors, they number greater than 10 per 10 high-power fields in the most mitotically active areas. Enlarged, pleomorphic nuclei are found in a third of the cases, and geographic necrosis is common. No satisfactory system has yet been derived for grading these tumors,[59] and almost every example should be treated as a sarcoma with a metastatic potential.[61]

The differential diagnosis of malignant PNST is long and includes fibrosarcoma, malignant

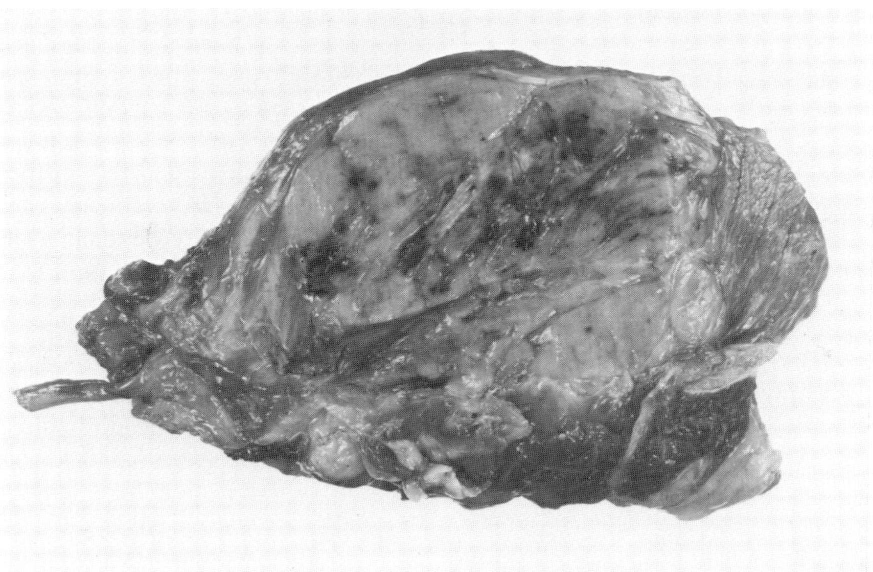

Fig. 9-17. Malignant PNST of the femoral nerve. There is gross evidence of necrosis.

fibrous histiocytoma (MFH), leiomyosarcoma, mono- and biphasic synovial sarcoma, hemangiopericytoma, sweat gland carcinoma, neuroblastoma, and melanoma. Similarities to the first four tumors lie in a similar woven pattern and, in the case of MFH, on the occasional presence of storiform and myxoid areas. Immunohistochemistry may be needed to distinguish these tumors from a PNST. An occasional malignant PNST will have areas simulating hemangioperi-

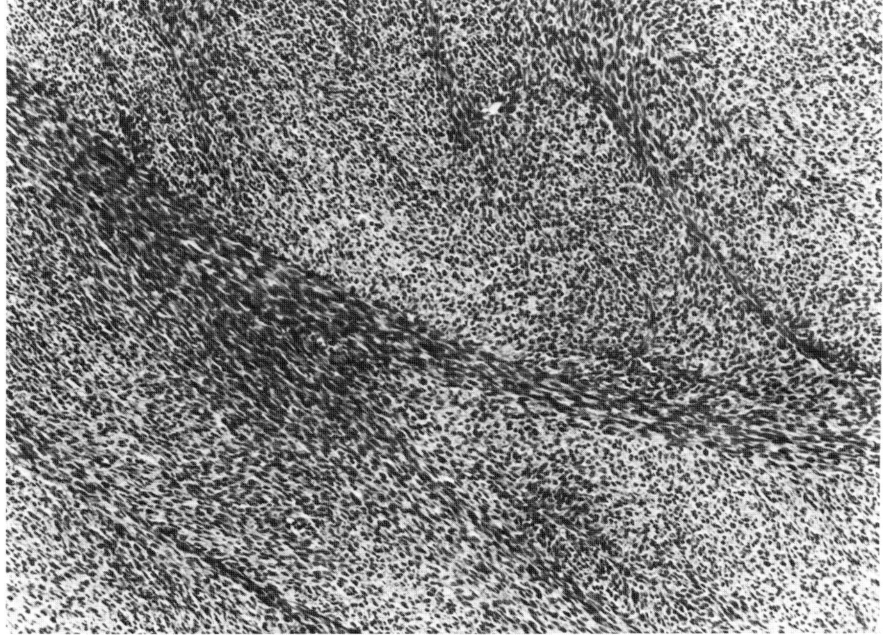

Fig. 9-18. Most common histologic pattern seen in malignant PNST.

cytoma, but this growth pattern is always limited.

The remaining tumors in this list of differential diagnosis owe their presence to the divergent differentiation exhibited by 15 to 28 percent of malignant PNST. Two main categories of differentiation are seen: epithelial and epithelioid cells, and mesenchymal cells. Less than 5 percent of malignant PNST are made up in part or purely of epithelioid cells,[68–70] which are characterized by abundant cytoplasm and sometimes prominent nucleoli. Some epithelioid areas may be myxoid. The purely and extensively epithelioid malignant PNST can mimic metastatic carcinoma, sweat gland carcinoma, amelanotic melanoma, and myxoid forms of MFH, soft tissue chondrosarcoma, and embryonal rhabdomyosarcoma. The fine points of distinguishing the purely and extensively epithelioid malignant PNST from these lesions is discussed at length by DiCarlo et al.[69] The epithelioid cells of about 50 percent of epithelioid MPNST express S-100 protein, and with a metastatic rate of 20 percent, it is this form of malignant PNST that metastasizes most frequently to regional lymph nodes.[70]

Epithelial glands may be found in some PNST, and the vast majority of such tumors are malignant[69] (Fig. 9-19). There is a predominance of females with NF-I in this group of cases. The glands are usually lined by a mixture of simple columnar cells and goblet cells.[71] Squamous metaplasia has been seen in some glands.[72] In 62.5 percent of the cases, neuroendocrine cells that stain most often for somatostatin and serotonin are distributed throughout the glands.[54] The gland lumens often contain carminophilic mucin, and in all cases the glandular epithelium expresses keratins. The glandular malignant PNST must be distinguished from the biphasic synovial sarcoma (BSS). The distinction between these tumors rests in part on the presence in the BSS of a transition from cells of the stroma to those of the glands, and an absence in the BSS of globlet and neuroendocrine cells.

A third type of epithelium seen in malignant PNST is neuroepithelium, which sometimes

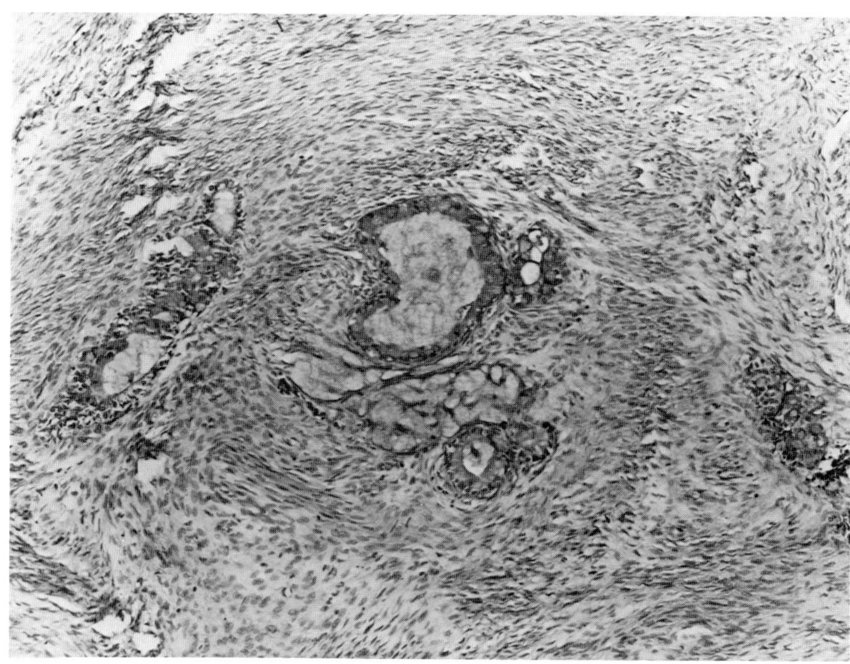

Fig. 9-19. Malignant glandular PNST with intraglandular mucin.

takes the form of Homer-Wright-type rosettes and small undifferentiated cells in an otherwise typical spindle cell tumor.[69] Rare malignant PNT are composed entirely of neuroepithelium. These are discussed in Chapter 10.

Mesenchymal tissues most frequently found in malignant PNST are chondrosarcoma and rhabdomyosarcoma.[72, 73] Malignant PNST containing rhabdomyosarcoma are referred to as malignant Triton tumors.[73, 74] Malignant PNST with osteosarcoma has been reported,[72] and this writer has seen one case with epithelial glands and rhabdomyosarcoma in addition to osteosarcoma.[71] The similarities between the malignant Triton tumor and a pleomorphic rhabdomyosarcoma and between a PNST with chondrosarcoma and a spindle cell chondrosarcoma are striking. Distinction of the malignant PNST from these various mimickers rests on identifying a nerve of origin, or antecedent neurofibroma, or even on an immunohistochemical evaluation. Malignant Triton tumors are highly malignant.[75]

OTHER TUMORS REGARDED AS OF PERIPHERAL NERVE SHEATH ORIGIN OR THAT MAY PRESENT AS A PERIPHERAL NERVE TUMOR

PERINEURIOMA

Perineurioma, an as yet incompletely defined tumor type of adults, is thought to be a neoplasm composed almost exclusively of cells having the characteristics of perineurial cells. The lesion was described in 1978 by Lazarus and Trombetta,[76] and a handful of other reports followed. In almost all cases, the diagnosis has rested on ultrastructural findings; one exception is the report by Weidenheim and Campbell[77] in which an example of this tumor was found not to express S-100 protein. What is needed for final proof of the cell type is evidence that the tumor cells also express epithelial membrane antigen. This writer agrees with Weidenheim and Campbell that the category of perineurioma

should not include the entity of LHN (see the section on LHN above). Perineuriomas are circumscribed tumors that closely resemble neurofibromas microscopically. The constituent cells are uniformly spindle shaped with thin, elongated processes. They are fasciculated, may whorl and pinwheel, and are separated by a variable amount of intercellular collagen.

Until recently, all reported cases of perineurioma were benign. In 1989 Hirose et al.[55] reported a malignant tumor that had the immunohistochemical profile and some of the fine structural features of perineurial cells. It is not clear whether this neoplasm is a malignant form of the tumor described by Lazarus and Trombetta.

DERMAL NERVE SHEATH MYXOMA (NEUROTHEKEOMA)

A benign multilobulated myxoid tumor described by Harkin and Reed in 1969,[9] dermal nerve sheath myxoma presents as a solitary cutaneous lesion most often on the face and upper extremities of young females.[30, 78] There are two histologic forms, and both are usually lobulated: one is composed of loosely arranged stringy syncytial-like and stellate cells with some epithelioid cells, embedded in an abundant myxoid matrix (Fig. 9-20); the other is composed of more closely arranged epithelioid or plump nevoid cells, separated by a less conspicuous myxomatous matrix. The latter is referred to as a *neurothekeoma*.[30] Some neurothekeomas are so cellular as to simulate intradermal or Spitz nevi. Immunohistochemical findings have been variable, ranging from no expression of S-100 protein to focal expression of S-100 protein. Recently the expression of S-100 protein in the stellate and plump cells within myxoid lobules, associated with the expression of EMA in cells surrounding the lobules[25] has been reported. In this last study the epithelioid cells of two more cellular examples failed to stain for S-100 protein. Fine structural studies support a nerve sheath origin for this tumor.[79]

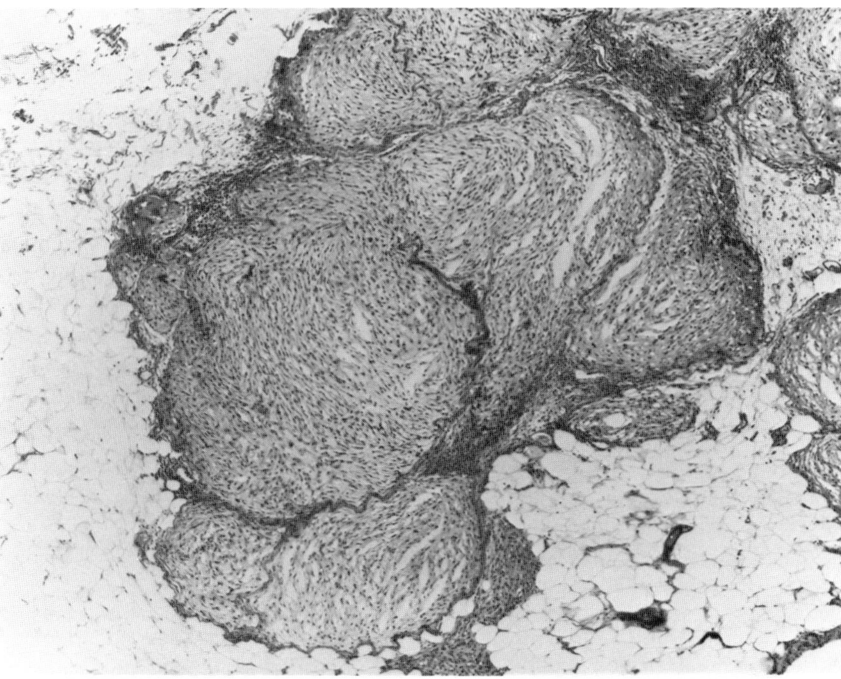

Fig. 9-20. Nerve sheath myxoma with subcutaneous extension.

GRANULAR CELL TUMOR

The granular cell tumor, described in 1926 by Abrikossoff, and thought by him to be of myogenic origin, is now regarded as a nerve sheath tumor. The granular cell tumor commonly occurs in the tongue, skin, and breast, but also in such sites as the upper respiratory tract, gastrointestinal tract, urinary bladder, and muscle. A similar lesion, probably of astrocytic origin, occurs in the posterior lobe and stalk of the pituitary.[80] The evidence for a nerve sheath origin includes the occasional intimate involvement of peripheral nerves, immunoreactivity for S-100 protein[81] and Leu-7 antigen,[82] and a fine structure consistent with the Schwann cell.[83] There is disagreement about the presence of immunoreactive myelin basic protein in the lesions. Although most granular cell tumors are benign, at least 21 clinically malignant cases were reported between 1945 and 1981.[84] A granular cell leiomyosarcoma should be ruled out before making a diagnosis of malignant granular cell tumor.

Granular cell tumors are characterized histologically by stellate, roughly circumscribed, or infiltrative collections of polyhedral cells with an abundant granular, eosinophilic cytoplasm, well-defined cell membranes, and usually round, dark nuclei. Small eosinophilic bodies may sometimes be seen in the cytoplasm on routinely stained material. The cytoplasm stains with the periodic acid-Schiff reaction with or without diastase, and it routinely expresses carcinoembryonic antigen. Approximately half of the malignant granular cell tumors have cytologically malignant characteristics. Ultrastructural features to look for in granular cell tumors are large numbers of autophagosomes, residual bodies, ceroid-lipofuscin inclusions, angulate bodies, and cell processes lined by basement membrane.[83]

NEUROTROPIC MELANOMA (NEUROID MELANOMA)

With neurotropic melanoma we are not referring to a primary PNST, but rather to a subgroup of desmoplastic melanomas that histologically have a neuromalike fasciculated growth and an affinity for growth along peripheral nerves. In their initial report in 1979, Reed and Leonard[85] pointed out that this lesion was most commonly associated with lentigo maligna melanoma, but could also occur in association with what they referred to as a "minimal deviation melanoma," and also with a dermal melanoma lacking clear intraepidermal melanoma (a de novo group). A majority of lesions present in the head and neck (on sun-exposed surfaces) of males, and the peak incidence is in the sixth and seventh decades. Reed and Leonard's cases involved cutaneous nerves, and they thought the melanoma cells had neuroid features. They believed the neuroid features of the tumor represented an expression of Schwann cell characteristics by a neoplastic cell (melanoma cell) sharing a common lineage (the neural crest). Subsequent fine structural findings in some cases of many cell processes and some basement membrane[86] supported their contention of a nerve sheath differentiation. Of considerable interest in this regard is the report of presumed nerve sheath cell differentiation in six desmoplastic melano-

mas,[87] only four of which were neurotropic. This suggests that physical contact with nerves is not necessary for the development of neuroid features, thereby permitting a wider latitude for designating melanomas as neuroid. Nonetheless, the term *neurotropic melanoma* should be reserved for those cases involving peripheral nerves. We have seen tumors identical to neurotropic melanomas growing along and in nerves of the head and neck (Fig. 9-21), and in the intracranial portion of the trigeminal nerve, in patients without a known cutaneous melanoma. It is likely that some tumors reported as malignant PNST of the head[88] are really neurotropic melanomas.

Microscopically the neurotropic melanoma grows as curved fascicles of somewhat plump spindle cells containing oval nuclei, often prominent nucleoli, and a pale eosinophilic to gray cytoplasm. Most tumors have cells that express S-100 protein. The tumor grows along the perineurium of nerves and into the endoneurium, disrupting the nerve fibers. The disease is characterized by multiple local recurrences, progressive proximal extension along nerves, and

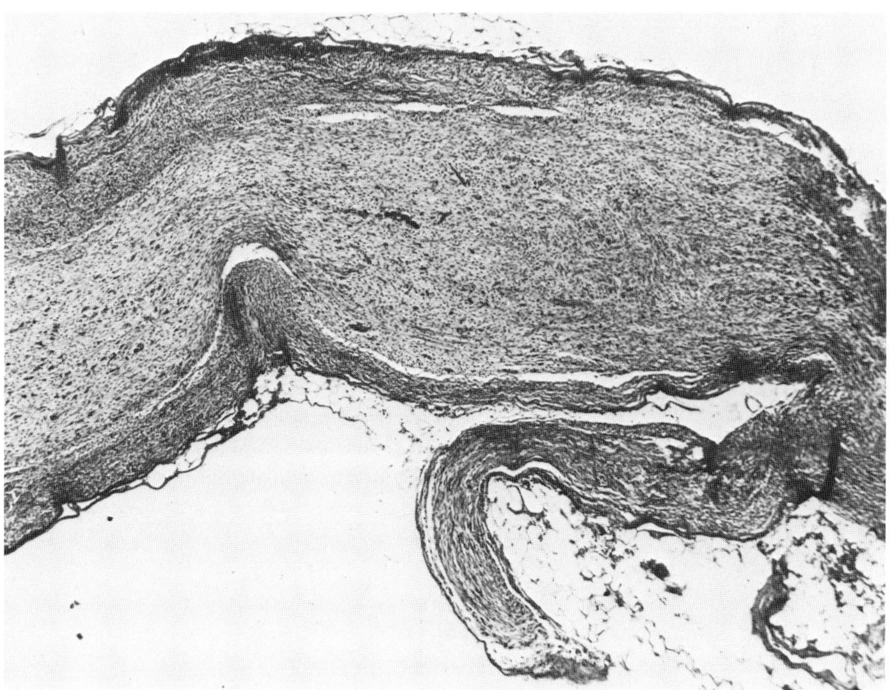

Fig. 9-21. Neurotropic melanoma involving a cranial nerve.

distant metastasis. Of 16 patients followed by Reed and Leonard, 56 percent of the patients died with tumor.

REFERENCES

1. Shanthaveerappa TR, Bourne GH: Perineural epithelium: a new concept of its role in the integrity of the peripheral nervous system. Science 154:1464, 1966
2. Weston JA: The migration and differentiation of neural crest cells. Adv Morphogenet 8:41, 1970
3. Le Douarin NM: Cell recognition based on natural morphological nuclear markers. Med Biol 52:281, 1974
4. Bunge MB, Wood PM, Tynan LB, et al: Perineurium originates from fibroblasts: demonstration in vitro with a retroviral marker. Science 243:229, 1989
5. Weiss SW, Langeloss JM, Enzinger FM: Value of S-100 protein in the diagnosis of soft tissue tumors with particular reference to benign and malignant schwann cell tumors. Lab Invest 49:299, 1983
6. Perentes E, Nakagawa Y, Ross GW, et al: Expression of epithelial membrane antigen in perineurial cells and their derivatives. An immunohistochemical study with multiple markers. Acta Neuropathol 75:160, 1987
7. Barrett R, Cramer F: Tumors of the peripheral nerves and so-called "ganglia" of the peroneal nerve. Clin Orthop 27:135, 1963
8. Cobb CA, Moiel RH: Ganglion of the peroneal nerve. Neurosurgery 41:255, 1974
9. Harkin JC, Reed RJ: Tumors of the Peripheral Nervous System. Atlas of Tumor Pathology. 2nd series, fascicle 3. Armed Forces Institute of Pathology, Washington, DC, 1969
10. Scotti TM: The lesion of Morton's metatarsalgia (Morton's toe). Arch Pathol Lab Med 63:91, 1957
11. Graham WD, Johnson CD: Plantar digital neuroma. Lancet 2:470, 1957
12. Woodruff JM, Horten BC, Erlandson RA: Pathology of peripheral nerves and paragangliomas. In Silverberg SG (ed): Principles and Practice of Surgical Pathology. 2nd Ed. Churchill Livingstone, New York, 1990
13. Silverman TA, Enzinger FM: Fibrolipomatous hamartoma of nerve. A clinicopathologic analysis of 26 cases. Am J Surg Pathol 9:7, 1985
14. Louhima I, Rapola J: Intraneural muscular hamartoma: report of two cases in small children. J Pediatr Surg 7:696, 1972
15. Markel SF, Enzinger FM: Neuromuscular hamartoma—a benign "Triton tumor" composed of mature neural and striated muscle elements. Cancer 49:140, 1982
16. Bonneau R, Brochu P: Neuromuscular choristoma. A clinco-pathologic study of two cases. Am J Surg Pathol 7:521, 1983
17. Williams ED, Pollock DJ: Multiple mucosal neuromata with endocrine tumors: a syndrome allied to von Recklinghausen's disease. J Pathol 91:71, 1966
18. Khairi MRA, Dexter RN, Burzynski, et al: Mucosal neuroma, pheochromocytoma and medullary thyroid carcinoma: MEN type III. Medicine 54:89, 1975
19. Carney JA, Sizemore GW, Tyce GM: Bilateral adrenal medullary hyperplasia in multiple endocrine neoplasm, type 2. The precursor of endocrine neoplasia, type 2b. Mayo Clin Proc 50:3, 1975
20. Carney JA, Hayles AB: Alimentary tract manifestations of multiple endocrine neoplasia, type 2b. Mayo Clin Proc 52:543, 1977
21. Reed RJ, Fine RM, Meltzer HD: Palisaded, encapsulated neuromas of the skin. Arch Dermatol 106:865, 1972
22. Hart WR, Thompson NW, Hildreth DH, Abell MR: Hyperplastic pacinian corpuscles: a cause of digital pain. Surgery 70:730, 1971
23. Schuler FA III, Adamson JE: Pacinian neuroma, an unusual cause of finger pain. Plast Reconstr Surg 62:576, 1978
24. Aziza A, Bilboa JM, Rosai J: Immunohistochemical detection of epithelial membrane antigen in normal perineurial cells and perineuroma. Am J Surg Pathol 12:678, 1988
25. Theaker JM, Fletcher CDM: Epithelial membrane antigen expression by the perineurial cell: further studies of peripheral nerve lesions. Histopathology 14:581, 1989
26. Mitsumoto H, Wilbourn AJ, Goren H: Perineurioma as the cause of localized hypertrophic neuropathy. Muscle Nerve 3:403, 1980
27. Lallemand RC, Weller RO: Intraneural neurofibromas involving the posterior interosseous nerve. J Neurol Neurosurg Psychiatry 36:991, 1973
28. Bilbao JM, Khoury NJS, Hudson AR, Briggs SJ: Perineurioma (localized hypertrophic neuropathy). Arch Pathol Lab Med 108:557, 1984

29. Stout AP: The peripheral manifestations of the specific nerve sheath tumor (neurilemoma). Am J Cancer 24:751, 1935
30. Gallagher RL, Helwig NB: Neurothekeoma—a benign cutaneous tumor of neural origin. Am J Clin Pathol 74:759, 1980
31. Erlandson RA, Woodruff JM: Peripheral nerve sheath tumors: an electron microscopic study of 43 cases. Cancer 49:273, 1982
32. Woodruff JM, Godwin TA, Erlandson RA, et al: Cellular schwannoma. A variety of schwannoma sometimes mistaken for a malignant tumor. Am J Surg Pathol 5:733, 1981
33. Burns DK, Silva FG, Forde KA, et al: Primary melanocytic schwannoma of the stomach. Cancer 52:1432, 1983
34. Fisher ER, Wechsler H: Granular cell myoblastoma—a misnomer. Cancer 15:936, 1962
35. Shishiba T, Niimura M, Ohtsuka F, Tsuru N: Multiple cutaneous neurilemomas as a skin manifestation of neurilemomatosis. J Am Acad Dermatol 10:744, 1984
36. Riccardi VM, Eichner JE: Neurofibromatosis: Phenotype, Natural History and Pathogenesis. John Hopkins Univ. Press, Baltimore, 1986
37. Carstens, PH, Schrodt GR: Malignant transformation of a benign encapsulated neurilemoma. Am J Clin Pathol 51:144, 1969
38. Slooff JL: Pathological anatomical findings in the cerebellopontine angle. Adv Otorhinolaryngol 34:89, 1984
39. Woodruff JM, Marshall ML, Godwin TA, et al: Plexiform (multinodular) schwannoma. A tumor simulating the plexiform neurofibroma. Am J Surg Pathol 7:691, 1983
40. Fletcher CDM, Davies SE: Benign plexiform (multinodular) schwannoma: a rare tumor unassociated with neurofibromatosis. Histopathology 10:971, 1986
41. Iwashita T, Enjoji M: Plexiform neurilemoma: a clinicopathological and immunohistochemical analysis of 23 tumors from 20 patients. Virchows Arch [A] 411:305, 1987
42. Weiss SW, Gnepp DR, Bratthauer GL: Palisaded myofibroblastoma. A benign mesenchymal tumor of lymph node. Am J Surg Pathol 13:341, 1989
43. Suster S, Rosai J: Intranodal hemorrhagic spindle-cell tumor with ''amianthoid'' fibers. Report of six cases of a distinctive mesenchymal neoplasm of the inguinal region that simulates Kaposi's sarcoma. Am J Surg Pathol 13:347, 1989
44. Deligdish L, Loewenthal M, Friedlaender E: Malignant neurilemoma (schwannoma) in the lymph nodes. Int Surg 49:226, 1968
45. Enzinger FM, Weiss SW: Soft Tissue Tumors. 2nd Ed. p. 734. CV Mosby, St. Louis, 1988
46. Fletcher CDM, Davies SE, McKee PH: Cellular schwannoma: a distinct pseudosarcomatous entity. Histopathology 11:21, 1987
47. Killeen RM, Davy CL, Bauserman SC: Melanocytic schwannoma. Cancer 62:174, 1988
48. Fu Y, Kaye GI, Lattes R: Primary malignant melanocytic tumors of the sympathetic ganglia, with an ultrastructural study of one. Cancer 36:2029, 1975
49. Danoff A, Jormark S, Lorber D, Fleischer N: Adrenocortical micronodular dysplasia, cardiac myxomas, lentigines, and spindle cell tumors. Arch Intern Med 147:443, 1987
50. Carney JA, Gordon H, Carpenter PC, et al: The complex of myxomas, spotty pigmentation, and endocrine overactivity. Medicine 64:270, 1985
51. Carney JA: Psammomatous melanotic schwannoma: a distinctive, heritable tumor with special associations, including cardiac myxoma and the Cushing syndrome. Am J Surg Pathol 14:206, 1990
52. Watabe K, Kumanishi T, Ikuta F, Oyake Y: Tactile-like corpuscles in neurofibromas: immunohistochemical demonstration of S-100 protein. Acta Neuropathol 61:173, 1983
53. Weiser G: An electron microscope study of ''pacinian neurofibroma.'' Virchows Arch [A] 366:331, 1975
54. Christensen WN, Strong EW, Bains MS, Woodruff JM: Neuroendocrine differentiation in the glandular peripheral nerve sheath tumor. Pathologic distinction from the biphasic sarcoma with glands. Am J Surg Pathol 12:417, 1988
55. Hirose T, Sumitomo M, Kudo E, et al: Malignant peripheral nerve sheath tumor (MPNST) showing perineurial cell differentiation. Am J Surg Pathol 13:613, 1989
56. Guccion JG, Enzinger FM: Malignant schwannoma associated with von Recklinghausen's neurofibromatosis. Virchows Arch [A] 383:43, 1979
57. Foley KM, Woodruff JM, Ellis FT, Posner J: Radiation induced malignant and atypical PNST. Ann Neurol 7:311, 1980
58. Ducatman B, Scheithauer BW: Postirraadiation neurofibrosarcoma. Cancer 51:1028, 1983
59. Ducatman BS, Scheithauer BW, Piepgras DG, et al: Malignant peripheral nerve sheath tumors. A clinicopathologic study of 120 cases. Cancer 57:2006, 1986

60. Ricci A, Parham DW, Woodruff JM: Malignant peripheral nerve sheath tumors arising from ganglioneuromas. Am J Surg Pathol 8:19, 1984

61. Hruban RA, Shiu MH, Seine RT, Woodruff JM: Malignant peripheral nerve sheath tumors of the buttock and lower extremity: A study of 46 cases. Cancer 66:1253, 1990

62. Perentes E, Rubinstein LJ: Immunohistochemical recognition of human nerve sheath tumors by anti-Leu 7 (HNK-1) monoclonal antibody. Acta Neuropathol 68:319, 1985

63. Wick MR, Swanson PE, Scheithauer BW, Manivel JC: Malignant peripheral nerve sheath tumor. An immunohistochemical study of 62 cases. Am J Clin Pathol 87:425, 1987

64. Perentes E, Rubinstein LJ: Recent applications of immunoperoxidase histochemistry in human neuro-oncology. An update. Arch Pathol Lab Med 111:796, 1987

65. Daimaru Y, Hashimoto H, Enjoji M: Malignant peripheral nerve-sheath tumors (malignant schwannomas). An immunohistochemical study of 29 cases. Am J Surg Pathol 9:434, 1985

66. Matsunou H, Shimoda T, Kakimoto S, et al: Histopathologic and immunohistochemical study of malignant tumors of peripheral nerve sheath (malignant schwannoma). Cancer 56:2269, 1985

67. Sorensen SA, Mulvihill JJ, Nielsen A: Long-term follow-up of von Recklinghausen neurofibromatosis. N Engl J Med 314:1010, 1986

68. Enzinger FM, Weiss SW: Soft Tissue Tumors. 2nd Ed. p. 798. CV Mosby, St. Louis, 1988

69. DiCarlo EF, Woodruff JM, Bansal M, Erlandson RA: The purely epithelioid malignant peripheral nerve sheath tumor. Am J Surg Pathol 10:478, 1986

70. Lodding P, Kindblom L, Angervall L: Epithelioid malignant schwannoma. A study of 14 cases. Virchows Arch [A] 409:433, 1986

71. Woodruff JM: Peripheral nerve tumors showing glandular differentiation (glandular schwannomas). Cancer 37:2399, 1976

72. Ducatman BS, Scheithauer BW: Malignant peripheral nerve sheath tumors with divergent differentiation. Cancer 54:1049, 1984

73. Woodruff JM, Chernik NL, Smith MC, et al: Peripheral nerve tumors with rhabdomyosarcomatous differentiation (malignant "Triton" tumors). Cancer 32:426, 1973

74. Daimaru Y, Hashimoto H, Enjoji M: Malignant-

"Triton" tumors: a clinicopathologic and immunohistochemical study of nine cases. Hum Pathol 15:768, 1984

75. Brooks JSJ, Freeman M, Enterline HT: Malignant "Triton" tumors. Natural history and immunohistochemistry of nine new cases with literature review. Cancer 55:2543, 1985

76. Lazarus SS, Trombetta LD: Ultrastructural identification of a benign perineurial cell tumor. Cancer 41:1823, 1978

77. Weidenheim KM, Campbell WC: Perineurial cell tumor. Immunocytochemical and ultrastructural characterization. Relationship to other peripheral nerve tumors with a review of the literature. Virchows Arch [A] 408:375, 1986

78. Pultizer DR, Reed RJ: Nerve sheath myxoma (perineurial myxoma). Am J Dermatol 7:409, 1985

79. Angervall L, Kindblom L, Haglid K: Dermal nerve sheath myxoma. A light and electron microscopic, histochemical and immunohistochemical study. Cancer 53:1752, 1984

80. Harland WA: Granular-cell myoblastoma of the hypophyseal stalk. Cancer 6:1134, 1953

81. Stefansson K, Wollmann RL: S-100 protein in granular cell tumors (granular cell myoblastoma). Cancer 49:1834, 1982

82. Smolle J, Konrad K, Kerl H: Granular cell tumors contain myelin-associated glycoprotein. Virchows Arch [A] 406:1, 1985

83. Erlandson RA: Diagnostic Transmission Electron Microscopy of Human Tumors. Masson, New York, 1981

84. Robertson AJ, McIntosh W, Lamont P, Guthrie W: Malignant granular cell tumor (myoblastoma) of the vulva: a report of a case and review of the literature. Histopathology 5:69, 1981

85. Reed RJ, Leonard DD: Neurotropic melanoma. A variant of desmoplastic melanoma. Am J Surg Pathol 3:301, 1979

86. Warner TFCS, Hafez GR, Finch RE, Brandenberg JH: Schwann cell features in neurotropic melanoma. J Cutan Pathol 8:177, 1981

87. DiMaio SM, Mackay B, Smith JL, Dickersin GR: Neurosarcomatous transformation in malignant melanoma. An ultrastructural study. Cancer 50:2345, 1982

88. David DJ, Speculand B, Vernon-Roberts B, Sach RP: Malignant schwannoma of the inferior dental nerve. Br J Plast Surg 31:323, 1978

10

Peripheral Primitive Neuroectodermal Tumors

Andrea O. Cavazzana, Ambrogio S. Fassina, and Vito Ninfo

Primitive neuroectodermal tumors (PNET) constitute a controversial and poorly defined class of tumors of neuroectodermal origin occurring in the central nervous system (CNS) and peripheral sites.[1] Although the term *PNET* has been criticized as an oversimple definition for lesions located in the CNS,[2] it appears the most appropriate to indicate a family of extracranial and extraspinal small round cell tumors of neural crest origin.

EMBRYOLOGY

The neural crest is a transitory embryonal structure located on the top of the neural ridges, between the dorsolateral ectoderm and the neural tube. Cells composing this structure show a capacity for migration and multipotential development; depending on their relative position, cells migrate along precise pathways to reach their final destination, where they differentiate into a variety of phenotypes (Fig. 10-1).[3] In fact, the neural crest gives origin to the sensory, parasympathetic, and sympathetic ganglia of the peripheral nervous system (PNS); skin melanocytes; Schwann cells; and neuroendocrine cells, such as adrenal medulla cells, type I paraganglia cells, and calcitonin-producing "C" cells of the thyroid. Moreover, the cephalic portion of the neural crest yields mesenchymal derivates (*mesectoderm*), including the membranous bones of the face and the connective tissues of the buccal and pharyngeal regions, and also contributes to the skeletal muscles of the face, jaw, and tongue.[4]

According to their different anatomoclinical settings and biological characteristics, peripheral PNET can be conveniently classified in three major categories: neuroblastomatous tumors, non-neuroblastomatous tumors, and PNET with "divergent differentiation" (Table 10-1). Retinoblastoma and olfactory neuroblastoma are excluded from this group, and can be more properly allocated to the central PNET category.

Despite their anatomoclinical differences, these tumors share many aspects, from in vitro growth characteristics to morphologic and immunocytochemical features.

In vitro, peripheral PNET show long cellular processes (*neurites*) that form a delicate network among the cellular bodies (Fig. 10-2). This well-known phenomenon occurs early, generally within 24 hours of tumor explant. Due to its reproducibility and regularity, this finding has been considered highly characteristic and diagnostic of tumors of neural origin.[5–7]

ULTRASTRUCTURE

According to the extent of their neural commitment and the areas sampled, these tumors show a wide spectrum of ultrastructural features.[8–16] In undifferentiated tumors, cells have a very primitive appearance, characterized by round nuclei with regular, smooth borders, finely distributed chromatin, and absent or inconspicuous nucleoli. Cytoplasm is scarce, with a few intracytoplasmic organelles such as mitochondria, free ribosomes, and a small Golgi apparatus. Pools of glycogen are a common

229

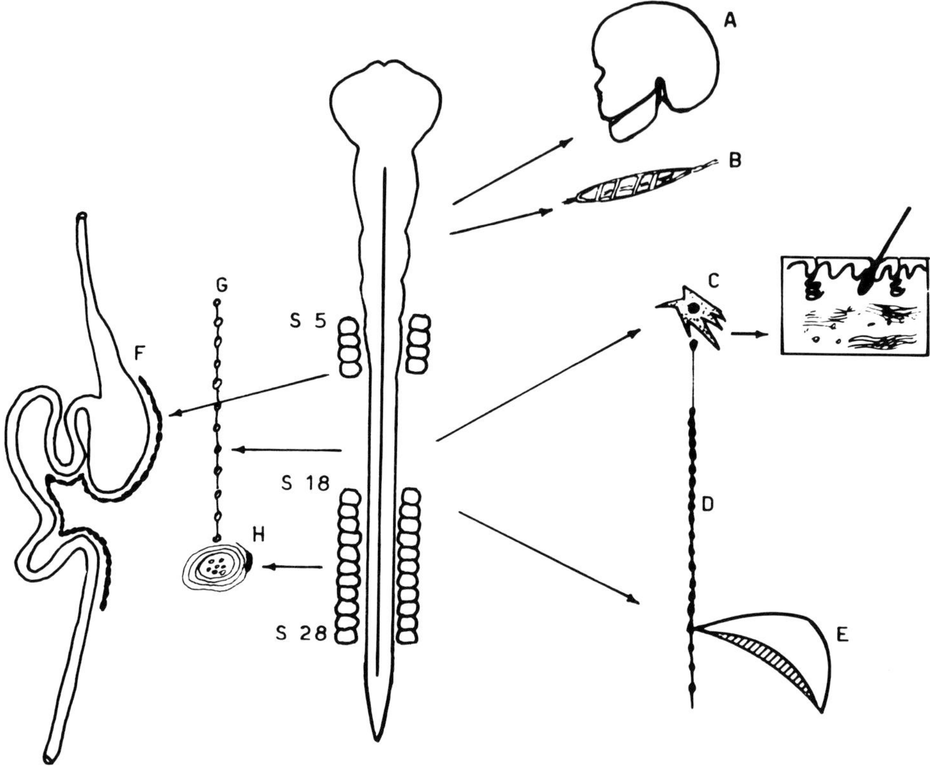

Fig. 10-1. Principal phenotypes originating from the neural crest. In the cranial region the neural crest contributes to the facial arch skeleton (*A*) and striated muscles of the face, jaw, and tongue (*B*) (mesectoderm). At the trunk level, the neural crest gives rise to sympathetic (*D*), parasympathetic (*G*), and enteric (*F*) ganglia, adrenomedullary cords (*E*), Schwann cells (*H*), and skin melanocytes (*C*).

observation (Fig. 10-3), although they are also found in more differentiated forms.[17,18] As neural differentiation proceeds, the cells show a more complex intracytoplasmic organization, with a well-developed Golgi apparatus, a dis-

Table 10-1. Classification of Peripheral PNET

Neuroblastomatous tumors
  Neuroblastoma
  Ganglioneuroblastoma
  Ganglioneuroma

Non-neuroblastomatous tumors
  Peripheral neuroepithelioma, including malignant small
    cell tumor of thoracopulmonary origin (Askin's tumor)
  Intraosseous neuroectodermal tumors
  Ewing's sarcoma (?)

PNET with "divergent differentiation"
  Pigmented neuroectodermal tumor (retinal anlage tumor
    or prognoma)
  Peripheral medulloepithelioma
  Ectomesenchymoma

tinct cytoskeletal network, and a few dense core granules. Primitive intercellular junctions are occasionally observed, and true rosettes or rosettelike configurations can be recognized (Fig. 10-4). More differentiated tumors show long cellular processes containing an evident cytoskeleton composed of microtubules and arrays of intermediate filaments along which numerous neurosecretory granules are generally located (Fig. 10-5).

Neurosecretory granules and neuritic extensions are the morphologic markers of a neuroectodermal origin, even though their respective number and length may vary according to the tumor phenotype. Long neurites and numerous dense core granules are generally found in neuroblastoma, whereas shorter neurites and fewer pleomorphic granules characterize peripheral neuroepithelioma.

The production of extracellular matrix is gen-

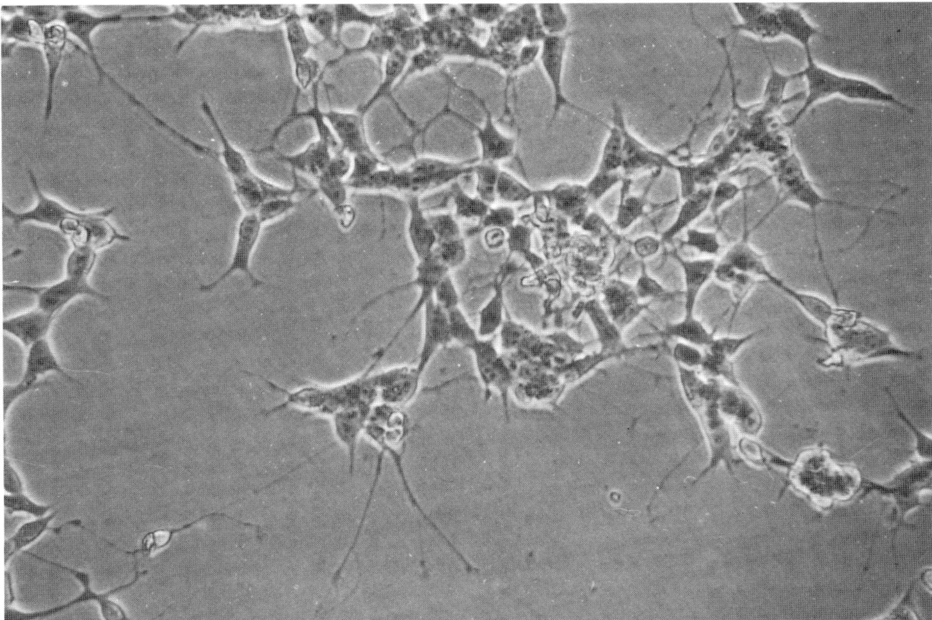

Fig. 10-2. Long and slender cytoplasmic processes (neurites) connecting cellular bodies are in vitro diagnostic hallmarks of PNET. (Phase contrast, × 200.)

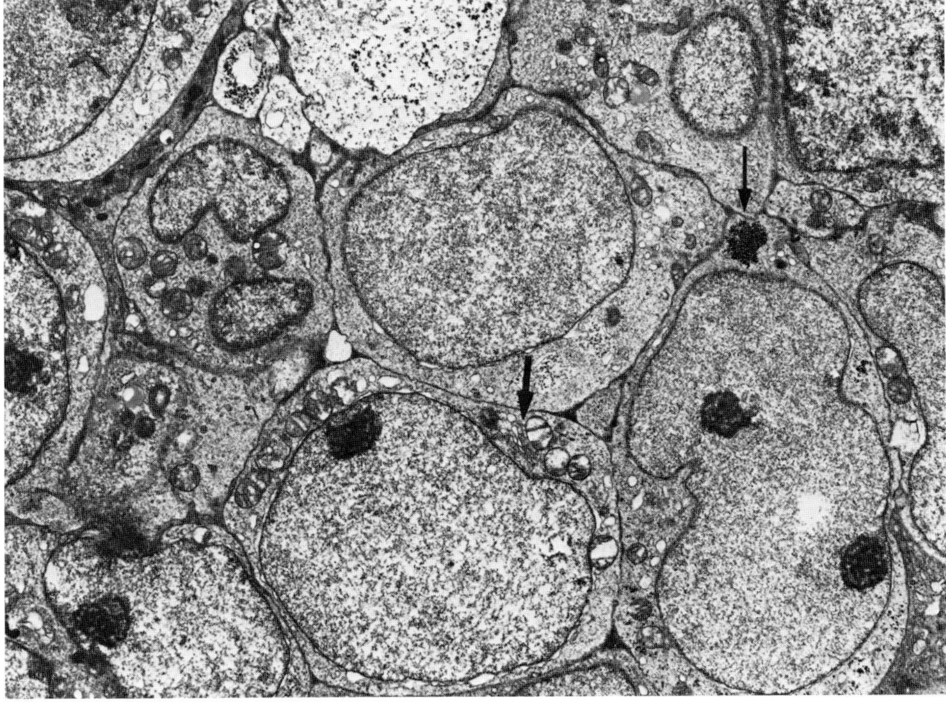

Fig. 10-3. Ultrastructurally PNET may have a very primitive appearance, with round or oval nuclei, scarce cytoplasm containing a few organelles, and a small Golgi apparatus (thick arrow). Pools of glycogen are frequently observed (thin arrow). (× 4,000.)

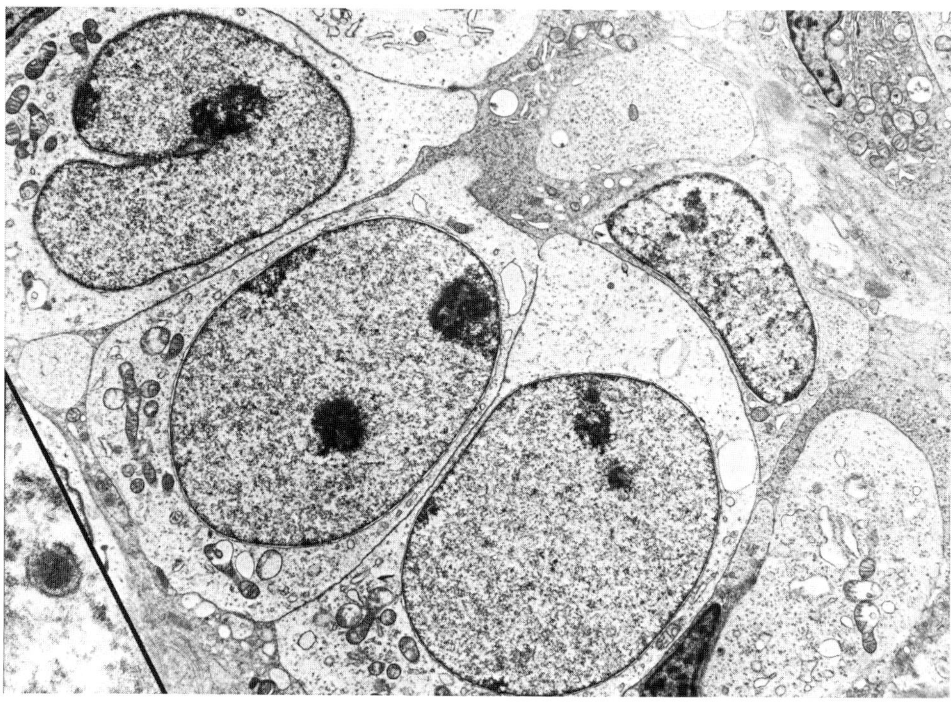

Fig. 10-4. A vague rosettelike configuration, more complex cytoplasms, and a few neurosecretory granules (insert) are observed in more differentiated forms of PNET. ($\times$ 4500; inset, $\times$ 12,000.)

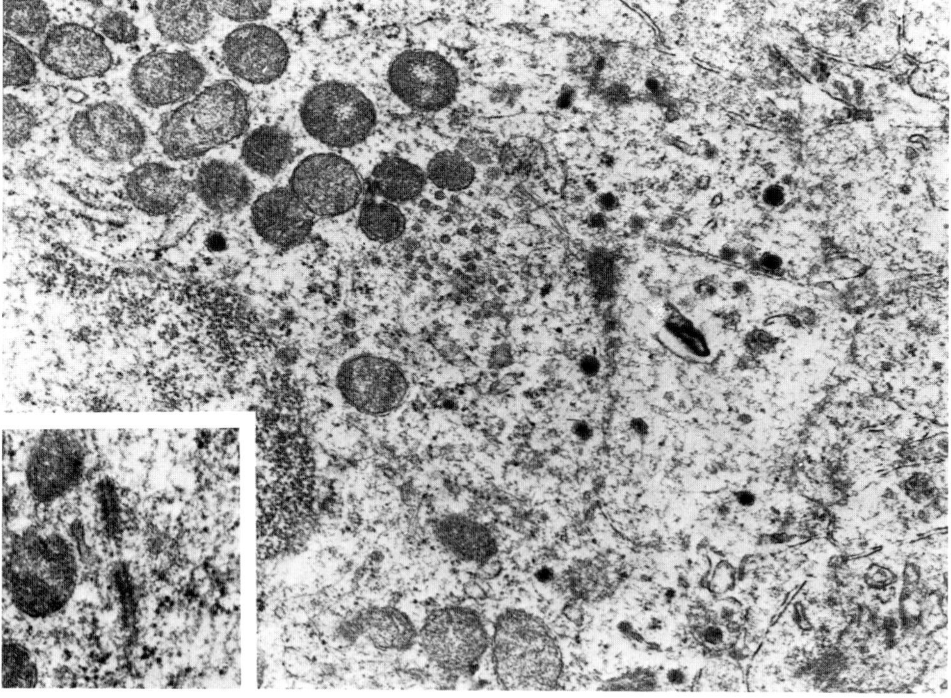

Fig. 10-5. Well-differentiated neuroblastoma shows long neuritic extensions containing numerous neurosecretory granules and neurotubules. Occasional primitive intercellular junctions are also observed (insert). ($\times$ 7000.)

erally scant, and a few profiles of basal lamina-like material and collagen fibers can be observed.[19]

IMMUNOCYTOCHEMISTRY

A large number of polyclonal and monoclonal antibodies have been successfully employed in the immunodiagnosis of peripheral PNET. Table 10-2 summarizes some of the most common neural markers routinely used in formalin-fixed, paraffin-embedded tissue sections.

S-100 PROTEIN

S-100 protein is an acidic protein present in three dimeric forms with a different subunit composition: α/α, α/β, and β/β.[20, 21] Although the α and β subunits show a broad distribution in various tissues,[22] cells of neuroectodermal origin such as Schwann cells and melanocytes express mainly the beta subunit.[23, 24] In neuroblastomatous tumors, S-100 reactivity is restricted to Schwann cells and elongated spindle cells of the stroma, whereas neuroblasts are neg-

**Table 10-2.
Immunocytochemical Markers
in PNET**

S-100 protein

HNK-1 (Leu-7)

NGF-receptor

NSE (γ/γ)

Synaptophysin

Chromogranin A
  NB + +
  PN −

NF (68, 160, 200 kd)

GFAP

Vimentin
  NB −/+
  PN + +

Keratin
  NB −
  PN −/+

ative (Fig. 10-6).[25–27] Single cell positivity is occasionally observed in non-neuroblastomatous PNET.[15,28]

HNK-1 (LEU-7)

The HNK-1 (Leu-7) monoclonal antibody, originally raised against a membrane antigen of a cultured T-cell line, is a specific marker for a lymphocyte population with natural killer activity.[29] Subsequent studies demonstrated that it recognizes an antigenic carbohydrate also present in a variety of glycoproteins and glycolipids involved in modulating intercellular adhesion.[30, 31] This antibody strongly reacts with myelinated tissue from both the CNS and PNS,[32] as well as with human tumors of neuroectodermal origin.[33, 34]

NERVE GROWTH FACTOR RECEPTOR

Positivity to anti-nerve growth factor (NGF)-receptor antibody has also been reported in peripheral PNET.[35, 36]

NEURON-SPECIFIC ENOLASE (NSE) (γ/γ Isoenzyme)

The enolase is a glycolytic enzyme composed of three different subunits: α, β, and γ.[37] The γ/γ isomer is highly expressed in neural tissues and derived tumors (Fig. 10-7)[38] and, therefore, was considered a reliable neural marker.[39, 40] Although it is now known that detectable enolase levels are present in many normal non-neural tissues,[41] it remains the single most reliable neural marker. Errors in interpretation can be obviated by using properly titered monoclonal antibodies to the isoenzyme γ/γ in conjunction with suitable negative controls (Fig. 10-8).

INTERMEDIATE FILAMENTS

Among the cytoskeletal components, intermediate filaments (IF) represent the most important class of proteins insofar as tumor typing

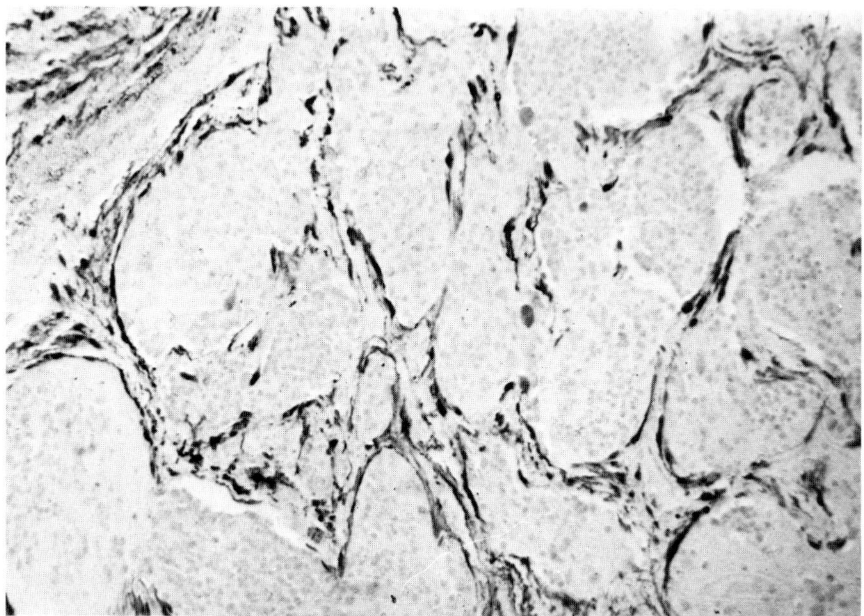

Fig. 10-6. The spindle cells of the vasculoconnective septa of neuroblastoma strongly react to anti-S-100 protein antibody. (ABC method, × 125.)

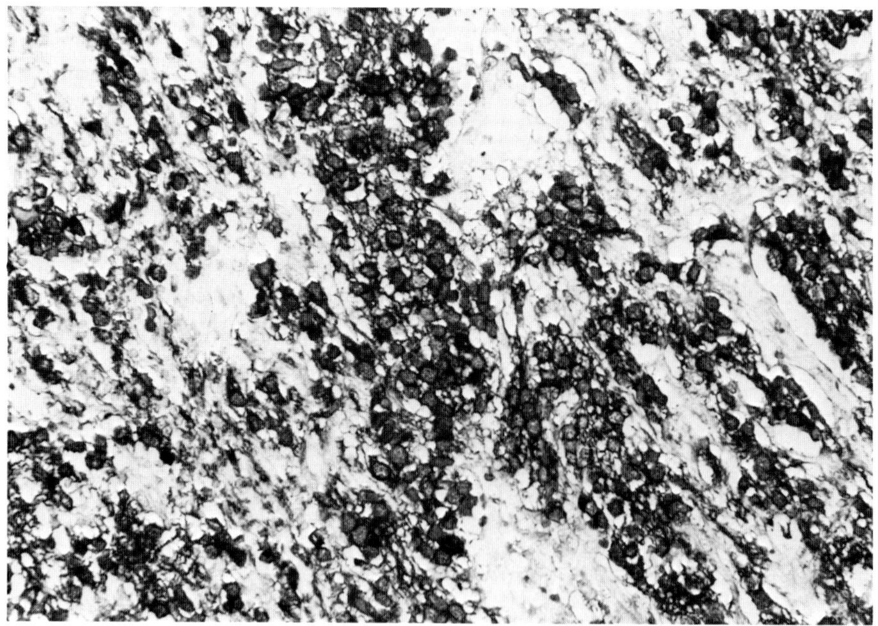

Fig. 10-7. Diffuse cytoplasmic positivity to NSE (γ/γ isoenzyme) in PNET. (ABC method, × 200.)

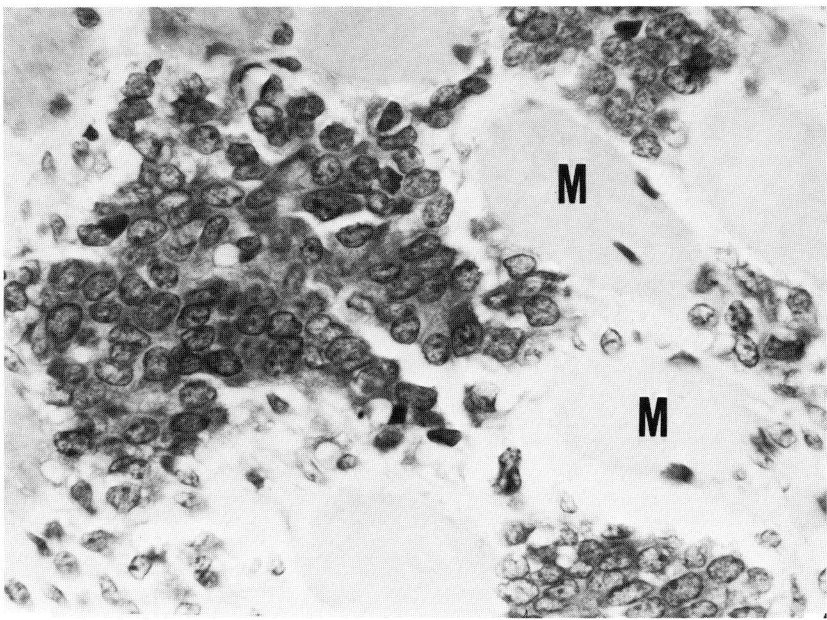

Fig. 10-8. Skeletal muscle infiltration by PNET. NSE reactivity is restricted to tumor cells, whereas muscle fibers (*M*) are negative. The negativity of skeletal fibers, rich in β/β or β/γ enolase, ensures the specificity of the reaction. (ABC method, × 250.)

and differential diagnosis are concerned.[42–44] Five classes of IF are recognized, and their expression is generally restricted to specific mature cell types,[45] such as vimentin in mesenchymal cells, desmin in muscle cells, keratin in epithelial cells, neurofilaments in neurons, and the glial fibrillary acidic protein (GFAP) in glial cells.

NEUROFILAMENTS

Neurofilaments (NF) are composed of three different subunits with molecular weights of about 68,000, 160,000, and 200,000[46] which are orderly expressed during neuron development.[47] Antibodies against each of these proteins, in both their phosphorylated and nonphosphorylated forms,[48] enabled demonstration of a different spatiotemporal NF distribution, according to the extent of neuronal differentiation.[49] The 68,000-d protein appears early in the perikaryon of developing neurons, whereas phosphorylated isoforms of the 160,000- and

200,000-d NF predominate along the neurites and dentrites of terminally differentiated neurons. This different expression of NF protein is partially conserved in neuroectodermal tumors. In neuroblastoma, primitive round neuroblasts are positive to only the 68-kd component, whereas differentiating neuroblasts with more abundant cytoplasm and gangliar cells show intense positivity to both 160,000- and 200,000-d NF.[50, 51]

GLIAL FIBRILLARY ACIDIC PROTEIN, VIMENTIN, AND CYTOKERATIN

GFAP reactivity was demonstrated in the fibrillar portions of highly differentiated neuroblastomatous tumors,[51] as well as in the cytoplasm of undifferentiated neuroblasts.[52, 53] Vimentin seems differently distributed in peripheral PNET. It was reported positive in the majority of non-neuroblastomatous PNET,[16, 28] whereas neuroblasts have low, if any, expression both in vitro and in vivo.[54, 55]

Pigmented neuroectodermal tumor of infancy[56] and a few cases of peripheral neuroepithelioma[28, 57] were also positive to cytokeratin.

NEUROENDOCRINE MARKERS

In addition to the neural profile, PNET also have some neuroendocrine aspects, which are evidenced by their positivity to pan-neuroendocrine markers such as synaptophysin and chromogranin. Synaptophysin, an integral membrane glycoprotein, was originally isolated from presynaptic vesicles of bovine neurons.[58, 59] Immunocytochemical studies indicate that synaptophysis is an independent marker of neural differentiation;[60] its expression, in fact, is not correlated with that of other neural markers, such as neurofilament triplet proteins or neurosecretory products. Neuroblastoma, ganglioneuroblastoma, and peripheral neuroepithelioma are all strongly positive to synaptophysin.[15, 51, 60, 61]

The acidic glycoproteins present in chromaffin granules have been collectively called *chromogranins*.[62] Three different glycoproteins,

A, B, and C, have thus far been identified;[63] chromogranin A is the most abundant,[64] and is commonly expressed in neuroblastomatous PNET (Fig. 10-9),[51, 61, 65–67] whereas non-neuroblastomatous tumors are consistently negative.[28, 66, 67]

NEUROBLASTOMA

Neuroblastoma (NB) is the third most common solid malignancy in childhood,[68] and its annual incidence ranges from 6.6 to 10.6 cases per million children under 15 years of age.[69–73] However, a mass screening program based on vanillylmandelic acid urinary excretion revealed a higher rate of 13.3 cases per million.[74] Nodules of undifferentiated neuroblasts, histologically indistinguishable from NB, are occasionally found in the adrenals of newborns deceased for unrelated reasons; the term *NB in situ* has been proposed for these unexpected nodules[75, 76] whose frequency is 40 times greater than expected. This discrepancy has been taken as evidence for spontaneous NB regression. On the

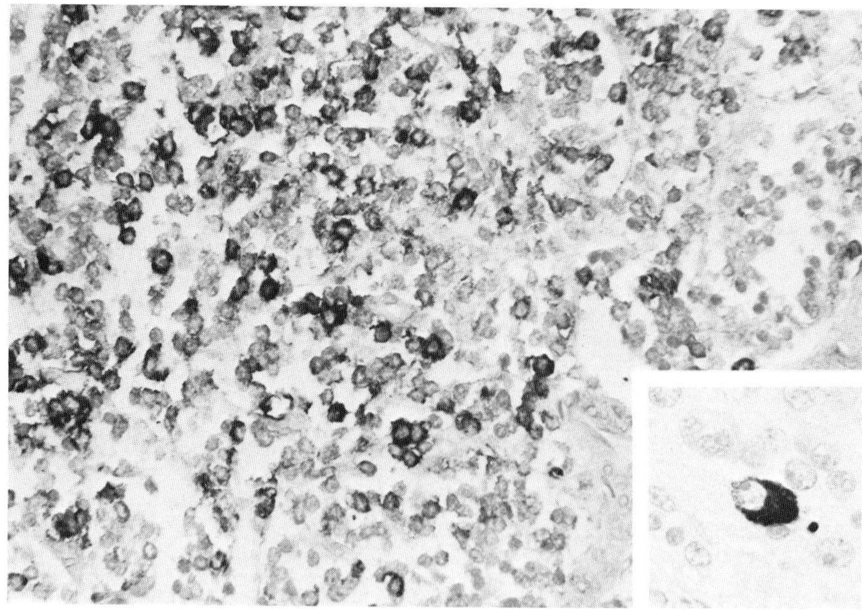

Fig. 10-9. Neuroblastoma cells show a strong positivity to anti-chromogranin A MoAb. Note the typical cytoplasmic granularity of the reaction (insert). (ABC method, × 200.)

other hand, the neoplastic nature of these nodules has been questioned, since similar neuroblastic nests are considered a normal part of fetal adrenal glands.[77]

Over 50 percent of cases are diagnosed within the first year of life,[78] with a median age at diagnosis of 2 years.[79] NB is uncommon after the first decade, and exceedingly rare in adulthood.

This tumor originates from neural crest cells that give rise to the adrenal medulla and the sympathetic ganglia. Therefore, the adrenal medulla, retroperitoneum, mediastinum, and head and neck are the most frequently involved regions.[78, 79] About one-third of the patients present with metastatic disease,[80] and in a small percentage of cases the primary site is not detected.

Macroscopically NB has a variegated appearance that parallels the degree of histologic differentiation. On the cut surface, tumors with undifferentiated histology are soft and pink with alternating foci of hemorrhagic and yellow necrotic areas. A firm, gray, homogeneous cut surface indicates a greater tumor differentiation.

Foci of dystrophic calcification are frequently seen.

HISTOLOGY

NB has a wide spectrum of histologic features, depending on the degree and amount of its cytologic differentiation. *Undifferentiated neuroblasts* are small round cells with round or oval nuclei containing finely dispersed chromatin (Fig. 10-10); cytoplasm is scarce, and the cellular borders ill defined. A condensed chromatin pattern, presence of evident nucleoli, and a larger eosinophilic cytoplasm with neuritic extensions are the hallmarks of *differentiating neuroblasts*. At the other end of the spectrum is the mature ganglion cell, which is recognized by a large eosinophilic, pear-shaped cytoplasm occasionally containing pyroninophilic granules in a juxtanuclear position (Nissl's substance); single or multiple, at times bizzare, nuclei with large nucleoli are present. Based on the relative amount of the above elements, NB can be subdivided into three major histologic subtypes; gan-

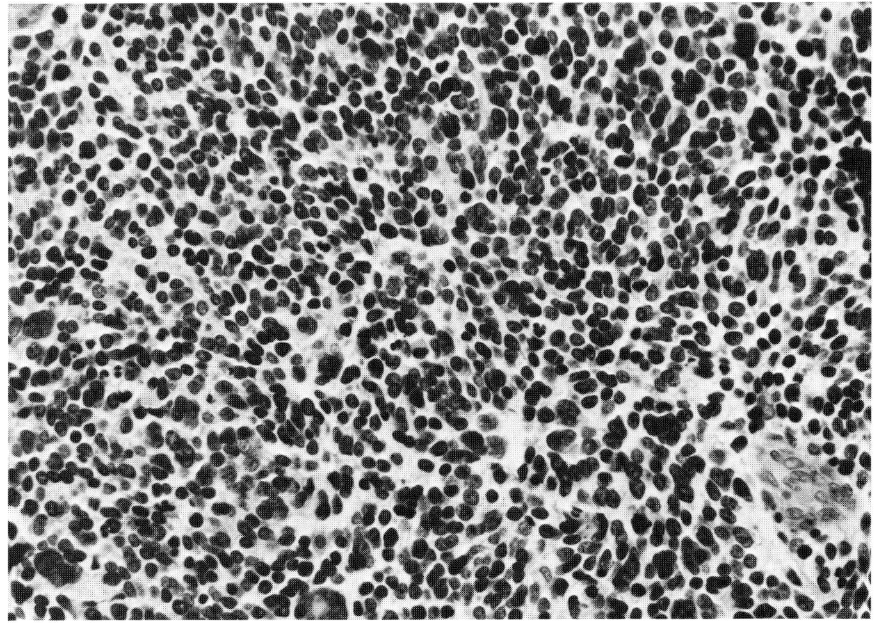

Fig. 10-10. A rather primitive uncommitted appearance of undifferentiated NB. The tumor is composed of a uniform population of small round cells with ill-defined cellular borders. (H&E, × 160.)

glioneuroblastoma (GNB), well-differentiated NB, and poorly differentiated NB.

Ganglioneuroblastoma

At low power, GNB shows a distinct nodular pattern. The tumoral nodules consist of differentiating neuroblasts intermixed with mono- or multi-nucleated mature ganglion cells embedded in a neurofibromatous or highly fibrillar background (Fig. 10-11). At least 5 percent mature ganglion cells are required for a diagnosis of GNB.[81] Scattered foci of calcification are commonly found. Broad fibrovascular septa, composed of spindle cells embedded in a collagenous stroma, surround the tumoral nodules.

Scattered ganglion cells in a neurofibromatous background are the diagnostic features of ganglioneuroma (Fig. 10-12). Occasionally discrete, well-demarcated foci of neuroblasts in different stages of differentiation can be observed in an otherwise typical ganglioneuroma. These cases are classified as *composite GNB*.

Well-Differentiated Neuroblastoma

Less than 5 percent ganglion cells and more than 50 percent differentiating neuroblasts define well-differentiated NB. The neuroblasts, immersed in a slightly fibrillar background, are arranged in a less-distinctive nodular pattern with thin fibrovascular septa. Homer-Wright rosettes with characteristic neurofibrillar cores are frequently observed, as well as areas of necrosis and hemorrhage (Fig. 10-13).

Poorly Differentiated Neuroblastoma

Poorly differentiated NB is typified by less than 50 percent differentiating neuroblasts. Areas composed of diffuse sheets or large nodules of small round cells with scarce cytoplasm and a few cytoplasmic processes are frequently seen. Tumors consisting almost entirely of small round cells are also referred to as *undifferentiated NB* (Fig. 10-10).

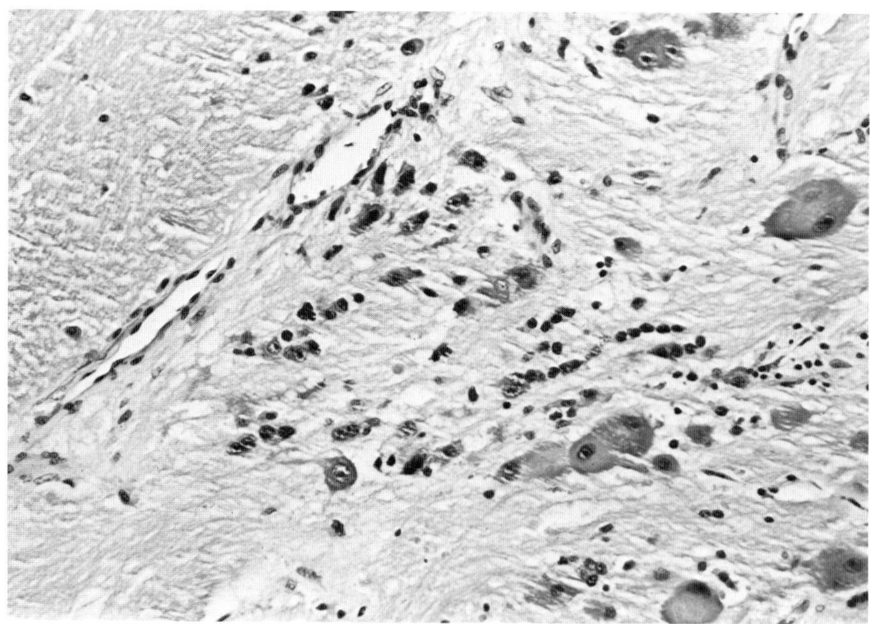

Fig. 10-11. Ganglion cells and differentiating neuroblasts characterize GNB. (H&E, × 160.)

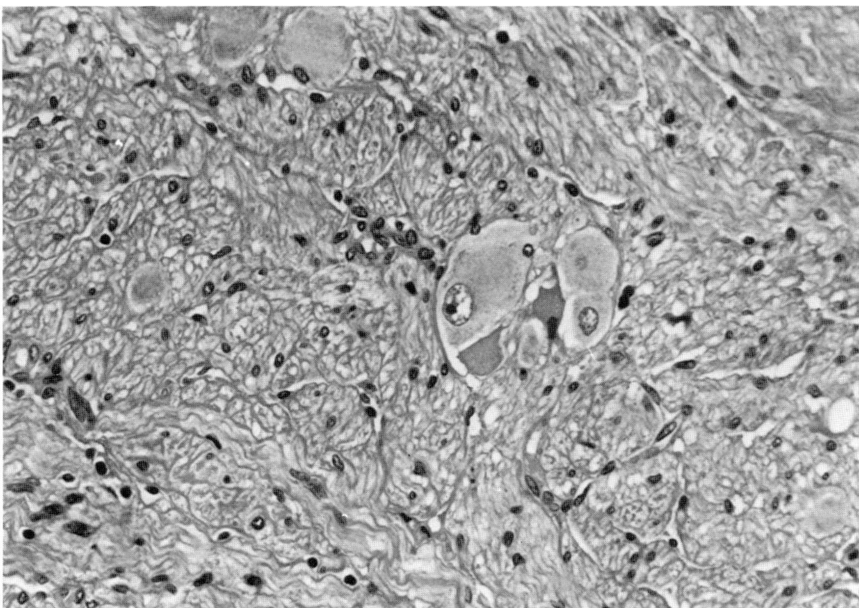

Fig. 10-12. Scattered ganglion cells in a neurofibromatous background is the hallmark of ganglioneuroma. (H&E, × 200.)

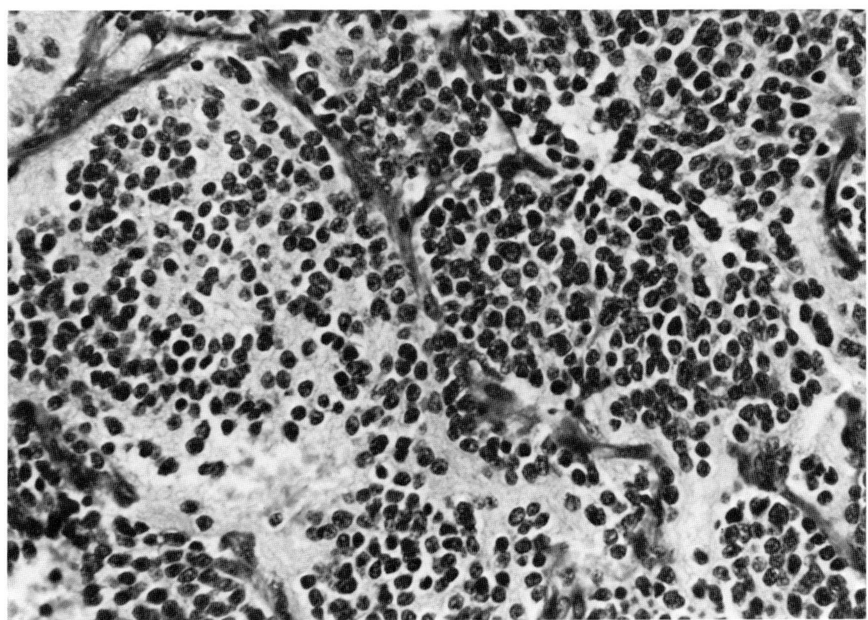

Fig. 10-13. Well-differentiated NB. The tumor nodules are composed of neuroblasts in different stages of differentiation immersed in an abundant fibrillar stroma. (H&E, × 200.)

PROGNOSIS

NB is a highly aggressive tumor with a tendency for early regional lymph node and visceral involvement; overall survival is about 60 percent at 2 years from diagnosis.[82, 83] The organs most frequently involved are the liver, lymph nodes, lungs, and bone marrow. Spontaneous or therapy-induced differentiation and/or regression of NB is known to occur in 2 to 4 percent of cases,[84, 85] and is more frequently observed in children under 1 year of age.[86] The final outcome in a patient with NB depends on several factors. The most important prognostic factors are summarized in Table 10-3.

Stage, Age, and Site

Extent of tumor spread, patient age at diagnosis, and site of the primary tumor are the most important prognostic factors.[70, 82, 83, 87, 88] According to Evans' staging system,[89] survival rates range from 80 to 90 percent for localized disease, to less than 20 percent for disseminated disease.[70, 82, 83, 87, 88] Children under 1 year of age, regardless of stage, fare better than older patients.[87, 90] Patients with localized disease and secondary involvement of one or more of several sites (i.e., liver, skin, lymphnodes, and bone marrow) constitute a separate group, identified as stage IV-S.[91, 92] This group of patients shows a highly spontaneous tumor regression rate (more than 50 percent of cases) and an excellent prognosis; 90 percent survival at 3 years has been reported for patients in stage IV-S, as opposed to 44 percent in a comparable group of patients in stage IV.[93]

Tumors arising in the abdomen, and particularly in the adrenal gland, have the poorest prognosis, whereas tumors originating above the diaphragm show better survival rates.[78, 79, 83, 94]

Histology

Various attempts have been made to correlate histology and prognosis on the basis of cytologic differentiation, neuropil formation, and presence of mature ganglion cells.[95–98] Tumors mainly composed of undifferentiated neuroblasts show a more aggressive course than differentiated tumors (Fig. 10–14). Shimada et al.[99] recently proposed a new classification based on the presence and amount of stroma in the neoplasia; two major, prognostically significant groups of NB were identified: "stroma rich" and "stroma poor." Stroma-rich tumors show a diffuse or nodular pattern, with the latter corresponding to the prognostically unfavorable composite GNB. The prognostically favorable stroma-rich tumors virtually comprehend all classic GNB and some well-differentiated NB. Age at diagnosis, degree of cytologic differenti-

Table 10-3. Prognostic Factors in Neuroblastoma

	Favorable	Unfavorable
Age	< 2 yrs	> 2 yrs
Site	Head and neck, thorax	Adrenal, retroperitoneum
Stage	I II IV-S	III IV
Ferritin	Low	High
NSE	< 100 ng/ml	> 100 ng/ml
Histology	GNB, well diff. NB	Composite GNB, poorly diff. NB
Chromosome 1 marker	Absent	Present
N-*myc* amplification	Absent	Present
DNA content	Near triploid	Near diploid, hypotetraploid

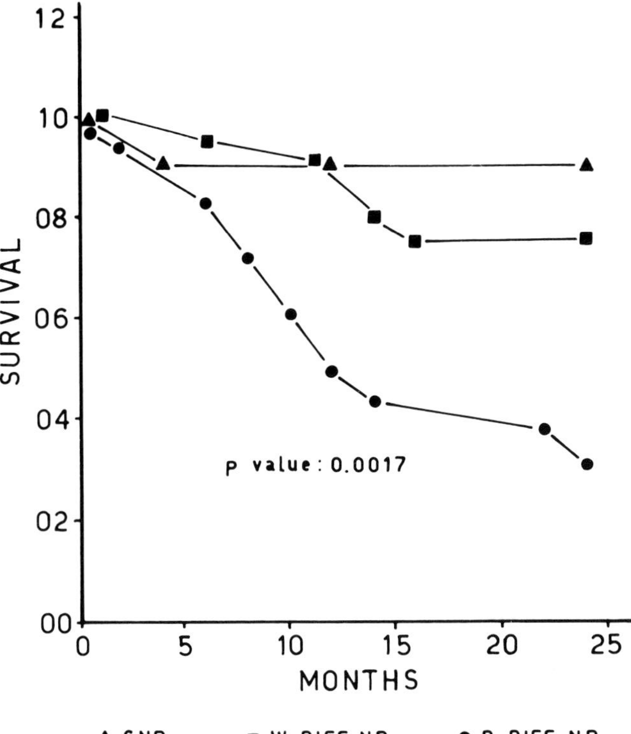

Fig. 10-14. Cumulative proportion survival in 55 cases diagnosed at the Institute of Pathologic Anatomy of Padua University. Significant differences in survival were observed between differentiated (GNB, well-differentiated NB) and poorly differentiated forms of NB.

ation, and the mitotic-karyorrexic index are other important parameters for prognostic evaluation of the stroma-poor group.[100]

Biological Markers

Urinary catecholamine metabolites, ferritin, and NSE have been successfully employed as diagnostic and prognostic markers. Since most NB are adrenergic, urinary catecholamine metabolites such as vanillylmandelic acid (VMA), homovanillic acid (HVA), vanillacetic acid and 3-methoxy-4-hydroxyphenylethylenglycol are found in the overwhelming majority of cases.[101, 102] The highest catecholamine excretion was reported in undifferentiated tumors.[103] High HVA levels are commonly associated with a poor prognosis,[103, 104] whereas a high VMA/HVA ratio in patients with disseminated disease correlates with a better prognosis.[101]

Serum ferritin is closely associated with tumor growth[105] and plays an important role in predicting the outcome of patients; high serum ferritin values are, in fact, associated with a poor prognosis.[82] Moreover, serum ferritin values are useful markers to evaluate the response to treatment as they return to normal with clinical remission.

A serum NSE level over 100 ng/ml has been reported to be of prognostic significance for disseminated disease (stage III and IV) in patients under 2 years of age.[106]

Genetics and Molecular Biology

A deletion or rearrangement of the short arm of chromosome 1 has been consistently described in NB.[107, 108] This abnormality is more commonly found in disseminated disease (stage

III and IV), and correlates with a poor prognosis.[109, 110] Other chromosomal abnormalities described in association with NB include homogeneous staining regions (HSR) and double minutes (DM).[111] These abnormalities are now recognized as morphologic expressions of genomic amplification of the N-*myc* oncogene.[112]

The N-*myc* copy number correlates with advanced disease and poor prognosis,[113, 114] even if gene amplification does not seem related to tumor progression, as originally thought.[115] N-*myc* amplification seems to occur exclusively in adrenal and retroperitoneal tumors, and is more commonly associated with undifferentiated NB.[116–119] On the other hand, lack of N-*myc* amplification does not exclude a poor prognosis.[117]

The DNA content of tumor cells was recently shown to be an important prognostic marker.[94, 120–122] Hyperdiploid tumors were associated with prolonged survival and good response to chemotherapy; diploid or near-diploid tumors occurred in advanced stages, and responded poorly to treatment. Hayashi et al.[110] recently showed that tumor ploidy and chromosomal pattern were closely associated: all near-diploid tumors showed chromosome 1 abnormalities. In the same study, none of the hyperdiploid and near-triploid cases was N-*myc* amplified, whereas such amplification occurred in only half of the near-diploid tumors. Thus, DNA content and chromosomal pattern appear to be better predictive factors of prognosis than N-*myc* amplification.

PERIPHERAL NEUROEPITHELIOMA

In 1918, A. P. Stout[123] described a tumor of the ulnar nerve in a 42-year-old man as "masses and strands of rather small rounded cells . . . separated by trabeculae of connective tissue." The tumor also showed structures closely resembling Flexner's rosettes. Stout initially suggested a primitive neuroepithelial origin for this tumor on the basis of its immature appearance in vitro.[124] The term *neuroepithelioma* was introduced by Bailey and Cushing[125] to identify malignant neuroectodermal tumors of the CNS with a putative primitive spongioblastic origin. Penfield, in 1932,[126] used the term *peripheral neuroepithelioma* (PN) to refer to peripheral nerve tumors such as those previously reported by Stout. In 1970, Abell described a case of PN arising in association with an intercostal nerve.[127] In 1973, at the 39th Annual Anatomic Pathology Slide Seminar of the American Society of Clinical Pathologists, Lattes[128] reported 17 cases of PN. Four were located in the trunk, and in one case the ribs were involved by tumor.

In 1979, Askin et al.[129] described a malignant small round cell tumor in the thoracopulmonary region of children and adolescents. Rib involvement was documented in six cases, and although an origin from an intercostal or intrathoracic peripheral nerve could not be proved, the ultrastructural observation of neurosecretory granules in three cases suggested a primitive neuroepithelial origin for this tumor. Subsequent immunocytochemical, ultrastructural, and cytogenetic studies[130–132] stressed the similarities between this tumor and PN, and it is now widely accepted that Askin's tumor is a topographic variant of PN.[133]

PN generally occurs in children and young adults, although any age may be affected; the median age is about 20 years.[15, 28, 128, 134, 135] The relative frequency is about 1 percent of all soft tissue sarcomas[134, 136] and about 6 percent of all pediatric malignant soft tissue tumors.[15] Trunk, extremities, and pelvis are the most commonly involved regions, whereas adrenal glands and sympathetic chains are always spared. Although association with a major nerve constitutes a useful diagnostic hallmark,[137–139] it is rarely observed and no longer required for diagnosis.[133]

HISTOLOGY

Microscopically PN is composed of a uniform population of small round cells, arranged in a lobular or diffuse pattern (Figs. 10-15 and 10-16). The nuclei are oval or round with mar-

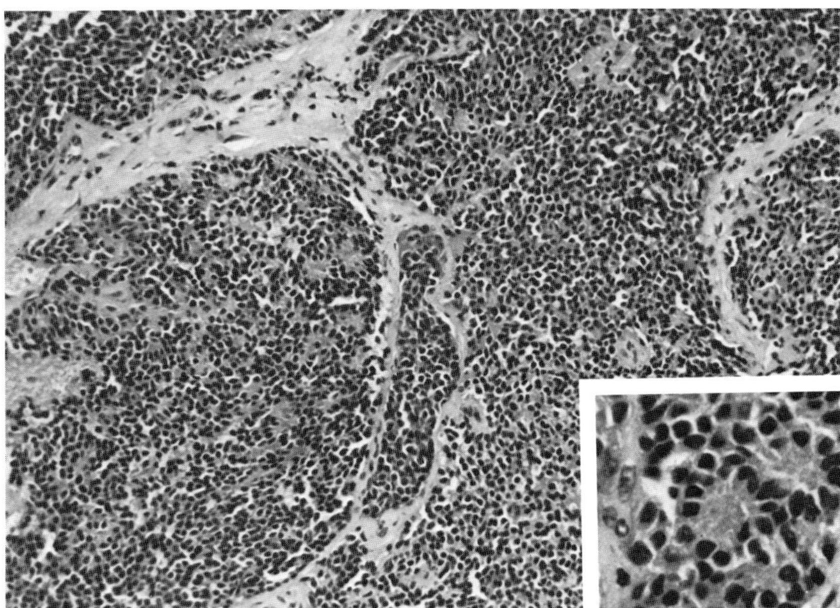

Fig. 10-15. Peripheral neuroepithelioma. The tumor is composed of nodules of uniform small round cells with numerous rosettes. (H&E, × 160: inset, H&E, × 250.)

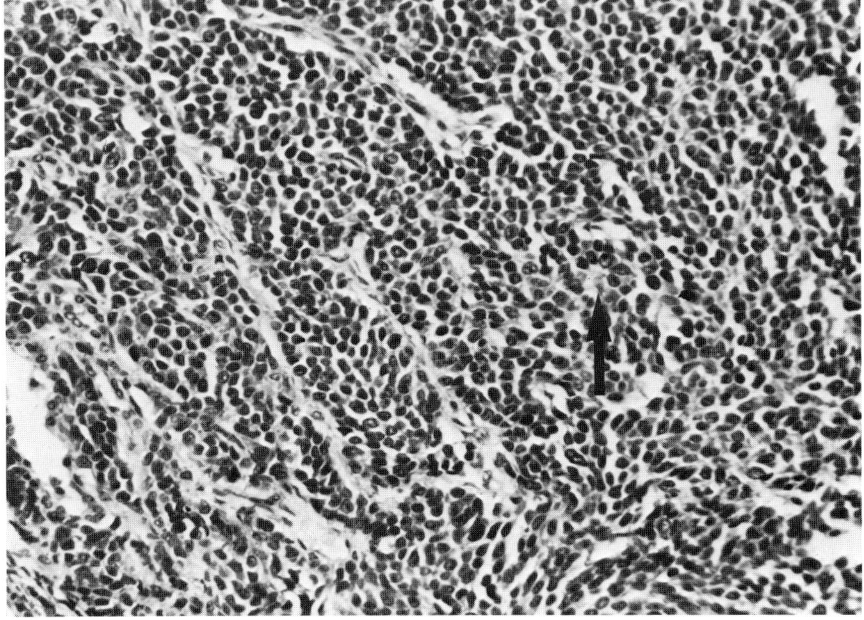

Fig. 10-16. Malignant small round cell tumor of the thoracopulmonary region (so-called Askin's tumor). The lobular pattern is less apparent and a few primitive rosettes are observed (arrow). (H&E, × 200.)

ginated chromatin, evident nuclear borders, and small nucleoli. Homer-Wright- or Flexner-type rosettes are frequently seen, as well as perivascular pseudorosettes. Mitotic figures are generally numerous. Tumor necrosis is a common finding despite high vascularization. Stroma is scarce or absent; a few delicate reticulin fibers are interspersed between cells in which a well-developed neurofibrillar stroma is usually absent. Undifferentiated areas with a blastematous Ewing-like appearance or a peripheral nerve sheathlike aspect are occasionally observed (Figs. 10-17 and 10-18). Glycogen has been found in 20 to 60 percent of cases,[15, 134, 135] and more abundantly in the undifferentiated areas.

PROGNOSIS

PN is a very aggressive tumor:[129, 134, 135] lungs, bone, and lymph nodes are the most common metastatic sites.[140] Two recent reports indicate that PN is an even more aggressive tumor than NB. A 56 percent disease-free survival at 3 years was reported for localized PN;[141] this figure is considerably lower than the 80 percent survival that is expected for a comparable group of patients with NB. In a similar manner, the use of combined therapy appears to be less effective in controlling PN than NB.[140]

NB AND PN: DIFFERENTIAL DIAGNOSIS

NB and PN are the two most representative and common examples of peripheral PNET. In the past, the two lesions were often confused, and were alternately called "classic" and "adult or peripheral" neuroblastoma,[14, 134, 142] with PN considered an unusual variant of NB arising in association with peripheral nerves.[137] Whereas PN and NB may be morphologically indistinguishable even on computed image system analysis,[143] they are nonetheless two distinct entities with different anatomoclinical and biologic characteristics.

NB is almost exclusively a tumor of infancy,

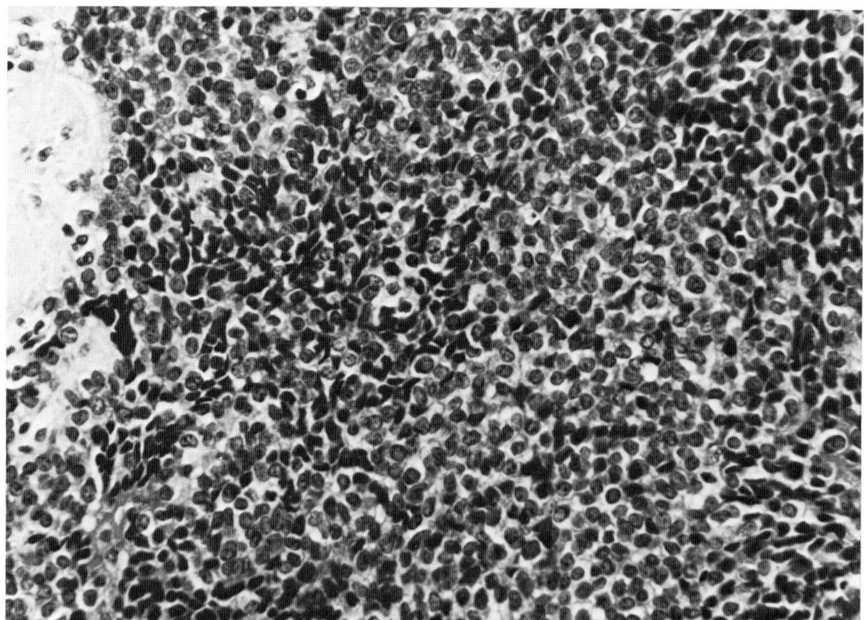

Fig. 10-17. Same case as in Figure 10-15. Undifferentiated, Ewing-like portion of the tumor. The presence of dark and light cells makes this portion morphologically indistinguishable from Ewing's sarcoma. (H&E, × 200.)

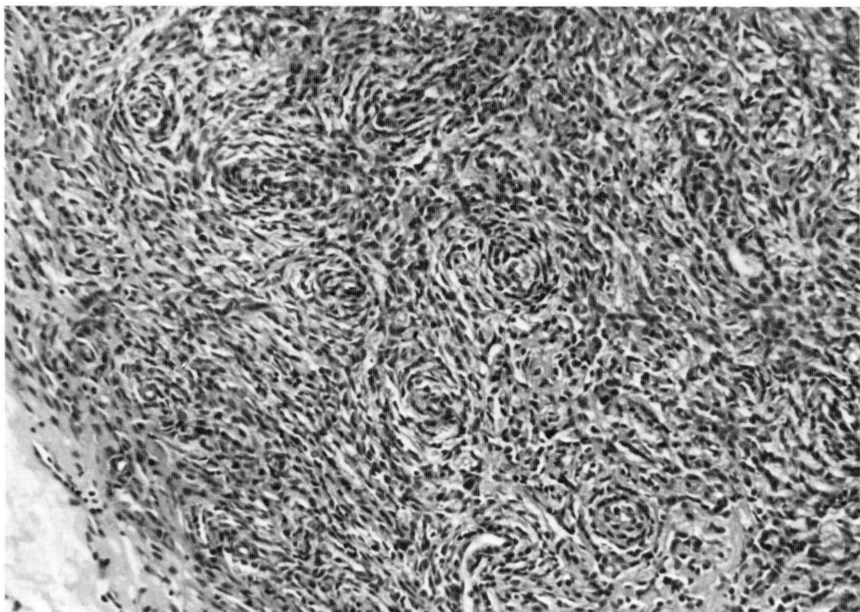

Fig. 10-18. Same case as in Figures 10-16 and 10-17. In another area of the tumor, spindle cells arranged in a tactoid pattern recall a malignant peripheral nerve sheath tumor. (H&E, × 160.)

whereas PN occurs mainly in adolescents and young adults, with a peak incidence in the second and third decades. If NB is the prototype of the adrenergic lineage, PN represents the cholinergic counterpart in the PNET family. An analysis of the neurotransmitter enzyme content in PN tumor cell lines showed high amounts of cholinergic neurotransmitters, whereas adrenergic neurotransmitters could not be demonstrated.[144] This finding correlates well with the lack of in vivo excretion of catecholamine metabolites on the one hand, and lack of chromogranin expression on the other. Chromogranin A expression, in fact, seems to be restricted to "secretory" PNET such as neuroblastomatous tumors.[66, 145]

A typical reciprocal chromosomal translocation 11:22 (q21:q12), first described in Ewing's sarcoma,[146, 147] was also recognized in PN and so-called Askin's tumor of the thoracopulmonary region.[148] No chromosome 1 short arm deletion and/or DM and HSR have thus far been observed in PN.

In a similar manner, major differences were found in the oncogenetic profile of these two tumors.[144, 149] No N-*myc* amplification and/or expression has been reported in PN cell lines or fresh specimens, whereas c-*myc* is invariably expressed in all PN tumor cell lines investigated to date. Major histocompatibility complex (MHC)-related molecules are also differently expressed in the two tumors. Neuroblasts and neurons of normal adult brain weakly express such molecules.[150, 151] Spindle cells in the stroma and a small proportion of neuroblasts (under 5 percent) express human leukocyte antigen (HLA) class I antigens and β_2-microglobulin,[28, 152] whereas the overwhelming majority of PN cells carry these antigens both in vitro and in vivo.[153, 154] The main differential characteristics of NB and PN are summarized in Table 10-4.

The diagnosis of PN thus rests primarily on anatomoclinical criteria. In an adolescent or young adult, a small round cell tumor arising outside the adrenal medulla and sympathetic ganglia and showing a lobular pattern, numerous rosettes, and a high mitotic rate is more likely PN rather than NB. The expression of MHC-related molecules, the absence of N-*myc* ampli-

**Table 10-4. Differential Diagnosis between Neuroblastoma (NB)
and Peripheral Neuroepithelioma (PN)**

	NB	PN
Age	<5 yrs	>10 yrs
Neurotransmitters	Adrenergic	Cholinergic
Metabolites excretion	Present	Absent
MHC	Absent	Present
Chromosomal abnormalities	del 1(q-), HSRs, DMS	rct 11:22
Oncogenes	N-*myc*	c-*myc*
Survival	LD, 80%	LD, 50%
	DD, 20%	DD, 10%

LD, localized disease; DD, disseminated disease.

fication and/or expression, and the presence of a rct 11:22 will subsequently confirm the diagnosis.

INTRAOSSEOUS PNET

PN frequently may involve adjacent bone, especially in regions where subcutaneous and muscle layers are thin and bones are superficial;[141] in the chest wall and pelvis, the ribs and iliac bones, in fact, are almost constantly involved. We have also observed primary bone PN in the tibia and femur;[28] histologically these tumors do not differ from their soft tissue counterparts.

Nevertheless, immunocytochemical and/or ultrastructural studies indicate that tumors composed of small undifferentiated round cells, lacking an overt neural differentiation, have "neural" characteristics.[155–157] As shown in Fig. 10-19, such tumors are often confused with Ewing's sarcoma at the light microscope; clearcut Homer-Wright rosettes are lacking, although rosettelike structures are often observed, and a lobular pattern is usually absent. However, positivity to neural markers, such as NSE, S-100 protein, and HNK-1, together with the ultrastructural observation of neurosecretory granules, neurotubules, and synapticlike buttons en-

able recognition of their neuroectodermal origin. The neural commitment of these tumors is further demonstrated by their spontaneous neural differentiation in vitro (Fig. 10-20).[155, 158, 159]

In the case illustrated in Fig. 10-19, cytogenetic analysis revealed a typical rct 11:22 (q12: q24), associated with deletion of the short arm of chromosome 1 (Fig. 10–21). This finding represents a unique combination of cytogenetic abnormalities, typical of both NB and PN; analysis of tumor cell DNA and RNA failed to show N-*myc* amplification or expression, and only c-*myc* expression was detected, even though N-*myc* product was present in another similar case.[158]

PNET of bone appear as a distinct entity, and thus should be distinguished from both PN and NB, which show a more overt neural differentiation, and Ewing's sarcoma of bone. The latter, however, presents a more challenging and somewhat controversial differential diagnosis, since it too has been ascribed a primitive neuroectodermal origin.[28, 155] In fact, it is still unclear whether PNET of bone and Ewing's sarcoma are two distinct entities or Ewing's sarcoma merely represents a misdiagnosed PNET. This dilemma may be resolved if the broad spectrum of morphologic features characterizing the different degrees of neural differentiation is considered. Small round undifferentiated

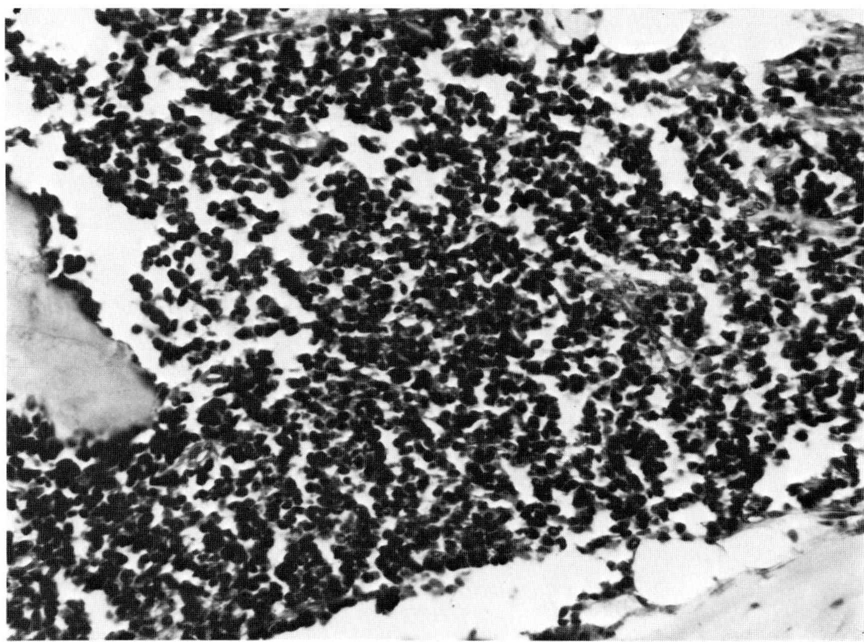

Fig. 10-19. Intraosseous PNET is composed of a uniform population of small round cells closely mimicking Ewing's sarcoma. (H&E, × 160.)

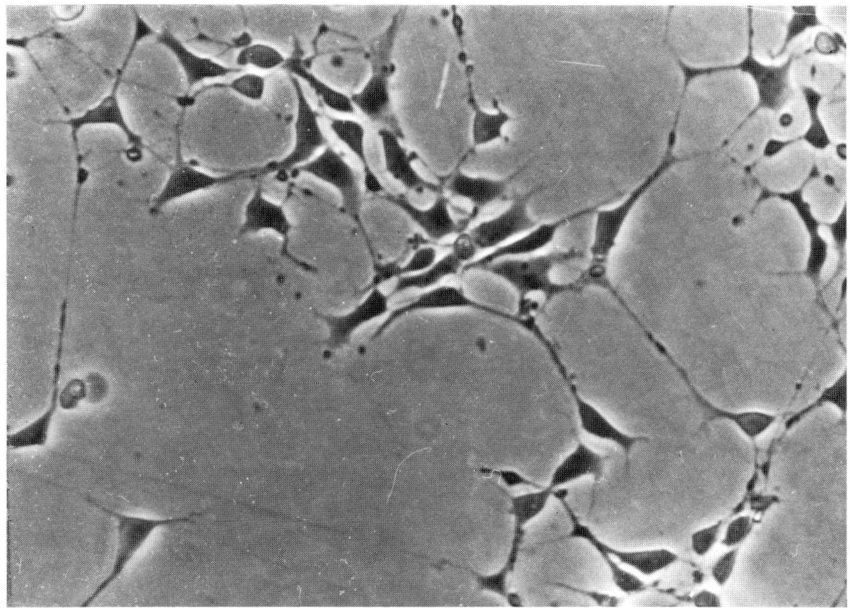

Fig. 10-20. After few days in culture, tumor cells of intraosseous PNET display characteristic and diagnostic features in support of the neuroectodermal origin of the tumor. (Phase contrast. × 200.)

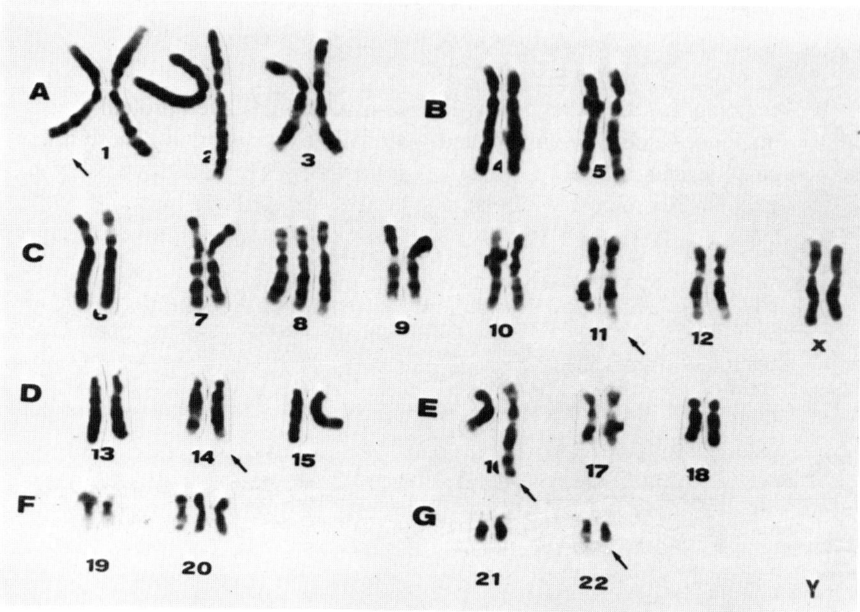

Fig. 10-21. Tumor cells of intraosseous PNET are characterized by a unique combination of cytogenetic abnormalities, including partial monosomy of chromosome 1 and rct 11:22.

cells showing large pools of glycogen are observed both in PN and NB,[18, 130, 157] so it is plausible that tumors made up almost exclusively of undifferentiated neuroectodermal cells can also occur. In this sense, Ewing's sarcoma could be considered the most immature form in the PNET family;[160] in fact, neural differentiation can only be induced in vitro[161] and no neural traits are detectable with conventional pathologic techniques (negativity to neural markers on routine immunocytochemistry and/or electron microscopy).[162, 163] For practical purposes, the diagnosis of Ewing's sarcoma should be reserved for small round cell tumors lacking both morphologic (rosettes, pseudorosettes, or neurosecretory granules) *and* immunocytochemical evidence of neural differentiation (negativity to all neural markers except vimentin). This distinction is not merely academic, since retrospective studies indicate that intraosseous PNET are associated with a poorer response to treatment than "classic" Ewing's sarcoma of bone.[163]

"DIVERGENT" DIFFERENTIATIONS OCCURRING IN PERIPHERAL PNET

Peripheral PNET may reveal a mixture of different phenotypes, including melanocytes, Schwann cells, ganglion cells, rhabdomyoblasts, and chondroblasts. The ability of primitive neoplastic neuroectodermal cells to differentiate into apparently unrelated phenotypes seems to reflect the pluripotentiality of their normal embryonic counterparts. In this sense, rhabdomyoblasts, lipoblasts, and chondroblasts do not represent a true divergent differentiation, since they belong to the spectrum of phenotypes arising from the neural crest.

Primitive neuroectodermal cells may undergo spontaneous differentiation in vivo into ganglion cells and Schwann cells (ganglioneuroma) as well as glial and ependymal cells.[164, 165] Melanocytes arise from the neural crest,[2] and it has been shown in vitro that interconversion from neuroblasts to melanocytes occurs either spontaneously[55] or after treatment with differentiating agents.[166] These studies lend experimental support to in vivo observations of melanocytic differentiation occurring in neural crest-derived tumors, such as melanotic schwannoma[167] and pigmented neuroectodermal tumor of infancy (retinal anlage tumor or progonoma). The latter is a rare tumor almost exclusively diagnosed within the first year of life; in more than 90 percent of the cases, the tumor arises in the head and neck, particularly in the maxilla; unusual sites include the uterus, ovary, skin, femur, thigh, mediastinum, and paratesticular region.[168, 169] On histology, it shows small alveolar spaces lined by heavily pigmented cuboidal cells, and nests of small round cells closely resembling those of an undifferentiated neuroblastoma (Fig. 10-22). Ultrastructurally premelanosomes, melanosomes, and neurosecretory granules have been described,[170–172] thus confirming the double, melanocytic, and neuroblastic differentiation occurring in this unusual lesion. Unexpectedly, and in apparent contrast to its melanocytic differentiation, the pigmented

cells were found to be S-100 negative and keratin positive.[56, 172] An abnormal urinary excretion of vanillylmandelic acid[170, 173, 174] and high serum levels of α-fetoprotein[174, 175] have occasionally been reported. These tumors generally follow a benign clinical course; less than 4 percent of the cases metastasize.[168–170]

Tumors co-expressing neural and mesenchymal phenotypes are generally referred to as *ectomesenchymomas*.[176] These infrequent tumors occur mostly in childhood,[177] although some adult cases have been described.[178] They are composed of neuroblasts, ganglion cells, Schwann cells, and mesenchymal cells of various types. A rhabdomyoblastic differentiation is present in more than 80 percent of the cases, although lipoblastic, chondroblastic, and melanocytic lineages of differentiation are also observed.[176–179] The clinical course is generally aggressive, but long-term survival rates have been reported.[180] Ectomesenchymomas should be distinguished from other soft tissue tumors that present a mixture of mesenchymal and neural derivates, such as malignant Triton tumor

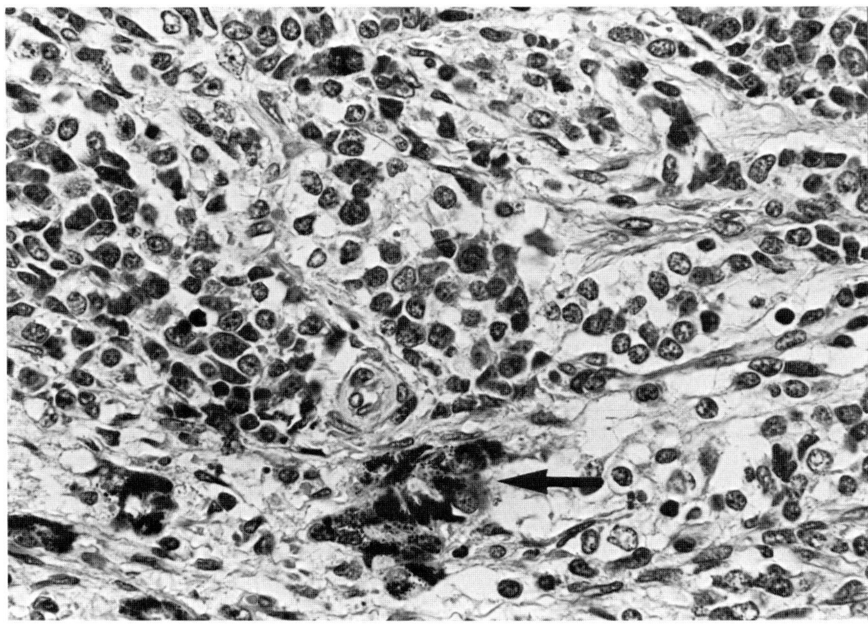

Fig. 10-22. The pigmented neuroectodermal tumor of infancy is easily recognized by the presence of small clusters of heavily pigmented cells (arrow). (H&E, × 250.)

and malignant mesenchymoma. Malignant Triton tumor is a highly malignant nerve sheath tumor (see Ch. 9) that generally affects older patients and is often associated with von Recklinghausen's disease.[181] It shows rhabdomyoblastic differentiation and lacks neuroblasts or typical ganglion cells. Malignant mesenchymoma, on the other hand, is a compound mesenchymal tumor composed of two or more cell types (other than fibroblasts) of mesodermal origin without neural crest derivates.[182]

PNET AND NON-PNET: DIFFERENTIAL DIAGNOSIS

The distinction of many small round cell tumors from PNET may be arduous: lymphoma, metastatic small cell carcinoma of the lung, neuroendocrine tumor of the skin, small cell osteosarcoma, and rhabdomyosarcoma are the most important differential diagnoses to be considered. The differential diagnosis and histogenetic controversies regarding extraosseous Ewing's sarcoma are discussed in Chapter 12. The distinctive features of peripheral PNET are given in Table 10-5.

The significance of glycogen in the differential diagnosis of small round cell tumors has greatly diminished, since both lymphomas[183]

and PNET[15, 17, 18] may contain it in variable amounts. Whereas rosettes or rosettelike structures are highly characteristic of neuroectodermal tumors, they may also be observed in follicular lymphomas[184] or primitive rhabdomyosarcomas (Fig. 10-23); in these cases, a positive reaction to the leukocyte common antigen (LCA)[185] and to muscle markers may help in clarifying the diagnosis.

In bones, other primitive or metastatic small round cell tumors may closely resemble a primitive neuroectodermal tumor. Malignant osteoid foci are commonly observed in small cell osteosarcoma, whereas metastatic small cell carcinoma of the lung tends to occur in older patients. NSE and neurofilaments have been reported positive in neuroendocrine tumors of the skin (Merkel cell tumors).[186, 187] Nonetheless, Merkel cell tumors can be identified by the characteristic peripheral subplasmalemmal distribution of neurosecretory granules[188] and by their intense perinuclear positivity to anti-cytokeratin antibodies.[189]

In summary, the neural crest origin of PNET may be morphologically overt or obscure. Morphologic evidence of the neural crest origin includes the presence of a distinct lobular pattern, Homer-Wright or Flexner rosettes, a fibrillar background, and the occurrence of schwannian and/or gangliar differentiation. In the absence

Table 10-5. Distinctive Features of Peripheral PNET

	Ewing	Intraosseous	PN	NB
Lobularity	−	−/+	+	+
Rosettes	−	−/+	+	+ +
Glycogen	+ +	+	+/−	−/+
Neurosecretory granules	−	+	+	+ +
Neurites	−	+/−	+	+ +
NSE	−	+	+ +	+ +
S-100 protein	−	+	+	+
NFTP	−	−/+	+	+ +
Chromogranin	−	−	−	+ +
MHC	+	+	+	−

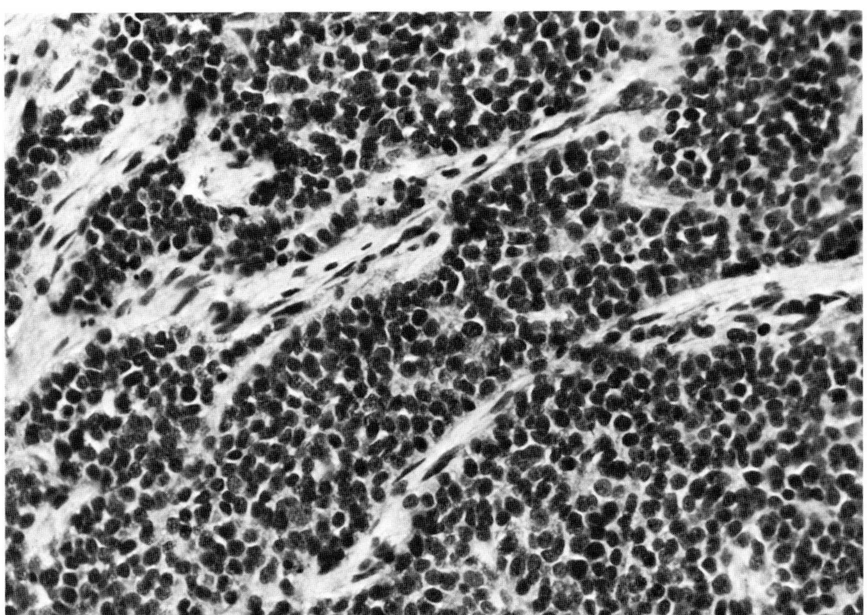

Fig. 10-23. Rosettelike structure in primitive rhabdomyosarcoma. (H&E, × 200.)

of the above-described features, PNET show a rather primitive, uncommitted appearance that is often inconclusive for diagnostic purposes. Immunocytochemical, ultrastructural, and whenever feasible, cytogenetic and molecular genetic studies are then of utmost importance to resolve and classify these cases correctly.

REFERENCES

1. Dehner LP: Peripheral and central primitive neuroectodermal tumors. A nosologic concept seeking a consensus. Arch Pathol Lab Med 110:997, 1986
2. Rubinstein LJ: Embryonal central neuroepithelial tumors and their differentiating potential: a cytogenetic view of a complex neurooncological problem. J Neurosurg 62:795, 1985
3. Le Douarin NM: Cell line segregation during peripheral nervous system ontogeny. Science, 231:1515, 1986
4. Le Lievre C, Le Douarin NM: Mesenchymal derivates of the neural crest: analysis of chimaeric quail and chick embryos. J Embryol Exp Morphol 34:125, 1975
5. Murray MR, Stout AP: Distinctive characteristics of sympathicoblastoma cultivated in vitro. A method for prompt diagnosis. Am J Pathol 23:429, 1947
6. Reynolds PC, German DC, Weimberger AG, Smith RG: Catecholamine fluorescence and tissue culture morphology. Techniques in the diagnosis of neuroblastoma. Am J Clin Pathol 75:275, 1981
7. Navarro-Fos S, Cavazzana AO, Noguera R, et al: Valor de las tecnicas de cultivos celulares y biologia molecular en el diagnostico diferencial de los sarcomas de celulas redondas de la infancia y adolescencia. Oncologia 3, XI:133, 1988
8. Misugi K, Misugi N, Newton WA: Fine structural study of neuroblastoma, ganglioneuroblastoma and pheocromocytoma. Arch Pathol 86:160, 1968
9. MacKay B, Luna MA, Butler JJ: Adult neuroblastoma. Electron microscopic observations in 9 cases. Cancer 37:1334, 1976
10. Taxy JB: Electron microscopy in the diagnosis of neuroblastoma. Arch Pathol Lab Med 104:355, 1980
11. Ghadially FN: Diagnostic Electron Microscopy of Tumours. Butterworths II ed. pp: 234–237, 1985
12. Romansky SG, Crocker DW, Shaw KN: Ultra-

structural studies on neuroblastoma. Evaluation of cytodifferentiation and correlation of morphology and biochemical survival data. Cancer 42:2392, 1978

13. Mierau GW: Extraskeletal Ewing's sarcoma (peripheral neuroepithelioma). Ultrastruct Pathol 9:91, 1985

14. Nesland JM, Sobrinho-Simoes MA, Johannessen JV: Primitive neuroectodermal tumor (peripheral neuroblastoma). Ultrastruct Pathol 9:59, 1985

15. Schmidt D, Harms D, Burdach S: Malignant peripheral neuroectodermal tumours of childhood and adolescence. Virchows Arch [A] 406:351, 1985

16. Bolen JW, Thorning D: Peripheral neuroepithelioma. A light and electron microscopic study. Cancer 46:2456, 1980

17. Triche TJ, Ross WE: Glycogen containing neuroblastoma with clinical and histopathological features of Ewing's sarcoma. Cancer 41:1425, 1978

18. Yunis EJ, Walpusk JA, Agostini RM, et al: Glycogen in neuroblastomas. Am J Surg Pathol 3:313, 1979

19. Llombart-Bosch A, Lacombe MJ, Contesso G, Peydro-Olaya A: Small round blue cell sarcoma of bone mimicking atypical Ewing's sarcoma with neuroectodermal features. Cancer 60: 1570, 1987

20. Isobe T, Okuyama T: The amino-acid sequence of the alpha subunit in bovine brain S100-a protein. Eur J Biochem 116:79, 1981

21. Isobe T, Okuyama T: The amino-acid sequence of S100 protein (PAP l-b Protein) and its relation to calcium bindings proteins. Eur J Biochem 89:379, 1978

22. Haimoto H, Hosoda S, Kato K: Differential distribution of immunoreactive S100-alpha and S100-beta proteins in normal nonnervous human tissues. Lab Invest 57:489, 1987

23. Stefansson K, Wollmann R, Jerkovic M: S-100 protein in Soft-Tissue tumors derived from Schwann cells and melanocytes. Am J Pathol 106:261, 1982

24. Baumal R, Kahn HJ, Marks A: Role of antibody to S100 protein in diagnostic pathology. Lab Invest 59:152, 1988

25. Misugi K, Aoki I, Kikyo S, et al: Immunohistochemical study of neuroblastoma and related tumors with anti-S-100 protein antibody. Pediatr Pathol 3:217, 1985

26. Pelc S, Gompel C, Simonet ML: S-100 protein expression in satellite and Schwann cells in neuroblastoma. Virchows Arch [B] 51:487, 1986

27. Shimada H, Aoyama C, Chiba T, Newton WA: Prognostic subgroups for undifferentiated neuroblastoma: immunohistochemical study with anti-S-100 protein antibody. Hum Pathol 16:471, 1985

28. Cavazzana AO, Ninfo V, Montesco M, et al: Peripheral neuroepithelioma: morphologic and immunologic criteria for diagnosis (Abstr). Mod Pathol 1:17, 1988

29. Abo T, Balch CM: Differentiation antigen of human NK and K cells identified by a monoclonal antibody (HNK-1). J Immunol 127:1024, 1981

30. Kruse J, Keilhauer G, Faissner A, Timpl R, Schachner M: The J1 glycoprotein—a novel nervous system cell adhesion molecule of the L2/HNK-1 family. Nature 316:146, 1985

31. Holley JA, Yu RK: Localisation of glycoconjugates recognized by the HNK-1 antibody in mouse and chick embryos during early neural development. Dev Neurosci 9:105, 1987

32. McGarry RC, Helfand SL, Quarles RH, Roder JC: Recognition of myelin-associated glycoprotein by the monoclonal antibody HNK-1. Nature 306:376, 1983

33. Caillaud JM, Benjelloun S, Bosq J, et al: HNK-1-defined antigen detected in paraffin-embedded neuroectodermal tumors and those derived from cells of the amine precursor uptake and decarboxylation system. Cancer Res 44:4432, 1984

34. Perentes E, Rubinstein LJ: Immunohistochemical recognition of human neuroepithelial tumors by anti-Leu 7 (HNK-1) monoclonal antibody. Acta Neuropathol (Berl) 69:227, 1986

35. Petrosio PM, Brooks JJ: Expression of nerve growth factor receptor in paraffin-embedded soft tissue tumors. Am J Pathol 132:152, 1988

36. Marchetti D, Perez-Polo RJ: Nerve growth factor receptors in human neuroblastoma cells. J Neurochem 49:475, 1987

37. Schmechel DE: Gamma-subunit of the glycolytic enzyme enolase: nonspecific or neuron specific? Lab Invest 52:239, 1985

38. Marangos PJ, Polak JM, Pearse AGE: Neuron-specific enolase. A probe for neurons and neuroendocrine cells. Trends Neurosci 5:193, 1982

39. Dhillon AP, Rode J, Leathem A: Neuron-spe-

cific enolase: an aid to the diagnosis of melanoma and neuroblastoma. Histopathology 6:81, 1982

40. Tsokos M, Linnoila RI, Chandra RS, Triche TJ: Neuron-specific enolase in the diagnosis of neuroblastoma and other small, round-cell tumors in children. Hum Pathol 15:575, 1984

41. Haimoto H, Takahashi Y, Koshikawa T, et al: Immunohistochemical localization of gamma-enolase in normal human tissues other than nervous and neuroendocrine tissues. Lab Invest 52: 257,1985

42. Lazarides E: Intermediate filaments: a chemically heterogeneous, developmentally regulated class of protein. Ann Rev Biochem 51:219, 1982

43. Altmannsberger M, Weber K, Holscher A, et al: Antibodies to intermediate filaments as diagnostic tools. Human gastrointestinal carcinomas express prekeratin. Lab Invest 46:520, 1982

44. Osborn M, Weber K: Tumor diagnosis by intermediate filament typing: a novel tool for surgical pathology. Lab Invest 48:372, 1983

45. Altmannsberger M, Osborn M, Schauer A, Weber K: Antibodies to different intermediate filament proteins are cell-specific markers in paraffin-embedded human tissues. Lab Invest 45:427, 1981

46. Schlaepfer WW, Freeman LA: Neurofilament proteins of rat peripheral nerve and spinal cord. J Cell Biol 78:653, 1978

47. Lee V, Wu H-L, Schaepfer WW: Monoclonal antibodies recognize individual neurofilament triplet proteins. Proc Natl Acad Sci USA 79:6089, 1982

48. Sternberger LA, Sternberger NH: Monoclonal antibodies distinguish phosphorylated and nonphosphorylated forms of neurofilaments in situ. Proc Natl Acad Sci USA 80:6126, 1983

49. Shaw G, Weber K: Differential expression of neurofilament triplet proteins in brain development. Nature 298:277, 1982

50. Mukai M, Torikata C, Iri H, et al: Expression of neurofilament triplet proteins in human neural tumors. An immunohistochemical study of paraganglioma, ganglioneuroma, ganglioneuroblastoma and neuroblastoma. Am J Pathol 122:28, 1986

51. Molenaar WM, Baker DL, Pleasure D, et al: The neuroendocrine and neural profiles of neuroblastomas, ganglioneuroblastomas and ganglioneuromas. Am J Pathol 136, 2:375, 1990

52. Carlei F, Polak JM, Ceccamea A, et al: Neuronal and glial markers in tumors of neuroblastic origin. Virchows Arch [A] 404:313, 1984

53. Schmidt D, Keil W, Harms D: Neuron-specific enolase, protein S-100, neurofilaments, glial fibrillary acidic protein and vimentin as markers for cytodifferentiation in neuroblastoma. Progr Surg Pathol 8:33, 1988

54. Osborn M, Altmannsberger M, Shaw G, et al: Various sympathetic derived human tumors differ in neurofilament expression. Use in diagnosis of neuroblastoma, ganglioneuroblastoma and pheochromocytoma. Virchows Arch [B] 40:141, 1982

55. Ross RA, Ciccarone V, Meyers MB, et al: Differential expression of intermediate filaments and fibronectin in human neuroblastoma cells. Prog Clin Biol Res 271:277, 1988

56. Stirling RW, Powell G, Fletcher CDM: Pigmented neuroectodermal tumor of infancy: an immunohistochemical study. Histopathology 12:425, 1988

57. Dellagi K, Lipinskj M, Paulin D; et al: Characterization of intermediate filaments expressed by Ewing's sarcoma tumor cell lines. Cancer Res 47:1170, 1987

58. Wiedenmann B, Franke WW: Identification and localization of synaptophysin, an integral membrane glycoprotein of M 38,000 of presynaptic vesicles. Cell 45:1017, 1985

59. Wiedenmann B, Franke WW, Kuhn C, et al: Synaptophysin: a marker for neuroendocrine cells and neoplasms. Proc Natl Acad Sci (USA) 83:3500, 1986

60. Gould V, Wiedenmann B, Lee I, et al: Synaptophysin expression in neuroendocrine neoplasms as determined by immunocytochemistry. Am J Pathol 126:243, 1987

61. Hachitanda Y, Tsuneyoshi M, Enjoji M: Expression of pan-neuroendocrine proteins in 53 neuroblastic tumors. Arch Pathol Lab Med 113:381, 1989

62. Angeletti RH: Editorial. Chromogranins and neuroendocrine secretion. Lab Invest 55:387, 1986

63. Hagn C, Schmid KW, Fischer-Colbrie R, Winkler H: Chromogranin A, B, and C in human adrenal medulla and endocrine tissues. Lab Invest 55:405, 1986

64. O'Connor DT, Frigon RP: Chromogranin A, the major catecholamine storage vesicles soluble protein: multiple size forms, subcellular

storage, and regional distribution in chromaffin and nervous tissue elucidated by radioimmunoassay. J Biol Chem 259:3237, 1984

65. Lloyd RV, Jin L, Fields K: Detection of chromogranin A and B in endocrine tissues with radioactive and biotinylated oligonucleotide probes. Am J Surg Pathol 14:35, 1990

66. Pagani A, Sanfilippo B, Forni M, et al: Chromogranin expression at the mRNA and protein level in small round cell tumors of infancy and childhood. Proceedings of the Adriatic Society of Pathology, Split, Yugoslavia, June 23–24, 1990

67. Cooper MJ, Helman LJ, Evans AE, et al: Chromogranin A expression in childhood peripheral neuroectodermal tumors. Adv Neuroblastoma Res 2:175, 1988

68. Young JL, Miller RW: Incidence of malignant tumors in US children. J Pediatr 86:254, 1975

69. Pastore G, Magnani C, Zanetti R, Terracini B: Incidence of cancer in children in the province of Torino (Italy 1967–1978). Eur J Cancer Clin Oncol 17:1337, 1981

70. Carlsen NLT, Christensen J, Schoreder H, et al: Prognostic factors in neuroblastomas treated in Denmark from 1943 to 1980. Cancer 58:2726, 1986

71. Birch JM, Marsden HB, Swindel R: Incidence of malignant disease in childhood: a 24-year review of the Manchester Children's Tumour Registry data. Br J Cancer 42:215, 1980

72. Gale G, D'Angio G, Uri A, et al: Cancer in neonates: The experience at the Children's Hospital of Philadelphia. Pediatrics 70:409, 1982

73. Young JL, Gloeckler Ries L, Silverberg E, et al: Cancer incidence, Survival, and Mortality for children younger than 15 years. Cancer 58:598, 1986

74. Sawada T, Sugimoto T, Tanaka T, et al: Number and cure rate of neuroblastoma cases detected by the mass screening program in Japan: future aspects. Med Pediatr Oncol 15:14, 1987

75. Beckwith JB, Perrin EV: In situ neuroblastomas: a contribution to the natural history of neural crest tumors. Am J Pathol 43:1089, 1966

76. Guin GH, Gilbert EF, Jones B: Incidental neuroblastoma in infants. Am J Clin Pathol 51:126, 1968

77. Beckwitt Turkel S, Itabashi HH: The natural history of neuroblastic cells in the fetal adrenal gland. Am J Pathol 76:225, 1974

78. Jaffe N: Neuroblastoma: review of the literature and an examination of factors contributing to

its enigmatic character. Cancer Treatment Rev 3:61, 1976

79. Kinnier-Wilson LM, Draper GJ: Neuroblastoma, its natural history and prognosis: a study of 487 cases. Br Med J 3:301, 1974

80. Evans AE, D'Angio GJ, Koop CE: Diagnosis and treatment of neuroblastoma. Pediatr Clin North Am 23:161, 1976

81. Dehner LP: Pediatric Surgical Pathology. 2nd Ed. William & Wilkins, Baltimore, 1988

82. Evans AE, D'Angio GJ, Propert K, et al: Prognostic factors in neuroblastoma. Cancer 59:1853, 1987

83. Coldman AJ, Fryer CJH, Elwood JM, Sonley MJ: Neuroblastoma: Influence of age at diagnosis, stage, tumor site and sex on prognosis. Cancer 46:1896, 1980

84. McLaughlin JE, Urich H: Maturating neuroblastoma and ganglioneuroblastoma: a study of four cases with long survival. J Pathol 121:19, 1977

85. Jones PG, Campbell PE: Tumours of Infancy and Childhood. Blackwell Scientific Publications, Oxford, 1976

86. Stokes SH, Thomas PRM, Perez C, Vietti T: Stage IV-S Neuroblastoma. Results with definitive therapy. Cancer 53:2083, 1984

87. Breslow N, McCann B: Statistical estimation of prognosis for children with neuroblastoma. Cancer Res 31:2098, 1971

88. Thomas PRM, Lee JY, Fineberg BB, et al: An analysis of neuroblastoma at a single institution. Cancer 53:2079, 1984

89. Evans AE, D'Angio DJ, Newton WA, Randolph JA: Proposed clinical staging for children with neuroblastoma. Children's Cancer Study Group A. Cancer 27:374, 1971

90. Sutow WW, Gehan EA, Heyn RM, et al: Comparison of survival curves, 1956 versus 1962, in children with Wilms' tumor and neuroblastoma. Pediatrics 45:800, 1970

91. D'Angio GJ, Evans AE, Koop CE: Special pattern of widespread neuroblastoma with a favorable prognosis. Lancet 1:1046, 1971

92. Evans AE, Chatten J, D'Angio GJ, et al: A review of 17 IV-S neuroblastoma patients at the Children's Hospital of Philadelphia. Cancer 45:833, 1980

93. Nickerson HJ, Nesbit ME, Grosfeld JL, et al: Comparison of stage IV and IV-S neuroblastoma in the first year of life. Med Pediatr Oncol 13:261, 1985

94. Oppedal BR, Storm-Mathisen I, Lie SO,

Brandtzaeg P: Prognostic factors in neuroblastoma. Clinical, histopathologic, and immunohistochemical features and DNA ploidy in relation to prognosis. Cancer 62:772, 1988

95. Beckwith BJ, Martin RF: Observation on the histopathology of neuroblastoma. J Pediatr Surg 3:106, 1968

96. Makinen J: Microscopic patterns as a quide to prognosis of neuroblastoma in childhood. Cancer 29:1637, 1972

97. Hughes M, Marsden HB, Palmer MK: Histologic patterns of neuroblastoma related to prognosis and clinical staging. Cancer 34:1706, 1974

98. Sandstedt B, Jereb B, Eklund G: Prognostic factors in neuroblastoma. Acta Pathol Microbiol Immunol Scand (Sect A) 91:365, 1983

99. Shimada H, Chatten J, Newton WA, et al: Histopathologic prognostic factors in neuroblastic tumors: definition of subtypes of ganglioneuroblastoma and an age-linked classification of. neuroblastoma. J Natl Cancer Inst 73:405, 1984

100. Chatten J, Shimada H, Sather HN, et al: Prognostic value of histopathology in advanced neuroblastoma. A report from the Childrens Cancer Study Group. Hum Pathol 19:1187, 1988

101. Laug W, Siegel S, Shaw K, et al: Initial urinary catecholamine metabolite concentrations and prognosis in neuroblastoma. Pediatrics 62:77, 1978

102. Gitlow SE, Bertani LM, Rausen A, et al: Diagnosis of neuroblastoma by qualitative and quantitative determinations of catecholamine metabolites in urine. Cancer 25:1377, 1980

103. Gitlow SE, Bertani L, Strauss L, et al: Biochemical and histological determinants in the prognosis of neuroblastoma. Cancer 32:898–905, 1973

104. LaBrosse EH, Comoy E, Bohvon C: Catecholamine metabolism in neuroblastoma. J Natl Cancer Inst 57:633, 1976

105. Hann HL, Levy HM, Evans AE: Serum ferritin as a guide to therapy in neuroblastoma. Cancer Res 40:1411, 1980

106. Zeltzer PM, Marangos PJ, Evans AE, Schneider SL: Serum neuron-specific enolase in children with neuroblastoma: Relationship to stage and disease course. Cancer 57:1230, 1986

107. Brodeur GM, Sekhon GS, Goldstein MN: Specific chromosomal aberration in human neuroblastoma. Am J Hum Genet 27:20A, 1975

108. Brodeur GM, Sekhan GS, Goldstein MN: Chromosomal aberrations in human neuroblastomas. Cancer 40:2256, 1977

109. Franke F, Rudolph B, Christiansen H, et al: Tumour karyotype may be important in the prognosis of human neuroblastoma. J Cancer Res Clin Oncol 11:266, 1986

110. Hayashi Y, Kanda N, Inaba T, et al: Cytogenetic findings and prognosis in neuroblastoma with emphasis on marker chromosome 1. Cancer 63:126, 1989

111. Biedler JL, Ross RA, Shanske S, Spegler BA: Human neuroblastoma cytogenetics: Search for significance of homogeneously staining regions and double minute chromosomes. Progr Cancer Res Ther 12:81, 1980

112. Brodeur GM, Fong C, Morita M, et al: Molecular and clinical significance of N-myc amplification and chromosome lp monosomy in human neuroblastomas. Adv Neuroblastoma Res 2:3, 1988

113. Brodeur GM, Seeger RC, Schwab M, et al: Amplification of N-*myc* in untreated human neuroblastomas correlates with advanced disease stage. Science 224:1121, 1984

114. Tsuda H, Shimosato Y, Upton M, et al: Retrospective study on amplification of N-*myc* and c-*myc* genes in pediatric solid tumors and its association with prognosis and tumor differentiation. Lab Invest 59:321, 1988

115. Brodeur GM, Hayes FA, Green A, et al: Consistent N-*myc* copy number in simultaneous or consecutive neuroblastoma samples from a given patients tumor. Proc Am Soc Clin Oncol 5:13, 1986

116. Nakagawara A, Ikeda K, Tsuda T, et al: Amplification of N-*myc* oncogene in stage II and IV S neuroblastomas may be a prognostic indicator. J Pediatr Surg 22:415, 1987

117. Oppendal BR, Oien O, Jahnsen T, Brandtzaeg P: N-*myc* amplification in neuroblastomas: histopathological, DNA ploidy and clinical variables. J Clin Pathol 42:1148, 1989

118. Hayashi Y, Kanda N, Imaba T, et al: Cytogenetic findings and prognosis in neuroblastoma with emphasis on marker chromosome 1. Cancer 63:126, 1989

119. Hashimoto H, Daimaru Y, Enjoji M, Nakagawara A: N-*myc* gene product expression in neuroblastoma. J Clin Pathol 42:52, 1989

120. Look AT, Hayes FA, Nitschke R, et al: Cellular DNA content as a predictor of response to chemotherapy in infants with unresectable neuroblastoma. N Engl J Med 311:231, 1984

121. Gansler T, Chatten J, Varello M, et al: Flow cytometric DNA analysis of neuroblastoma. Cancer 58:2453, 1986

122. Taylor SR, Blatt J, Costantino JP, et al: Flow cytometric DNA analysis of neuroblastoma and ganglioneuroma. 110 years retrospective study. Cancer 62:749, 1988

123. Stout AP: A tumor of the ulnar nerve. Proc NY Pathol Soc 18:2, 1918

124. Stout AP, Murray MP: Neuroepitelioma of the radial nerve with study of its behavior in vitro. Rev Can Biol 1:651, 1942

125. Bailey P, Cushing H: A Classification of the Tumors of the Glioma Group on a Histogenetic Basis with a Correlated Study of Prognosis. JB Lippincott, Philadelphia, 1926

126. Penfield W: Tumors of the sheaths of the nervous system. p. 980. In Cytology and Cellular Pathology of the Nervous System. Paul B. Ebner, New York, 1932

127. Abell MR, Hart WR, Olson JR: Tumors of the peripheral nervous system. Hum Pathol 1:503, 1970

128. Lattes R: Proceedings of the Thirty-Ninth Annual Anatomic Pathology Slide Seminar of the American Society of Clinical Pathologists. p. 49. ASCP, Chicago, 1973

129. Askin FO, Rosai J, Sibley RK, et al: Malignant small cell tumor of the thoracopulmonary region in childhood. A distinctive clinicopathologic entity of uncertain origin. Cancer 43:2438, 1979

130. Linnoila RI, Tsokos M, Triche TJ, et al: Evidence for a neural origin and PAS-positive variants of the malignant small round cell tumor of the thoracopulmonary region (Askin's tumor). Am J Surg Pathol 10:124, 1986

131. Gonzalez-Crussi F, Wolfson SL, Misugi K, Nakajima T: Peripheral neuroectodermal tumors of the chest wall in childhood. Cancer 54:2519, 1984

132. Whang-Peng J, Triche TJ, Knutset T, et al: Cytogenetic characterization of selected small round cell tumor of childhood. Cancer Genet Cytogenet 21:185, 1986

133. Fletcher CDM: Peripheral nerve sheath tumors. A clinicopathologic update. Pathol Annu 25:53, 1990

134. Hashimoto H, Kiryu H, Enjoji M, et al: Malignant neuroepithelioma (peripheral neuroblastoma). A clinicopathologic study of 15 cases. Am J Surg Pathol 7:309, 1983

135. Llombart-Bosch A, Terrier-Lacombe MJ, Peydro-Olaya A, Contesso G: Peripheral neuroectodermal sarcomas of soft tissue (peripheral neuroepithelioma): a pathologic study of ten cases with differential diagnosis regarding other small, round-cell sarcomas. Hum Pathol 20:273, 1989

136. Hajdu SI: Pathology of Soft Tissue Tumors. Lea & Febiger, Philadelphia, 1979

137. Bolen JW, Thorning D: Peripheral neuroepithelioma: a light and electron microscopy study. Cancer 46:2456, 1980

138. Harper PG, Pringle J, Souhami RL: Neuroepithelioma. A rare malignant peripheral nerve tumor of primitive origin: report of two new cases and review of the literature. Cancer 48:2282, 1981

139. Nesbitt KA, Vidone RA: Primitive neuroectodermal tumor (neuroblastoma) arising in the sciatic nerve of a child. Cancer 37:1562, 1976

140. Marina NM, Etcubanas E, Parham DM, et al: Peripheral primitive neuroectodermal tumor (peripheral neuroepithelioma) in children. A review of the St. Jude experience and controversies in the diagnosis and management. Cancer 64:1952, 1989

141. Jurgens H, Bier V, Harms D, et al: Malignant peripheral neuroectodermal tumors. A retrospective analysis of 42 patients. Cancer 61:349, 1988

142. Aleshire SL, Glick AD, Cruz VE, et al: Neuroblastoma in adults: pathologic findings and clinical outcome. Arch Pathol Lab Med 109:352, 1985

143. Cavazzana AO, Santopietro R, Sforza V, et al: Morphometry adds to the differential diagnosis between peripheral neuroepithelioma and neuroblastoma. Mod Pathol (in press).

144. Thiele CJ, McKeon C, Triche TJ, et al: Differential proto-oncogene expression characterizes histologically indistinguishable tumors of the peripheral nervous system. J Clin Invest 80:804, 1987

145. Cooper MJ, Helman LJ, Evans AE, et al: Chromogranin expression in childhood peripheral neuroectodermal tumors. Progr Clin Biol Res 271:175, 1988

146. Turc-Carel, Philip I, Merger MP, et al: Chromosomal translocations in Ewing's sarcoma. N Engl J Med 309:497, 1983

147. Aurias A, Rimbaut C, Buffe D, Dubousset T, Mazabraud A: Chromosomal translocations in Ewing's sarcoma. N Engl J Med 309:496, 1983

148. Whang-Peng J, Triche TJ, Knutsen T, et al: Chromosomal translocation in peripheral neuroepithelioma. N Engl J Med 311:584, 1984

149. McKeon C, Thiele CJ, Ross RA, et al: Indistinguishable pattern of proto-oncogene expression in two distinct but closely related tumors: Ewing's sarcoma and neuroepithelioma. Cancer Res 48:4307, 1988

150. Lampson LA, Fisher CA, Whelan JP: Striking paucity of HLA-A,B,C, and Beta2-microglobulin on human neuroblastoma cell lines. J Immunol 130:2471, 1983

151. Lampson LA, Whelan JP, Fisher CA: HLA-A,B,C and Beta 2-microglobulin are expressed weakly by human cells of neuronal origin, but can be induced in neuroblastoma cell lines by interferon. Prog Clin Biol Res 175:379, 1985

152. Whelan JP, Chatten J, Lampson LA: HLA-class I and Beta 2-microglobulin expression in frozen and formaldehyde-fixed paraffin sections of neuroblastoma tumor. Cancer Res 45:5976, 1985

153. Cavazzana AO, Tirabosco R, Tollot M, et al: Prognostic factors in Neuroblastoma with regard to stromal component. Pathol Res Pract 185:35A, 1989

154. Reynolds PC, Tomayko MM, Donner L, et al: Biological classification of cell lines derived from human extra-cranial neural tumors. Prog Clin Biol Res 271:291, 1988

155. Jaffe R, Santamaria M, Yunis J, et al: The neuroectodermal tumor of bone. Am J Surg Pathol 8:885, 1984

156. Llombart-Bosch A, Lacombe MJ, Contesso G, Peydro-Olaya A: Small round blue cell sarcoma of bone mimicking atypical Ewing's sarcoma with neuroectodermal features. An analysis of five cases with immunohistochemical and electron microscopic support. Cancer 60:1570, 1987

157. Schmidt D, Mackay R, Ayala AG: Ewing's sarcoma with neuroblastoma-like features. Ultrastruct Pathol 3:143, 1982

158. Isayama T, Iwasaki H, Kikuchi M, et al: Neuroectodermal tumor of bone. Evidence for neural differentiation in a cultured cell line. Cancer 65:1771, 1990

159. Bagnara GP, Serra M, Giovannini M, et al: Establishment and characterization of a primitive neuroectodermal tumor of bone cell line (LAP-35). Int J Cell Cloning (in press)

160. Cavazzana AO, Magnani JL, Ross RA, et al: Ewing's sarcoma is an undifferentiated neuroectodermal tumor. Prog Clin Biol Res 271:487, 1988

161. Cavazzana AO, Miser JS, Jefferson J, Triche TJ: Experimental evidence for a neural origin of Ewing's sarcoma of bone. Am J Pathol 127:507, 1987

162. Triche TJ, Cavazzana AO: Small round cell tumors of bone. p. 119. In Unni KK (ed): Bone Tumors. Contemporary Issues in Surgical Pathology. Churchill Livingstone, New York, 1988

163. Schmidt D, Herrmann C, Harms D: Ewing's sarcoma and malignant peripheral neuroectodermal tumor: a retrospective analysis of 120 cases. Med Pediatr Oncol 17:282, 1989

164. Shuangshoti S: Primitive neuroectodermal tumor (neuroepithelial) tumor of soft tissue of the neck in a child: demonstration of neuronal and neuroglial differentiation. Histopathology 10:651, 1986

165. Nakamura Y, Becker LE, Mancer K, Gillespie R: Peripheral medulloepithelioma. Acta Neuropathol (Berl) 57:137, 1982

166. Tsokos M, Scarpa S, Ross RA, Triche TJ: Differentiation of human neuroblastoma recapitulates neural crest development. Study of morphology, neurotransmitter enzymes, and extracellular matrix proteins. Am J Pathol 128:484, 1987

167. Mennermeyer RP, Hammar SP, Tytus JS, et al: Melanotic Schwannoma: clinical and ultrastructural study of three cases with evidence of intracellular melanin synthesis. Am J Surg Pathol 1:3, 1979

168. Cutler LS, Chaudhry AP, Topazian R: Melanotic neuroectodermal tumor of infancy: an ultrastructural study, literature review, and re-evaluation. Cancer 48:257, 1981

169. Young S, Gonzalez-Crussi F: Melanocytic neuroectodermal tumor of the foot. Report of a case with multicentric origin. Am J Clin Pathol 84:371, 1985

170. Dehner LP, Sibley RK, Sauk JJ, et al: Malignant melanotic neuroectodermal tumor of infancy. A clinical, pathologic, ultrastructural and tissue culture study. Cancer 43:1389, 1979

171. Palacios JJN: Malignant melanotic progonoma. One case. Light and electron microscopic study. Cancer 46:529, 1980

172. Scheck O, Ruck P, Harms D, Kaiserling E: Melanotic neuroectodermal tumor of infancy

occurring in the left thigh of a 6-month-old female infant. Ultrastruct Pathol 13:23, 1989

173. Borg ED, Gorlin RJ: Melanotic neuroectodermal tumor of infancy. A neoplasm of neural crest origin. Report of a case associated with high urinary excretion of vanillmandelic acid. Cancer 19:196, 1966

174. Dourov N, Mayer R, de Martelaere F, et al: Melanotic neuroectodermal tumor of infancy with high levels of alpha-fetoprotein. J Oral Pathol 16:251, 1987

175. Ricketts RR, Majmudarr B: Epididymal melanotic neuroectodermal tumor of infancy. Hum Pathol 16(4):416, 1985

176. Naka A, Matsumoto S, Shirai T, Itoh T: Ganglioneuroblastoma associated with malignant mesenchymoma. Cancer 36:1050, 1975

177. Shuangshotj S, Kasantikul V, Suwangool P, Chittmittrapap S: Malignant neoplasm of mixed mesenchymal and neuroepithelial origin (ectomesenchymoma) of the thigh. J Surg Oncol 27:208, 1984

178. Kawamoto EH, Weidner N, Agostini RM, Jaffe R: Malignant ectomesenchymoma of soft tissue. Report of two cases and review of the literature. Cancer 59:1791, 1987

179. Karcioglu Z, Someren A, Mates SJ: Ectomesenchymoma: a malignant tumor of migratory neural crest (ectomesenchyme) remnants showing ganglionic, schwannian, melanocytic, and rhabdomyoblastic differentiation. Cancer 39:2486, 1977

180. Kodet R, Kasthuri N, Marsden HB, et al: Gangliorhabdomyosarcoma: a histopathologic and immunohistochemical study of three cases. Histopathology 10:181, 1986

181. Woodruff JM, Churnik NL, Smith MC, et al: Peripheral nerve tumors with rhabdomyosarcomatous differentiation (malignant "Triton" tumors). Cancer 32:426, 1973

182. Enzinger FM, Weiss SW: Soft Tissue Tumors. 2nd Ed. CV Mosby, St. Louis, 1988

183. Azar HA, Jaffe ES, Berard CW, et al: Diffuse large cell lymphomas (reticulum cell sarcomas, histiocytic lymphomas). Correlation of morphologic features with functional markers. Cancer 46:1428, 1980

184. Frizzera G, Gajl-Peczalska K, Sibley RK, et al: Rosette formation in malignant lymphoma. Am J Pathol 119:351, 1985

185. Kurtin PJ, Pinkus GS: Leukocyte common antigen. A diagnostic discriminant between hematopoietic and nonhematopoietic neoplasms in paraffin sections using monoclonal antibodies: Correlation with immunologic studies and ultrastructural localization. Hum Pathol 16:353, 1985

186. Gu J, Polak JM, Van Noorden S, et al: Immunostaining of neuron-specific enolase as a diagnostic tool for Merkel cell tumors. Cancer 52:1039, 1983

187. Miettinen M, Letho V-P, Virtanen I, et al: Neuroendocrine carcinoma of the skin (Merkel cell carcinoma): Ultrastructural and immunohistochemical demonstration of neurofilaments. Ultrastruct Pathol 4:219, 1983

188. Wick MR, Goellner JR, Scheithauer BW, et al: Primary neuroendocrine carcinomas of the skin (Merkel cell tumors). A clinical, histologic, and ultrastructural study of thirteen cases. Am J Clin Pathol 79:6, 1983

189. Heenan PJ, Cole JM, Spagnolo DV: Primary cutaneous neuroendocrine carcinoma (Merkel cell tumor). An adnexal epithelial neoplasm. Am J Dermatopathol 12:7, 1990

11

Clear Cell Sarcoma: A Tumor of Probable Neuroectodermal Origin

E. B. Chung

The evolving concepts of soft tissue tumor classification, previously described in Chapter 1, are well exemplified by clear cell sarcoma (CCS) of tendons and aponeuroses.

Since 1965, when Enzinger[1] reported 21 cases of CCS of tendons and aponeuroses, this tumor has been accepted as a clinicopathologic entity distinct from other soft tissue sarcomas. For almost 20 years CCS had been considered a tumor of unknown histogenesis, although synovial[2,3] and schwannian[4,5] origins have been considered.

Immunocytochemical and cytochemical studies[6–10] have now clearly demonstrated a neural crest origin for this lesion, and the term *malignant melanoma of soft parts* has been proposed.[6] CCS and melanoma, in fact, seem to share a common line of differentiation not only for their similar reactivity to S-100 protein[6,8] and other melanoma-associated proteins such as MHB-45[10,11] but also for the expression of melanin-related metabolic pathways involving tyrosinase and cholinesterase activities in both melanoma and CCS cells.[9,12]

CLINICAL FEATURES

The tumor mainly afflicts young adults between the ages of 20 and 40. The median age at diagnosis is 27 years. Females are affected more commonly than males.

The principal sites of the tumor are the extremities, especially the region of the foot and ankle (43 percent of cases). Next in frequency are the knee, thigh, and hand (36 percent). The head and neck region and the trunk are only rarely involved. The tumor is usually deep seated and, like epithelioid sarcoma, is often intimately bound to tendons and aponeuroses. The overlying skin is usually uninvolved, although many of the larger tumors extend into the subcutis and lower dermis.

The tumor presents as a slowly enlarging mass that causes tenderness or pain in about one-half of the cases. The duration of symptoms averages 2 years, and ranges from a few weeks to as long as 20 years. CCS that have been present for 5 or more years are not uncommon.

PATHOLOGIC FINDINGS

Grossly the tumor is circumscribed, but is seldom encapsulated or multilobulated. Frequently the mass is attached to tendons or aponeuroses. The tumor ranges in size from 1 cm to more than 10 cm, but in the majority of cases it measures 2 to 6 cm in diameter. The cut surfaces are gray-white and are accompanied by focal hemorrhage, necrosis, or cystic change. Foci of dark brown or black pigmentation are found in about 20 percent of cases.

Microscopically the tumor is composed of compact nests of fascicles of rounded or fusiform cells, often with clear cytoplasm, bordered and divided by fine fibrous tissue septa that merge with adjacent tendons or aponeuroses

259

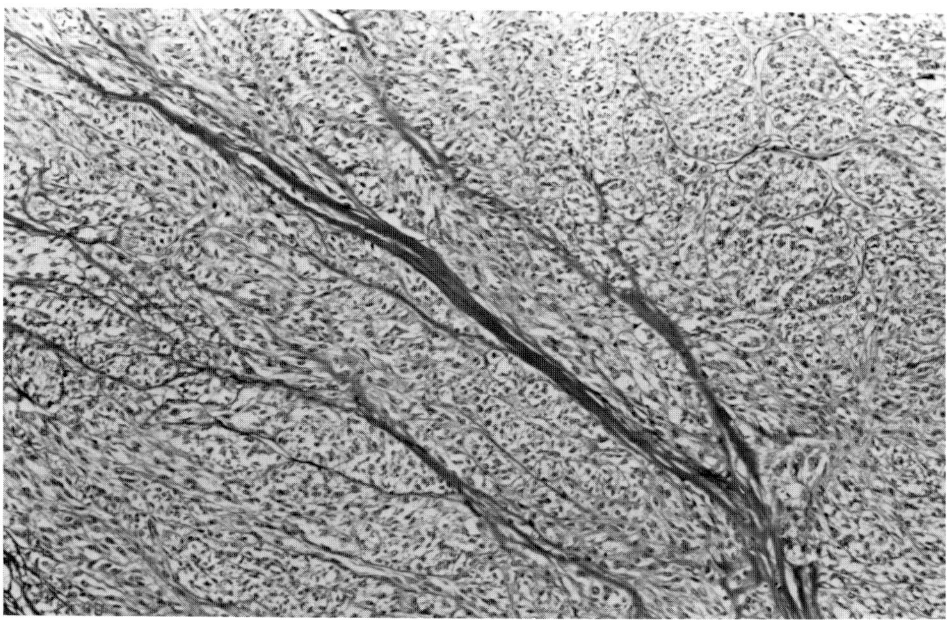

Fig. 11-1. Clear cell sarcoma showing nests and short fascicles of pale-staining tumor cells separated by fibrous septa. (H&E, ×125.)

(Fig. 11-1). The characteristic nestlike growth pattern can best be accentuated by a reticulin stain. The tumor cells are relatively regular and uniform, and have a round to oval nucleus with a central prominent nucleolus (Fig. 11-2A). They are often associated with multinucleated tumor giant cells having peripherally placed nuclei (Fig. 11-2B). Mitotic figures are usually scarce (less than 2 to 3 per 10 high-power fields).

Although the name implies that the neoplastic cells possess clear cell cytoplasm owing to the presence of large amounts of intracellular glycogen, in some cases they have more eosinophilic cytoplasm, resembling those of malignant melanoma. Indeed, intracellular melanin is detected with the Fontana stain in about one-half of the cases and with the Warthin-Starry preparation at pH 3.2 in nearly two-thirds of the cases. Immunocytochemically CCS shows a positivity to many neural markers, such as neuron-specific enolase, S-100 protein (Fig. 11-3), Leu-7, and synaptophysin, as well as to a melanoma marker such as MBH-45. Reactions to cytokeratin, desmin, and epithelial membrane antigen are always negative.

Ultrastructurally the tumor shows a remarkably uniform population of round or oval cells with abundant cytoplasm containing large amounts of glycogen, well-developed Golgi areas, and numerous melanosomes in various stages of development. A prominent and continuous basal lamina is frequently observed to surround small nests of cells.

DIFFERENTIAL DIAGNOSIS

In the past, some of these tumors were either diagnosed as synovial sarcoma or, alternatively, categorized under the tendosynovial sarcoma group. A distinction from synovial sarcoma is usually achieved by noting the presence of intracellular melanin (50 to 75 percent) and the absence of a biphasic cellular pattern and detectable cytoplasmic keratin.

Differentiation from a fibrosarcoma may be problematic if the neoplastic cells lack clear cytoplasm and if they bear smaller and less prominent nucleoli. However, the absence of nestlike cellular aggregates, S-100 protein nega-

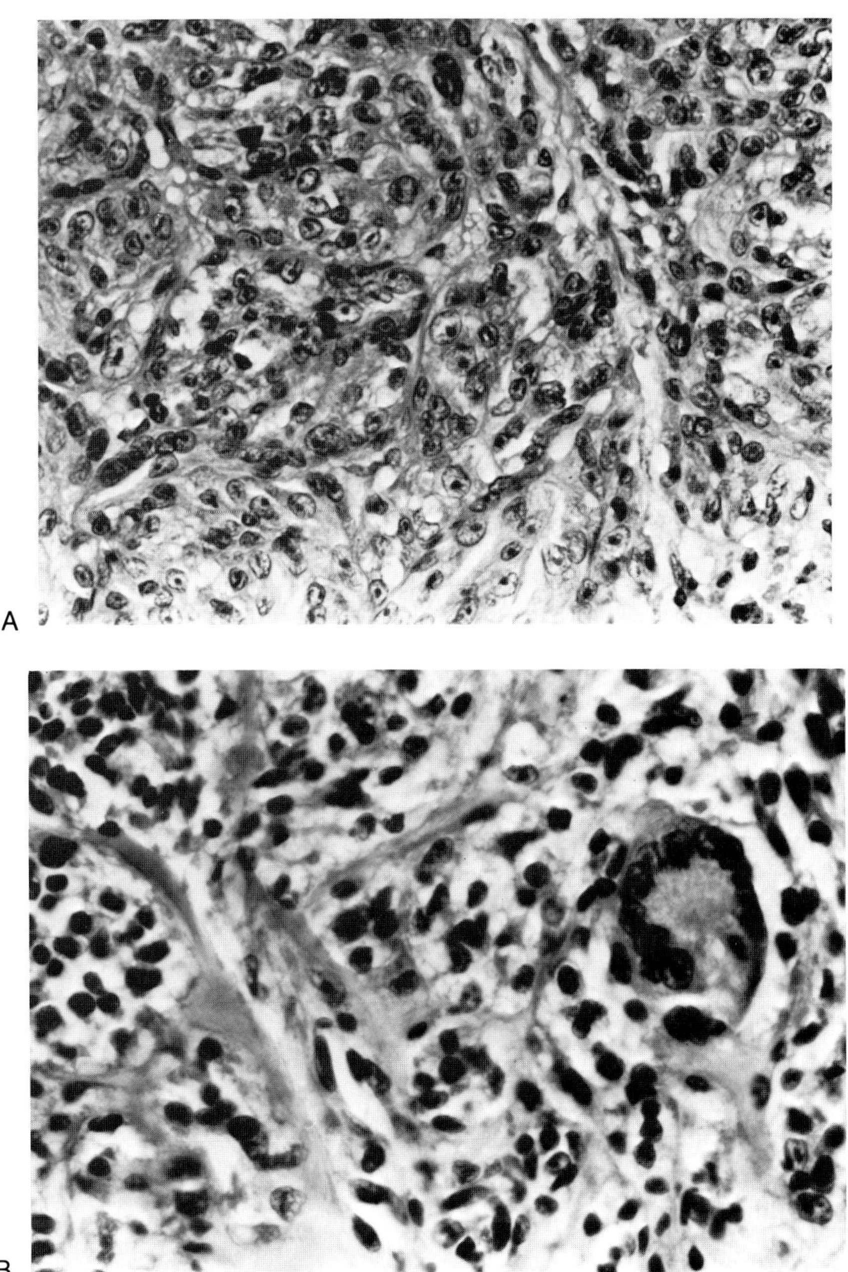

Fig. 11-2. Malignant melanoma of soft parts (clear cell sarcoma). **(A)** Tumor cells possessing round vesicular nuclei with a single prominent nucleolus. **(B)** Multinucleated tumor giant cell having peripherally placed nuclei. (H&E, ×500.)

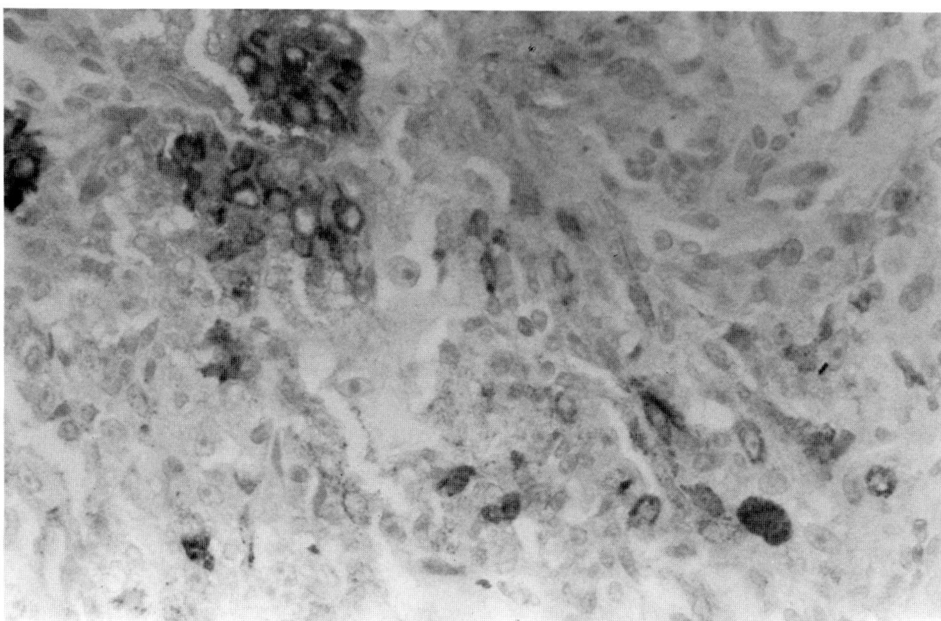

Fig. 11-3. Clear cell carcinoma displaying a strong immunoreactivity for S-100 protein. (×500.)

tivity, and a lack of intracytoplasmic glycogen in a fibrosarcoma may help in establishing a correct diagnosis. Other soft tissue tumors with an epithelioid or clear cell appearance enter the differential diagnosis, namely epithelioid malignant schwannoma, epithelioid sarcoma, and epithelioid leiomyosarcoma. Histochemical, immunocytochemical, and ultrastructural features are important to achieve the correct diagnosis.

The main differential diagnostic criteria are summarized in Table 11-1.

A more difficult task is to separate CCS from metastatic melanoma, with which the former shares many morphologic and immunocytochemical characteristics. A careful clinical examination of the patient is then required to rule out the possibility of a cutaneous or visceral melanoma.

Table 11-1. Distinctive Features of Epithelioid Sarcomas

	CCS	EMS	ES	EL
Histochemical				
Melanin	+ +	−	−	−
PAS positivity	+ +	−	−	+
Immunocytochemical				
S-100 protein	+ +	+/−	−	−
HMB-45	+	−	−	−
Keratin	−	−	+	+/−
Desmin	−	−	−	+ +
Electron microscopic				
Basal lamina	+ +	+/−	−	+/−
Glycogen	+ +	−	−	+
Melanosomes	+ +	−	−	−

PAS, periodic acid-Schiff; CCS, clear cell sarcoma; EMS, epithelioid malignant schwannoma; ES, epithelioid sarcoma; EL, epithelioid leiomyosarcoma.

PROGNOSIS

Although many of the tumors pursue a slow, indolent clinical course with a high rate of local recurrence and late metastasis, prognosis is generally poor (over 43 percent mortality), except for small and superficially located lesions. The most common sites of metastasis are the lung, regional lymph nodes, and bone. Thus, the treatment of choice appears to be a radical excision, including regional lymph node dissection or amputation if radical excision is not feasible. Since some of the tumors have recurred or metastasized 10 or more years after the initial excision, long-term follow-up is necessary before one can safely assume that the patient has been cured.

REFERENCES

1. Enzinger FM: Clear-cell sarcomas of tendons and aponeuroses. An analysis of 21 cases. Cancer 18:1163, 1965
2. Hajdu SI, Shiu MH, Fortner JG: Tendonsynovial sarcoma. A clinicopathologic study of 136 cases. Cancer 39:1201, 1977
3. Tsuneyoshi M, Enjoji M, Kubo T: Clear cell sarcoma of tendons and aponeuroses: a comparative study of 13 cases with a provisional subgrouping into the melanotic and synovial types. Cancer 42:243, 1978
4. Azumi N, Turner RR: Clear cell sarcoma of tendons and aponeuroses: electron microscopic findings suggesting Schwann cell differentiation. Hum Pathol 14:1084, 1983
5. Ohno T, Park P, Utsunomiya Y, et al: Ultrastructural study of a clear cell sarcoma suggesting schwannian differentiation. Ultrastruct Pathol 10:39, 1986
6. Chung EB, Enzinger FM: Malignant melanoma of soft parts. A reassessment of clear cell sarcoma. Am J Surg Pathol 7:405, 1983
7. Mukai M, Torikata C, Hiri H, et al: Histogenesis of clear cell sarcoma of tendons and aponeuroses. An electron microscopic, biochemical enzyme, histochemical, and immunohistochemical study. Am J Pathol 114:264, 1984
8. Kindblom LG, Lodding P, Angervall L: Clear-cell sarcoma of tendons and aponeuroses. Virchows Arch [A] 401:109, 1983
9. Mii Y, Miyauchi Y, Hohnoki K, et al: Neural crest origin of clear cell sarcoma of tendons and aponeuroses. Ultrastructural and enzyme cytochemical study of human and nude mouse-transplanted tumors. Virchows Arch [A] 415:51, 1989
10. Swanson PE, Wick MR: Clear cell sarcoma. An immunohistochemical analysis of six cases and comparison with other epithelioid neoplasms of soft tissue. Arch Pathol Lab Med 113:55, 1989
11. Papas-Corden P, Zarbo RJ, Grown AM, Crissman JD: Immunohistochemical characterization of synovial, epithelioid, and clear cell sarcomas. Surg Pathol 2:43, 1989
12. Hunter JAA, Paterson WD, Fairley D: Human malignant melanoma. Melanosomal polymorphism and the ultrastructural DOPA reaction. Br J Dermatol 98:381, 1978

<h1 style="text-align:center">12</h1>

Tumors of Uncertain Histogenesis

E. B. Chung and Vito Ninfo

Despite the considerable progress in the past three decades regarding the identification and diagnosis of soft tissue tumors, the histogenesis of some entities is still obscure. These lesions are collectively grouped under the conventional heading of tumors of uncertain histogenesis. A detailed discussion of each of these lesions is beyond the scope of this book, nevertheless pathologists should be aware of and familiar with some of the diagnostic problems these tumors present.

This chapter discusses the tumors listed in Table 12-1.

BENIGN TUMORS AND TUMORLIKE LESIONS

MYXOMA

Myxoma is a descriptive term for a group of lesions widely occurring in soft tissues, bone, and parenchymatous organs. Traditionally myxoma refers to hypocellular masses, mimicking primitive mesenchyme,[1] composed mainly of a loose extracellular matrix consisting of hyaluronic acid-rich mucopolysaccharides[2–4] produced in large amounts by spindle cells of probable fibroblastic origin. These tumors are poorly vascularized and secondary cystic changes are frequently observed. A degenerative rather than a true neoplastic process is probably involved in the pathogenesis of many of these lesions, such as cutaneous focal mucinosis, digital mucous cyst, meniscal cyst, and ganglion cyst.

Intramuscular myxomas deserve special attention because they can be easily overdiagnosed owing to their frequently large size and infiltrative growth pattern. These rare tumors generally occur in adults and usually affect the large muscles of the thigh, shoulder, and buttocks.[2–5] The great majority of intramuscular myxomas are solitary. Nearly all multiple myxomas are associated with fibrous dysplasia of bone, usually the monostotic type.[6, 7] Macroscopically they have a gelatinous appearance and are deceptively well circumscribed; at closer inspection, however, they merge imperceptibly into the surrounding muscle.

Microscopically they are composed of an abundant, poorly vascularized myxoid stroma containing a low number of bland spindle cells (Fig. 12-1). The matrix consists of hyaluronidase-sensitive acid mucopolysaccharides and a few scattered collagen fibers; small cystic spaces are commonly observed. At the periphery, the muscle fibers are often dissociated and surrounded by the mucoid material.

These tumors invariably follow a benign course, and recurrence is extremely rare.[3]

Due to its myxoid appearance and pseudoinfiltrative growth pattern, this neoplasm can easily be misdiagnosed as myxoid liposarcoma or myxoid malignant fibrous histiocytoma. However, the absence of a plexiform vascular pattern and lipoblasts and the absence of malignant pleomorphic cells, respectively, will rule out these sarcomas. Atrophic, multinucleated muscle fibers, frequently observed at the tumor periphery, can be mistaken for malignant rhabdomyoblasts, thus embryonal rhabdomyosarcoma sometimes enters the differential diagnosis.

265

Table 12-1. Tumors of Uncertain Histogenesis

Benign	Malignant
Myxoma	Alveolar soft part sarcoma
Parachordoma	Epithelioid sarcoma
	Extraosseous Ewing's sarcoma
	Malignant mesenchymoma
	Malignant rhabdoid tumor

Aggressive angiomyxomas are highly vascularized myxomatous tumors that occur chiefly in the pelvic and genital regions of adult women,[8, 9] although a few cases have also been described in men.[9] These tumors differ from ordinary myxoma by the presence of many vessels and numerous collagen fibers (Fig. 12-2). Pelvic myxoid leiomyoma can closely mimic an angiomyxoma, but the recognition of scattered smooth muscle fibers generally clarifies the diagnosis. Unlike ordinary myxoma, angiomyxoma tends to recur after surgical excision, but does not metastasize.

Myxoid hamartoma is a myxomatous tumor

recently described by Gonzalez-Crussi et al.[10] in the mesentery and omentum of young children; a well-developed vasculature and inflammatory background are its hallmarks. This rare tumor can closely simulate a myxoid liposarcoma or, alternatively, a botryoid rhabdomyosarcoma. Muscle markers, such as desmin and myoglobin, are negative in this lesion, and lipoblasts are always absent.

PARACHORDOMA

Parachordoma, a very rare benign tumor, is also known as *peripheral chordoma*. Originally described by Lyaskovsky,[11] it was later presented as a new clinicopathologic entity by Dabska[12] in 1977. Histologically it resembles a chordoid sarcoma or deep-seated chondroid syringoma. Some workers speculate that so-called chordoid sarcoma or extraskeletal myxoid chondrosarcoma may represent a poorly differentiated variant of parachordoma with prevailing myxoid areas.[13] Because of its rarity, this tumor

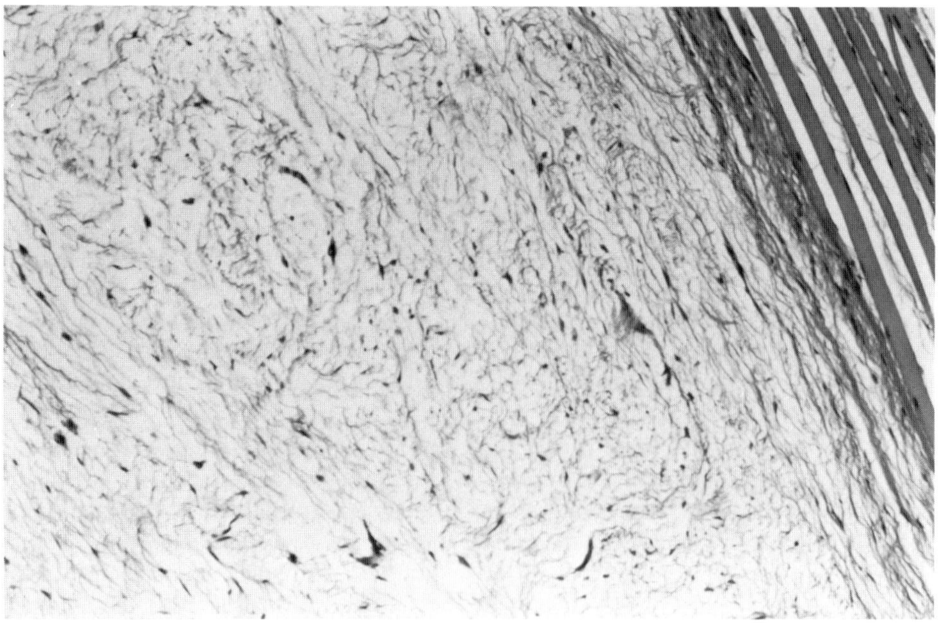

Fig. 12-1. Intramuscular myxoma surrounded by atrophic muscle fibers. Note the hypocellular myxomatous tissue with a virtual absence of vascular structures, and peripheral condensation of reticulin fibers. (H&E, × 125.)

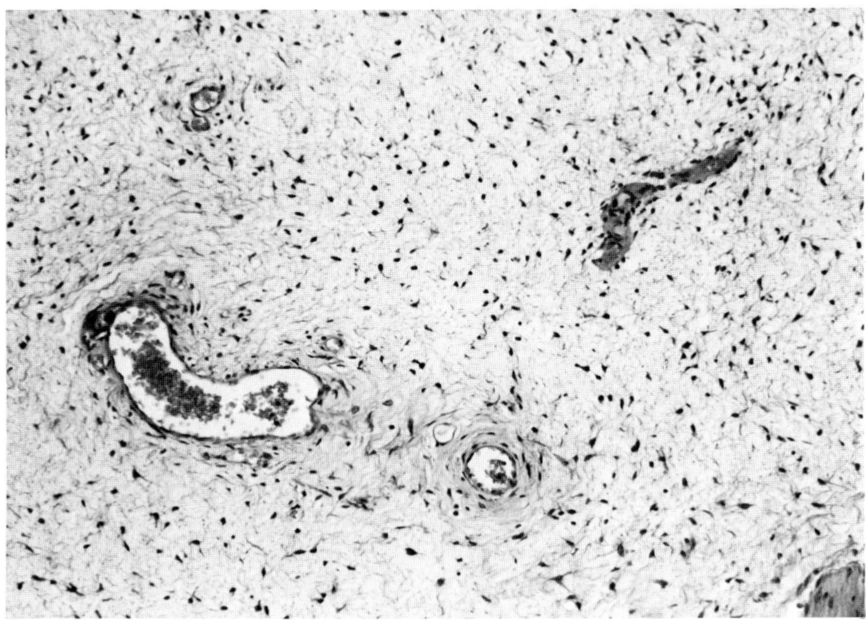

Fig. 12-2. Aggressive angiomyxoma of the pelvis in 52-year-old woman. Numerous dilated vascular structures are embedded in an abundant myxoid matrix. (H&E, × 125.)

may not be recognized, and may be readily confused with the aforementioned neoplasms.

Clinical Features

Parachordoma affects both children and adults, and occurs most commonly in the extremities or peripheral parts of the body. These tumors are usually deep seated and involve soft tissues adjacent to tendons, synovium, or bones.

Pathologic Findings

Grossly tumors are nodular or coarsely lobulated, and are often well demarcated, but not encapsulated. Histologically they consist of nests of pale-staining or vacuolated round cells of various size, resembling those of the notochord (Fig. 12-3). These cells are embedded in a myxoid, sometimes hyaline, matrix (Fig. 12-4), and contain glycogen (Fig. 12-5). The cell

nests may assume a pseudoacinar appearance (Fig. 12-4). The myxoid stroma contains abundant glycosaminoglycans that can be removed by pretreatment with hyaluronidase. Electron microscopic findings in parachordoma are essentially the same as those observed in chordomas of the axial skeleton. The physaliphorous cells in both tumors possess two types of intracytoplasmic vacuoles, namely glycogen-containing vacuoles and intracytoplasmic pseudoinclusions of intercellular substance.[13]

Differential Diagnosis

These tumors are most often confused with chordoma, extraskeletal myxoid chondrosarcoma, or chordoid sarcoma, and deep-seated mixed tumor of the skin or chondroid syringoma. Unlike tumors of chondroblastic and notochordal origin, the mucinous material in parachordoma is composed of hyaluronidase-sensitive acid mucopolysaccharides.

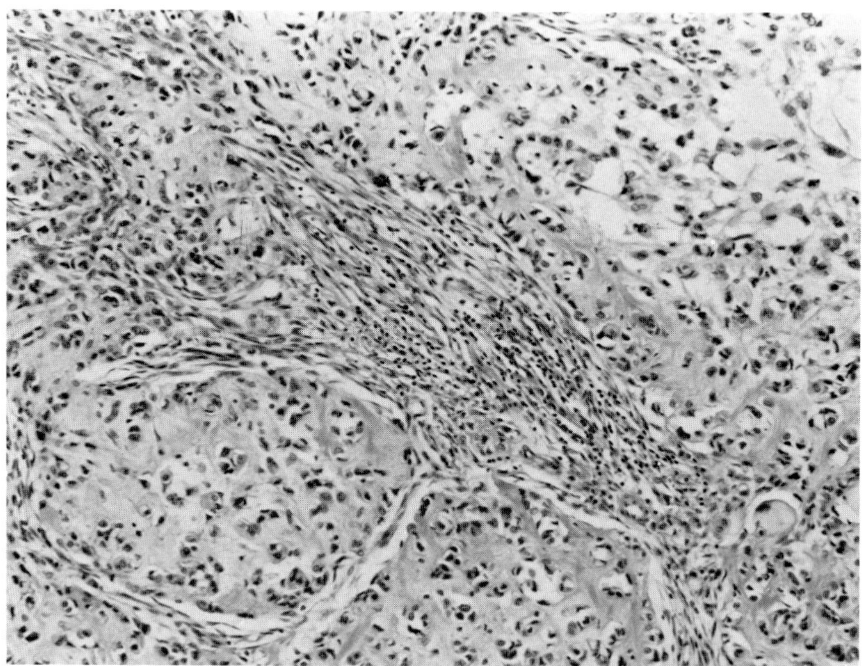

Fig. 12-3. Parachordoma showing nests of pale-staining cells surrounded by fibrovascular stroma. (H&E, × 125.)

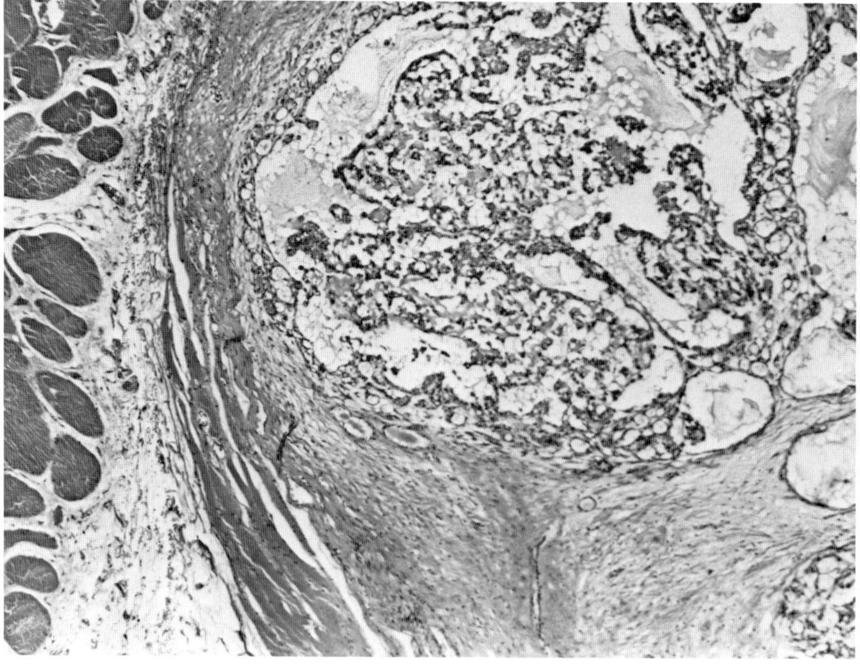

Fig. 12-4. Parachordoma exhibiting pseudocapsule and pseudoacinar structures. Aggregates of neoplastic cells are embedded in a myxoid and hyaline matrix. (H&E, × 50.)

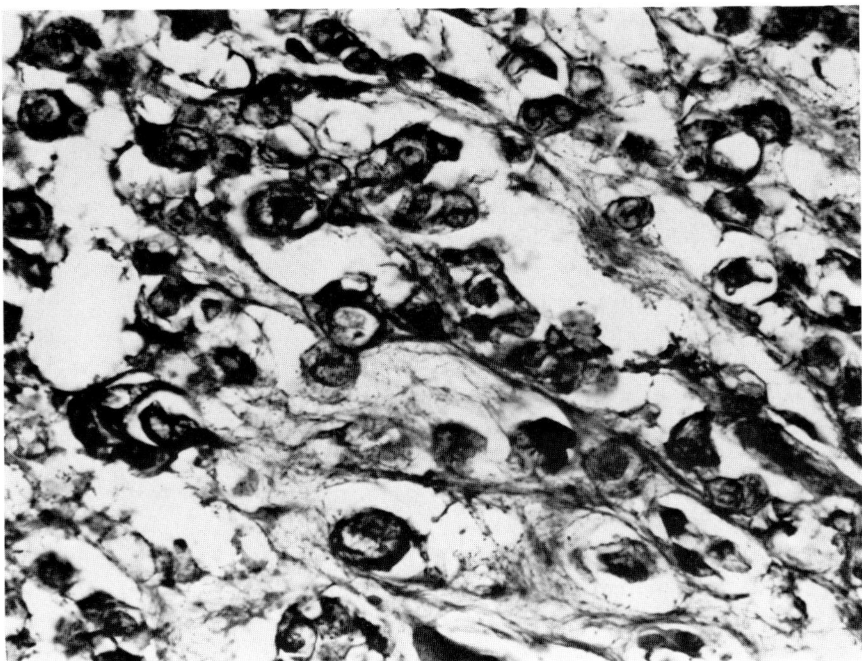

Fig. 12-5. Parachordoma. The pale-staining or vacuolated tumor cells often contain abundant glycogen. (PAS, × 500.)

Prognosis

Parachordoma follows a benign clinical course, however, the reported recurrence rate is about 37 percent. All recurrent lesions were cured by re-excision of the tumor.[12]

MALIGNANT TUMORS OF UNCERTAIN HISTOGENESIS

ALVEOLAR SOFT PART SARCOMA

The term *alveolar soft part sarcoma* (ASPS) was first coined in 1952 by Christopherson et al.[14] to designate a tumor that was previously referred to as *malignant organoid granular cell myoblastoma*[15, 16] and *malignant nonchromaffin paraganglioma*.[17] Although immunohistochemical, ultrastructural, and biochemical studies failed to provide conclusive evidence to support a paraganglionic, schwannian, or myogenic origin of this neoplasm,[18, 19] the myogenic origin is currently gaining more favor among pathologists[20–25]; nonetheless, the presence of myoglobin has not yet been reported.

Therefore, almost 37 years after its first description, controversy still surrounds the histogenesis of ASPS and its true nature is still obscure. Nonetheless, ASPS is a distinct clinicopathologic entity, representing less than 1 percent of all soft tissue sarcomas.[26] Its benign counterpart has never been reported.

Clinical Features

ASPS occurs chiefly in adolescents and young adults, with an approximate median age at diagnosis of 25 years.[19, 27] Female patients seem to outnumber males, especially among patients under 20 years of age.[18]

ASPS involves mainly the deep soft tissues of the extremities, particularly the thighs and buttocks, although there is a wide distribution of anatomic sites. In children, it is often located in the head and neck region, especially the orbit and tongue.[28] ASPS usually presents as a slow-growing painless mass, and hence, a metastasis in the lung or brain may be the first manifestation of the disease.[27]

Pathologic Findings

The tumor tends to be poorly circumscribed, and often exhibits areas of hemorrhage and necrosis. The histomorphologic picture is remarkably uniform, and is characterized by small ball-like organoid aggregates of polygonal, coarsely granular cells separated by thin-walled, cleftlike vascular spaces (Fig. 12-6). The typical alveolar pattern results from degeneration and detachment of central cells, and is well demonstrated by a reticulin stain. In children, the alveolar aspect is less evident, and a more solid growth pattern predominates. Many dilated blood vessels are found at the tumor periphery, and vascular invasion is usually readily observed. The neoplastic cells are relatively uniform, with large round nuclei and prominent nucleoli (Fig. 12-6). Mitoses are rare. The cells contain variable amounts of intracytoplasmic glycogen and pathognomonic periodic acid-Schiff (PAS)-positive, diastase-resistant crystalline material (Fig. 12-7). At the electron microscope, this material consists of unique rhomboid or rod-shaped membrane-bound crystals with characteristic linear and cross-hatched crystalloid patterns.[29]

Differential Diagnosis

The differential diagnosis includes mainly paraganglioma and granular cell tumor. Unlike paraganglioma, the cells in ASPS are frequently noncohesive, and often lack nuclear pleomorphism. Moreover, neurofilaments, [Met]enkephalin, [Leu]enkephalin, and neuron-specific enolase are negative in ASPS.[19, 24] The cells of granular cell tumor are less sharply defined and exhibit positive immunoreactivity for S-100 protein; they also lack PAS-positive, diastase-resistant crystalline material and the vascular

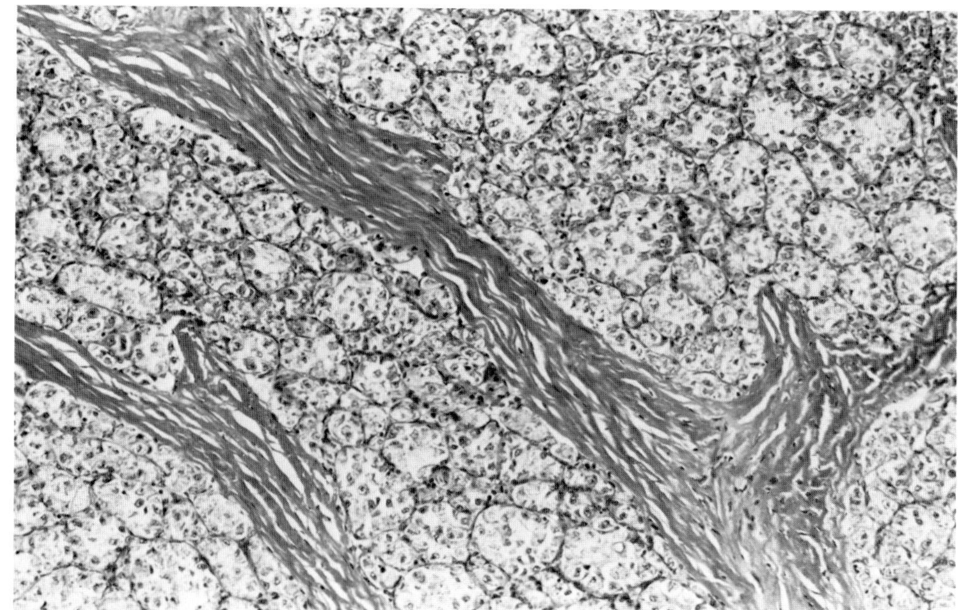

Fig. 12-6. Alveolar soft part sarcoma consisting of compact cell nests separated by thin-walled cleftlike vascular spaces. Groups of the cell balls are further divided by dense, fibrous septa. (H&E, × 125.)

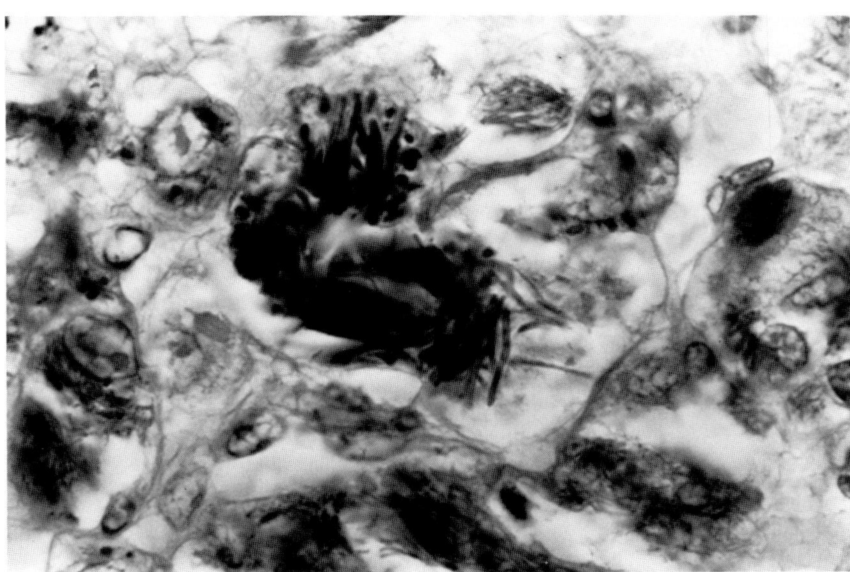

Fig. 12-7. Alveolar soft part sarcoma demonstrating characteristic intracellular crystalline material. (PAS with diastase, × 1250.)

endocrine pattern seen in ASPS. Furthermore, stainable glycogen is absent in both granular cell tumor and paraganglioma.

Alveolar rhabdomyosarcoma, along with metastatic adrenal cortical carcinoma, malignant melanoma, and clear cell sarcoma, should also be considered in the differential diagnosis. Unlike alveolar rhabdomyosarcoma, the alveoli in ASPS are not elongated, and are not separated by fibrous tissue. ASPS cells are much larger than myoblasts. Immunocytochemistry alone is not helpful in making this distinction, since many muscle markers are also expressed in ASPS.[21–23] Unlike ASPS, the neoplastic cells in the remaining tumors all reveal intracytoplasmic glycogen and express either positive epithelial markers (adrenal cortical carcinoma) or S-100 protein immunoreactivity (malignant melanoma and clear cell sarcoma).

Renal cell carcinoma bears a striking resemblance to ASPS, but can usually be distinguished by the absence of the characteristic PAS-positive crystalline material, the radiographic demonstration of a renal mass, and positive epithelial markers. Moreover, renal cell carcinoma is rarely encountered in a younger age group.

Prognosis

ASPS is a fully malignant neoplasm despite its deceivingly slow, protracted clinical course. Reported median survival of patients ranges from 6 years[18] to 6.5 years,[27] with survival rates of 77 percent at 2 years to 15 percent at 20 years.[18] Blood-borne metastases (68 percent) appear in the lungs, bone, and brain as late as 20 to 28 years following excision of the primary tumor.[14, 19] Chemotherapy and/or radiotherapy do not seem to improve the survival rates, and aggressive surgical excision with a long-term patient follow-up is therefore recommended.[18]

EPITHELIOID SARCOMA

Epithelioid sarcoma, a distinct entity first described by Enzinger[30] in 1970, has been accepted as a unique soft tissue sarcoma that typically pursues an indolent, relentless clinical course with multiple recurrences and late metastasis. This tumor is often mistaken for a granulomatous process, synovial sarcoma, and squamous cell carcinoma. The histogenesis of epithelioid sarcoma remains uncertain, however, primitive mesenchymal cells, histiocytes, fibroblasts, and synovial cells have all been implicated.[31–34]

Clinical Features

Epithelioid sarcoma chiefly affects young adults, with a median age of 26 years[31] to 27 years[35]; tumors involve the dermis, subcutis, or deeper soft tissues, particularly the fascial planes, aponeuroses, and tendon sheaths of the distal extremities. In children and adolescents, however, tumor may occur in such locations as the pelvis, head, and neck, which are rarely affected in adults.[33] This tumor typically grows in a multinodular manner, frequently with central necrosis of the tumor nodules and ulceration of the overlying skin. Hence, clinical appearance alone will allow its recognition.[36, 37]

Pathologic Findings

The tumors present grossly as firm, often multinodular masses with irregular outlines. The cut surface is gray-tan, glistening, and usually mottled with yellow to brown areas owing to necrosis and hemorrhage. At the light microscope, the tumor is characterized by a nodular growth pattern with central necrosis (Fig. 12-8), and consists of irregular nodular masses of large acidophilic polygonal cells, which merge imperceptibly with peripheral spindle-shaped cells, associated with dense fibrocollagenous tissue (Fig. 12-9).

The lesion is frequently accompanied by siderophages, and the tumor nodules are often surrounded by a cuff of lymphocytes and plasma cells. Some cases show broad areas of hyalinization in which the neoplastic cells appear to radiate from a central scarred zone. Foci of dystrophic calcification and occasional osteoid or bone formation may be observed.

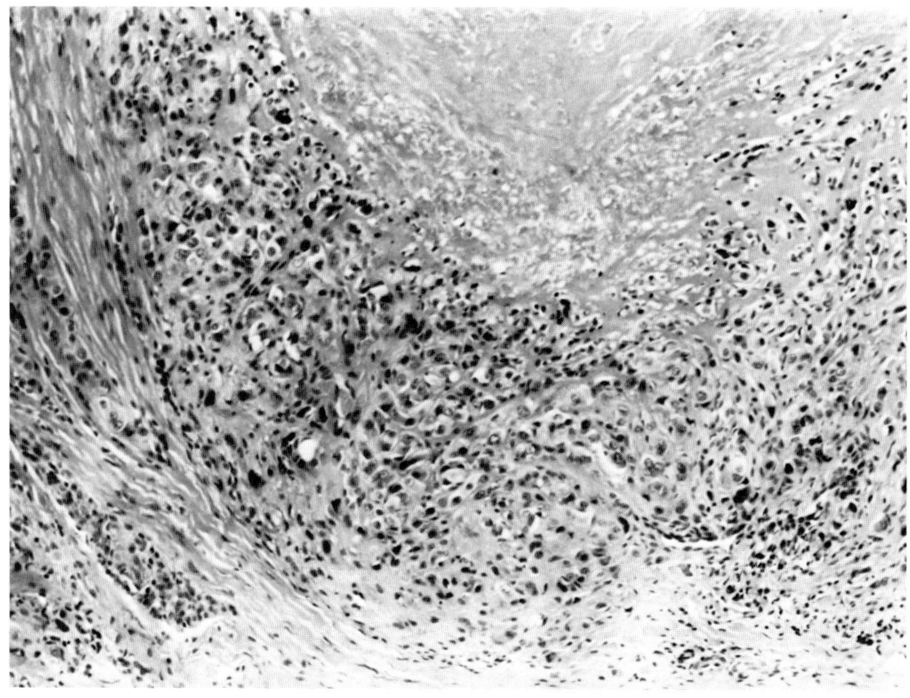

Fig. 12-8. Epithelioid sarcoma displaying a nodular growth pattern and central necrosis of the tumor nodule. (H&E, × 125.)

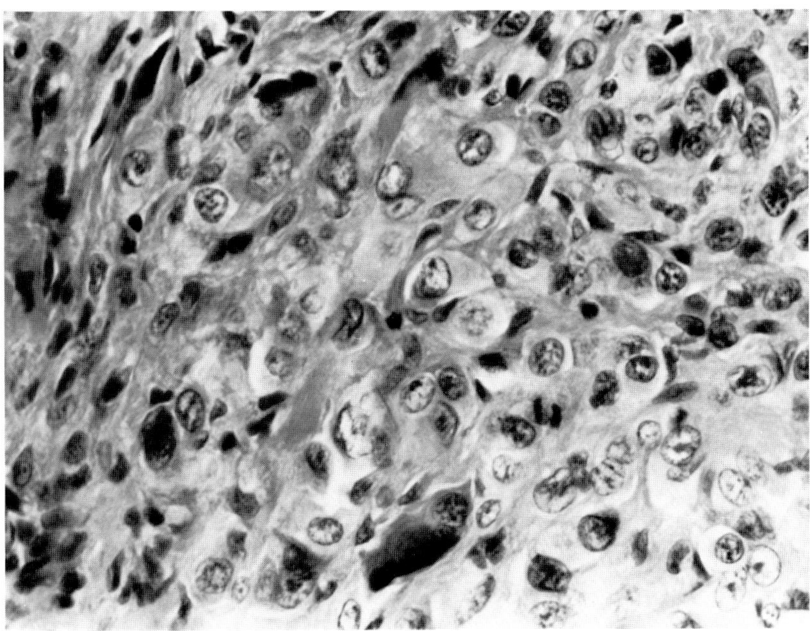

Fig. 12-9. Epithelioid sarcoma. Note the epithelioid appearance of the tumor cells which are intimately associated with spindle-shaped cells. (H&E, × 500.)

If the clinical presentation is atypical, diagnosis by light microscopy alone may be difficult. Although not pathognomonic for this entity, a strong globular, paranuclear reactivity to both antikeratin and antivimentin antibodies is commonly observed in the polygonal epithelioid cells (32–35, 37) (Fig. 12-10). At the ultrastructural level, this peculiar pattern reflects the presence of whorls of intermediate filaments filling the entire cytoplasm and pushing the nucleus to the periphery.[35]

Differential Diagnosis

In the initial stage, epithelioid sarcoma is often misinterpreted as a necrotizing infectious granuloma or necrobiotic granuloma, including granuloma annulare, necrobiosis lipoidica, and rheumatoid nodule. Epithelioid sarcoma cells are more eosinophilic than palisading histiocytes and the nuclei are more vesicular. Moreover, individual tumor nodules are more sharply defined than nodules of necrobiotic granuloma.

At times, the lesion is confused with squamous cell carcinoma, malignant melanoma, synovial sarcoma, and angiosarcoma.

The absence of pearl formation or dysplasia and dyskeratosis in the adjacent epithelium usually permits differentiation from an ulcerating squamous cell carcinoma. Unlike melanoma, it does not stain for S-100 protein. Although epithelioid sarcoma and synovial sarcoma share some similarities, dermal involvement and ulceration are more common in the former, where transition from epithelioid cell to spindle cell areas is also more gradual. The prominent fascicular or whorled growth pattern seen in synovial sarcoma is rarely encountered in epithelioid sarcoma. Moreover, intracytoplasmic mucin, noted in synovial sarcoma, is not seen in epithelioid sarcoma.[31]

Prognosis

The tumor pursues a slow indolent clinical course with a high tendency toward repeated local recurrences (63 to 77 percent) and late

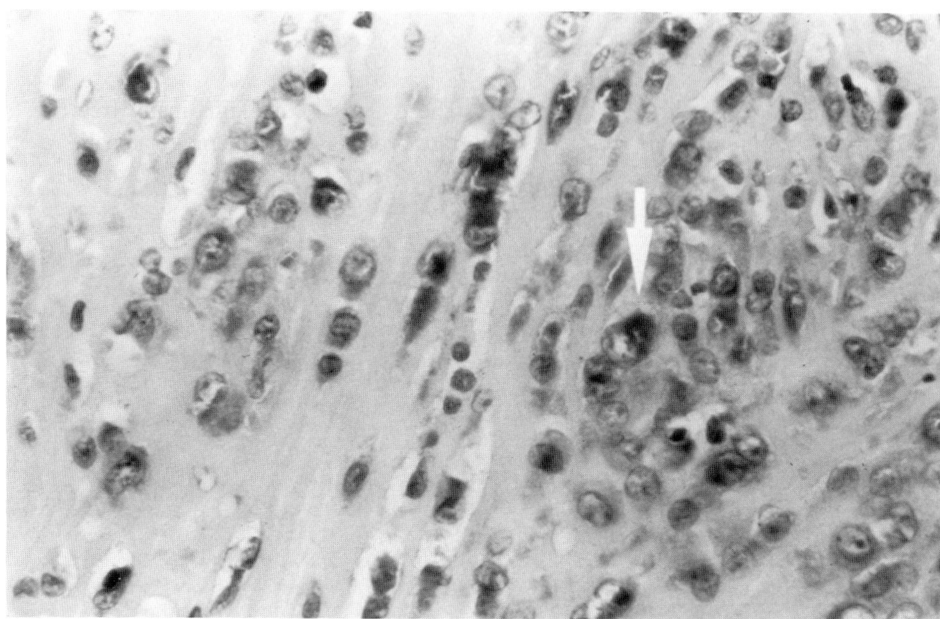

Fig. 12-10. Epithelioid sarcoma exhibiting strongly positive cytokeratin reactivity. (Monoclonal antibody anti-keratin AE1-AE3, × 500.)

metastases (45 percent) to lymph nodes and lungs.[31, 36] A more aggressive course is associated with a proximal or axial tumor location, increased size and depth, hemorrhage, necrosis, mitotic figures, and vascular invasion.[31, 36] Unlike most other soft tissue sarcomas, radical excision should include regional lymph node dissection in view of the high frequency of lymph node involvement.[36]

EXTRAOSSEOUS EWING'S SARCOMA

Primary tumors morphologically indistinguishable from Ewing's sarcoma of bone are known to occur in soft tissues.[38–41] It is still unclear whether these merely represent the soft tissue counterpart of the bone tumors or a distinct entity. This is not a question of semantics, since a primitive neuroectodermal origin for the osseous counterpart is now gaining wide acceptance,[42–44] whereas contradictory evidence regarding the histogenesis of extraosseous Ewing's sarcoma (EOE) was recently reported. A rhabdomyoblastic origin has been presumed, at least for some EOE, on the basis of ultrastructural[45] or in vitro[46] findings. On the other hand, the co-expression of epithelial, mesenchymal, and neural types of intermediate cytoskeleton filaments has suggested a blastematous rather than sarcomatous origin for Ewing's sarcoma, regardless of its location.[47]

A specific chromosomal abnormality involving chromosome 11 and 22 (t[11;22]-[q24;q21]),[48, 49] originally described in Ewing's sarcoma of bone and peripheral neuroepithelioma, was recently also reported in EOE.[50] Moreover, positivity to neural markers such as neuron-specific enolase and S-100 protein and ultrastructural detection of neurosecretory granules[51, 52] have been reported as well. These findings strongly suggest a close histogenetic relationship either between skeletal and extraskeletal Ewing's sarcoma on one hand, or peripheral primitive neuroectodermal tumors and EOE on the other.[51, 52]

Clinical Features

In general, the tumor presents clinically as a rapidly growing deep-seated mass. Like its bony counterpart, the tumor affects mainly adolescents and young adults (median age 20 years), and most commonly involves the soft tissues of the lower extremities and the paravertebral region. The preoperative duration of symptoms is usually less than 1 year, and catecholamine determinations are within normal limits.[39]

Pathologic Findings

Like the bony counterpart, EOE is composed of lobules of closely packed round cells with ill-defined cellular borders (Fig. 12-11). The nuclei show a blastemic appearance with finely dispersed chromatin and small nucleoli. Two types of cells are commonly recognized in the tumor lobules and light and dark cells. Light cells are characterized by a pale cytoplasm that is frequently vacuolated owing to the presence of large amounts of intracytoplasmic glycogen (Figs. 12-12 and 12-13). Dark cells are scattered in the lobules and show more irregular nuclei with condensed chromatin and scarce cytoplasm. The number of mitoses varies, but mitotic figures are rare. Areas of hemorrhage and necrosis are frequently encountered. Pseudorosettes are commonly observed, although Homer-Wright rosettes have also been described.[52]

Ultrastructurally the tumor resembles Ewing's sarcoma of bone and is characterized by a uniform population of round or oval cells. The cytoplasm contains many free ribosomes, rare profiles of rough endoplasmatic reticulum, mitochondria, and large pools of glycogen. A few primitive intercellular junctions may be observed.

Differential Diagnosis

Due to the undifferentiated round appearance of the tumor cells, the differential diagnosis includes all other "small round cell tumors," mainly malignant lymphoma, rhabdomyosarcoma, neuroblastoma, and neuroepithelioma.

Malignant lymphoma rarely shows the great uniformity in cell shape and size seen in EOE, and generally lacks sizable amounts of intracytoplasmic glycogen. Rhabdomyosarcoma may also display packed areas, but nuclei are more irregular with evident nucleoli. In these areas, scattered larger cells with eosinophilic cytoplasm are not uncommon, and a certain degree of spindling can also be observed. Desmin, α-actin, and myosin are generally positive in rhabdomyosarcoma.

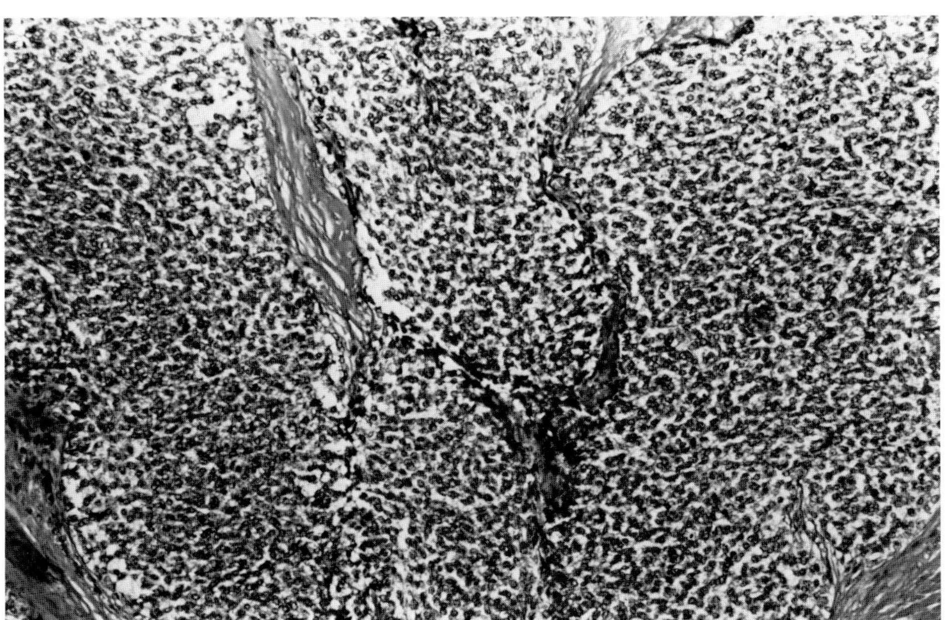

Fig. 12-11. Extraskeletal Ewing's sarcoma showing clusters and sheets of uniform round cells, separated by strands of fibrous tissue and thin-walled vascular channels. (H&E, × 125.)

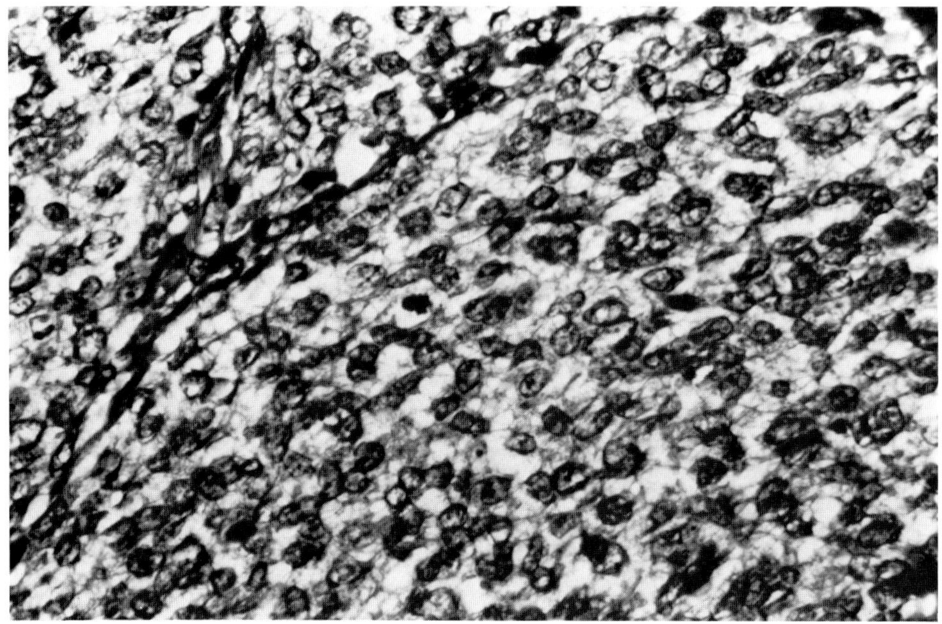

Fig. 12-12. Extraskeletal Ewing's sarcoma. The neoplastic cells have vesicular nuclei and an ill-defined pale-staining or vacuolated cytoplasm. (H&E, × 500.)

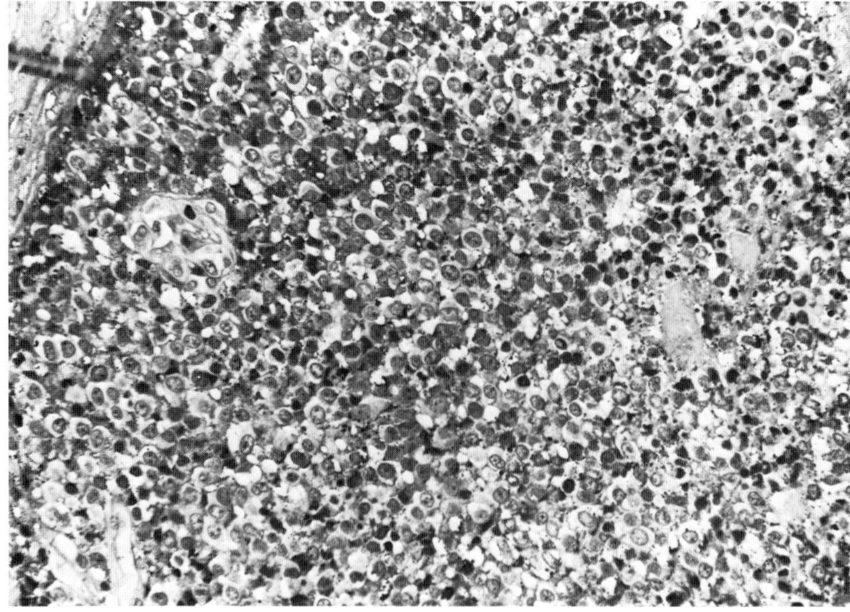

Fig. 12-13. Extraskeletal Ewing's sarcoma demonstrating abundant intracellular glycogen. (PAS, × 250.)

Peripheral primitive neuroectodermal tumors pose a more difficult differential diagnostic problem since they can bear a close resemblance to EOE. When classic Homer-Wright rosettes are absent, it may be impossible to draw a sharp line of distinction between these two tumors on morphologic criteria alone. Ultrastructural and immunocytochemical studies are of utmost importance in these cases. The presence of neurosecretory granules at the electron microscope and positivity to one or more neural markers[53] preclude a diagnosis of EOE.

Therefore, it seems convenient to retain the term EOE for undifferentiated small round cell tumors lacking any morphologic or immunocytochemical features of differentiation.

MALIGNANT MESENCHYMOMA

The term *mesenchymoma*, for mixed tumor of mesenchymal derivatives, was first coined by Stout[54] in 1948. Today, most benign mesenchymomas are categorized as developmental anomalies or hamartomas, the rest having been shown to be either an overgrowth of a certain tissue element (e.g., intramuscular hemangioma with overgrowth of adipose tissue) or expression of metaplastic features within a differentiated tumor of mesenchymal origin, such as lipoma with chondroid or osseous metaplasia.

Exactly what constitutes a malignant mesenchymoma may be debatable, although Stout originally defined it as a malignant tumor showing two or more unrelated differentiated tissue types in addition to a fibrosarcomatous element.[55] To avoid a meaningless "wastebasket" category, this diagnosis should be made only if each of the two or more tissue elements is sufficiently differentiated to permit clear recognition of its histological type.[56]

Malignant mesenchymoma should be distinguished from immature teratoma with multiple sarcomatous elements, malignant mixed mesodermal tumors of the genitourinary tract, tumors containing metaplastic cartilage or bone, and so-called collision tumor or carcinosarcoma.

Based on Stout's original definition, this entity should include tumors showing co-existence of rhabdomyosarcomatous and liposarcomatous elements, or combinations of leiomyosarcoma and liposarcoma and other types of sarcoma. Similarly a specific type of sarcoma together with areas of malignant cartilaginous or osseous tissue may be designated as malignant mesenchymoma. The most readily recognizable predominant pattern is usually that of rhabdomyosarcoma or liposarcoma, and less commonly, that of malignant fibrous histiocytoma or malignant schwannoma.

It is, however, preferred to diagnose this group of tumors according to the predominant tissue element, reflecting the reason for classifying it as malignant mesenchymoma (i.e., liposarcoma with areas of cartilaginous differentiation (malignant mesenchymoma). Mixed mesenchymal tumors are excluded, as these are considered distinct and separate entities that encompass malignant schwannoma with rhabdomyoblastic differentiation (malignant Triton tumor) and rhabdomyosarcoma with ganglionic elements (ectomesenchymoma).

The histogenesis of these heterogeneous tumors remains uncertain. It appears reasonable to speculate that they arise from primitive and uncommitted mesenchymal cells that have undergone multiple lines of differentiation.

Clinical Features

The clinical setting and presentation vary greatly. Most tumors occur in patients older than 55 years, and only a few affect children and young adults. Malignant mesenchymomas are generally deep seated, and in the majority of cases present as a stationary tumor of relatively long duration with a recent rapid increase in size. The two major sites of tumor involvement are the retroperitoneum and thigh.[56]

Pathologic Findings

There is a great variability in pathologic findings. Some reports describe large and bulky tumors that appear to be pseudoencapsulated and lobulated.[57] The cut surface is fleshy, gelatinous, and yellow-gray, and often mottled with areas of hemorrhage, necrosis, and cystification; a gritty sensation on cutting has been reported.

As noted above, on histology, combinations of rhabdomyosarcomatous and liposarcomatous patterns in the same tumor or the presence of co-existing leiomyosarcoma and liposarcoma may be observed. The neoplasms may be composed of other clearly recognizable types of sarcoma, such as rhabdomyosarcoma, malignant fibrous histiocytoma, or malignant schwannoma, together with more or less prominent areas of malignant cartilaginous or osseous tissue (Figs. 12-14 and 12-15).

Differential Diagnosis

Depending on the histologic type of tissue elements and growth patterns present within the tumors, the differential diagnosis also varies widely.

Prognosis

The outcome is usually related to the prevalent mesenchymal components, therefore, survival varies considerably from case to case. Prognosis is best with basically liposarcomatous neoplasms, and appears worst with those showing a prominent rhabdomyosarcomatous component. The mode of therapy must be selected on the basis of the predominant and least differentiated histologic type.[56]

MALIGNANT RHABDOID TUMOR

Malignant rhabdoid tumor (MRT) was initially described in 1978 by Beckwith and

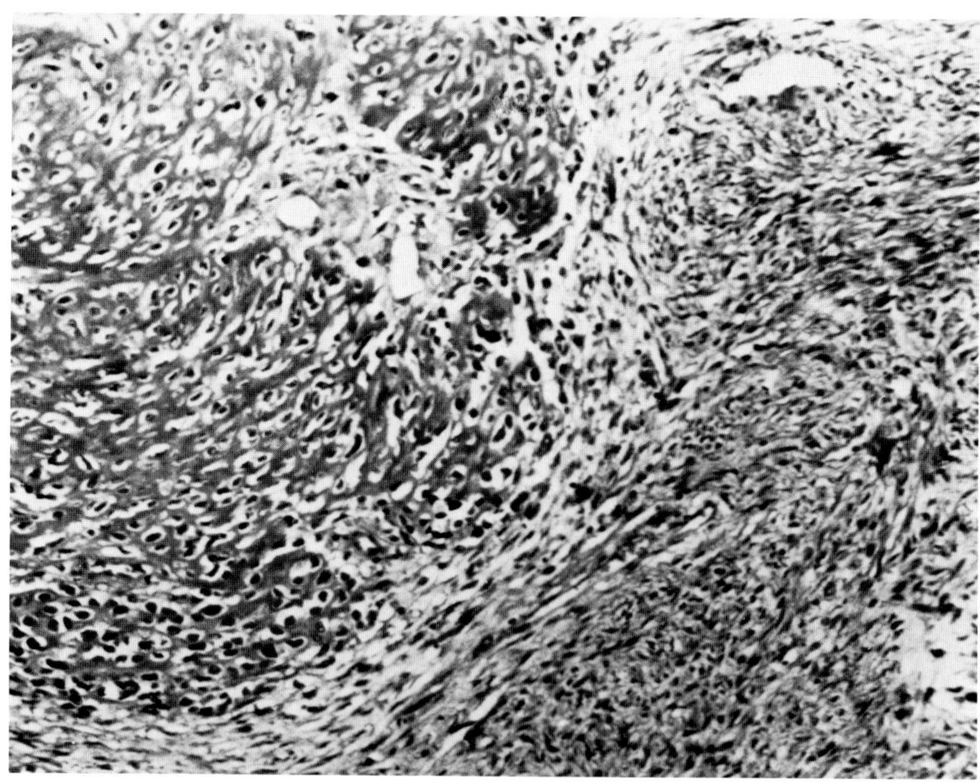

Fig. 12-14. Malignant mesenchymoma of the retroperitoneum (Masson trichrome, × 125.)

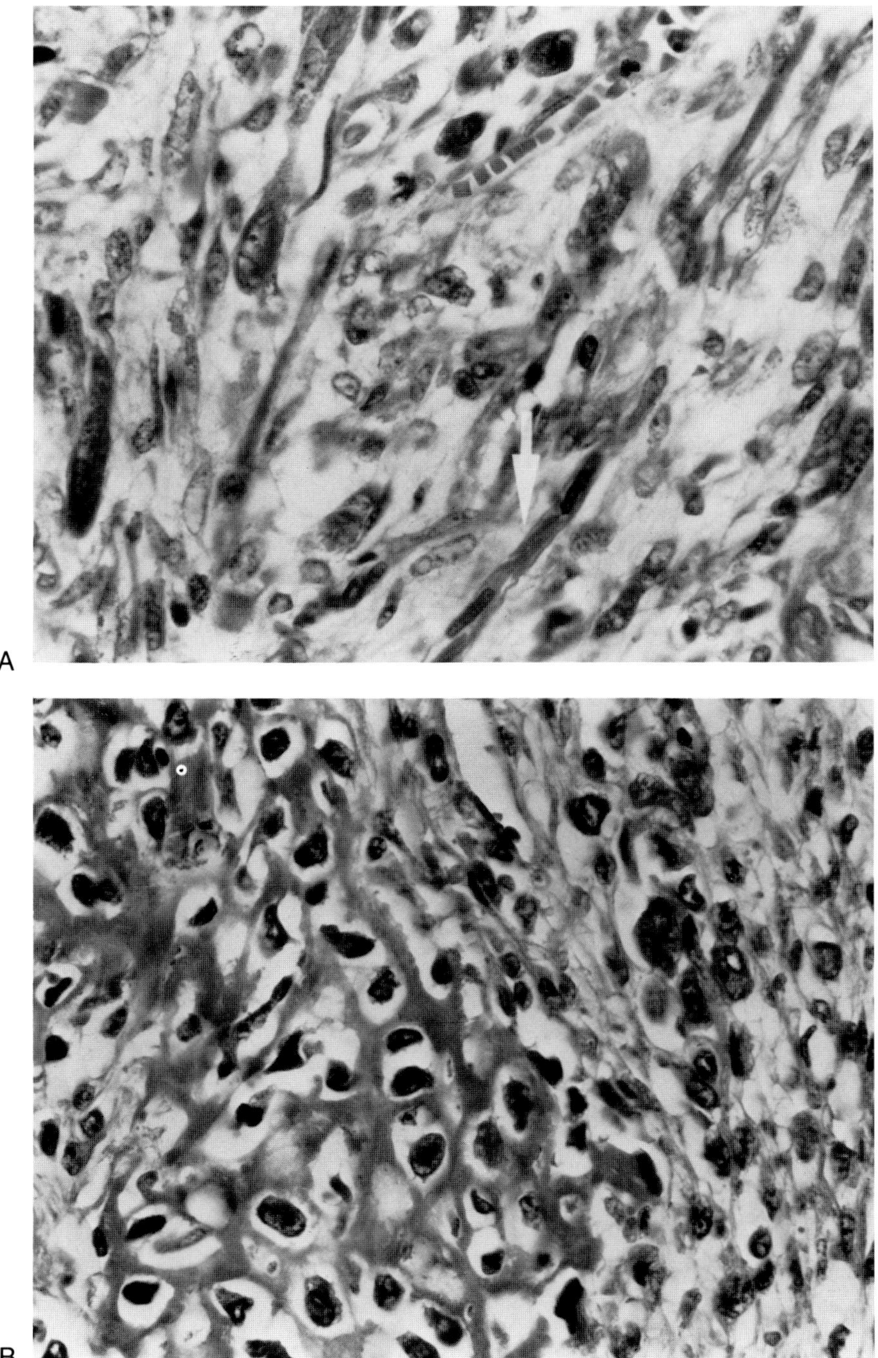

Fig. 12-15. High-power views of the same tumor shown in Fig. 12-14. (**A**) Rhabdomyosarcomatous pattern. Note the cross striations (arrow). (**B**) Osteosarcomatous pattern. (Masson trichrome, × 500.)

Palmer[58] as an unfavorable variant of Wilms' tumor under the heading of "rhabdomyosarcomatoid pattern" because of its superficial resemblance to rhabdomyosarcoma. Ultrastructural findings, however, failed to demonstrate a myogenous differentiation, and hence the term *rhabdoid tumor* was coined instead by Haas et al.[59] in 1981.

Extrarenal forms of this tumor are very uncommon, however, they have been described in both soft tissues and parenchymatous organs (such as heart or brain).[60–64]

The histogenesis of malignant rhabdoid tumor remains obscure, and possible myogenic,[58, 65, 66] neural crest,[59] histiocytic,[67] mesenchymal[62] and epithelial origins[68] have been advanced. The co-expression in tumor cells of different classes of intermediate filaments, such as vimentin, desmin, and cytokeratin, suggested a multipotential blastematous origin of the tumor.[60 61, 64, 68, 69] Nonetheless, the recognition of this rare tumor is important[69] because its poor prognosis requires appropriate and more aggressive therapy.

Clinical Features

Extrarenal MRT occurs most commonly in infants and children younger than 15 year of age. This tumor accounts for less than 10 percent of all childhood lesions, and is also rarely encountered in adults.[63] Soft tissue MRT occurs more often in the trunk than in the extremities, with a slight preference for the paravertebral region. There appears to be no sex predilection, although some series show a male preponderance.[61] Curiously extrarenal rhabdoid tumor associated with brain tumors has often been reported.[70]

Pathologic Findings

Grossly the tumors are poorly circumscribed and the usually gray-white and fleshy cut surface often shows foci of hemorrhage and necrosis.

Microscopically the tumor is composed of sheets of round or polygonal cells with vesicular nuclei with prominent nucleoli and abundant pink cytoplasm (Fig. 12-16). In general, there

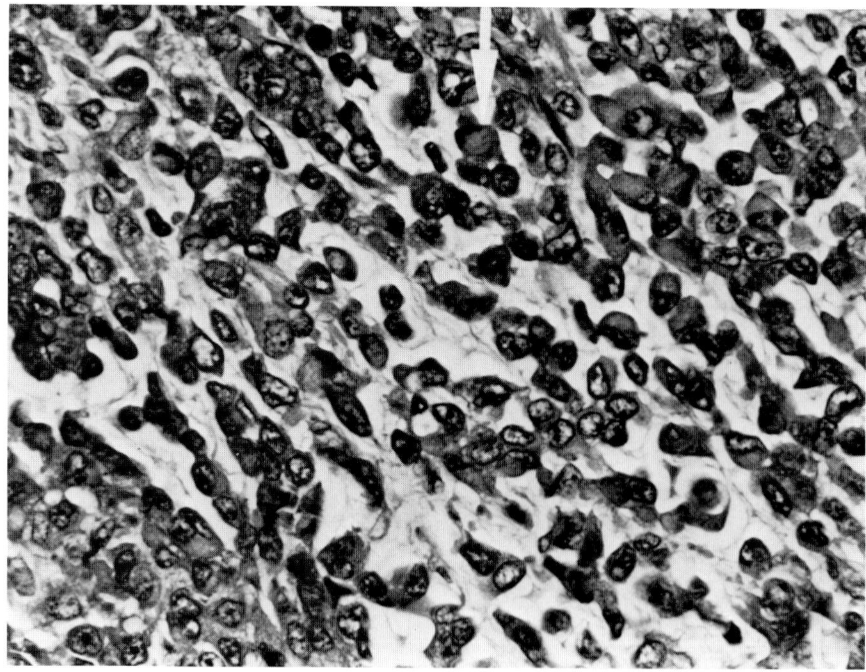

Fig. 12-16. Malignant rhabdoid tumor arising in the chest wall of a 4-month-old girl. Note the hyaline inclusions (arrow). (H&E, × 500.)

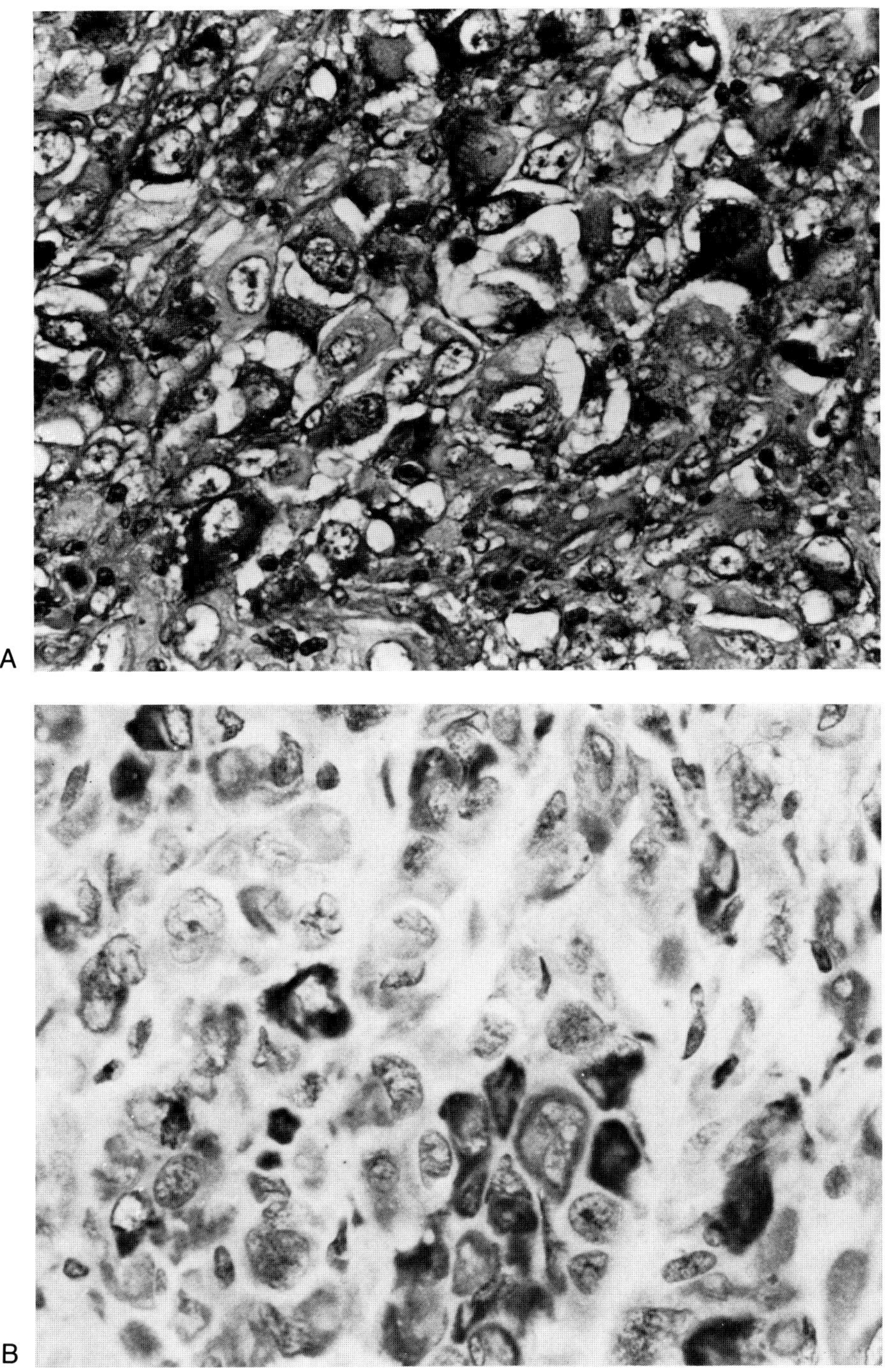

Fig. 12-17. Malignant rhabdoid tumor. **(A)** PAS-positive hyaline inclusions or globules. **(B)** Expression of immunoreactive cytokeratin. (× 500.)

is little, if any, evidence of neoplastic cell spindling. Tumor cells frequently contain acidophilic and PAS-positive hyaline inclusions or globules (Fig. 12-17A), and express both immunoreactive keratin (Fig. 12-17B) and vimentin. At the electron microscope, the intracellular acidophilic hyaline material is shown to consist of compact whorls of intermediate filaments (Fig. 12-18).

Differential Diagnosis

The typical hyaline paranuclear inclusions and co-expression of vimentin and keratin have been considered diagnostic hallmarks, but unfortunately, these features are not exclusively found in MRT. Epithelioid cells with eosinophilic perinculear inclusions are commonly found in other soft tissue tumors, such as epithelioid sarcoma, synovial sarcoma, mesenchymal myxoid chondrosarcoma, malignant mesothelioma[71] and epithelioid neurofibroma.[72] As in MRT, keratin and vimentin co-expression is usually detected in epithelioid sarcoma and sy-

novial sarcoma. Nevertheless, tumor cell spindling is a rare finding in MRT, and is more commonly encountered in epithelioid and synovial sarcoma. Moreover, the clinical course is remarkably different; MRT is a highly aggressive tumor compared to the indolent course of epithelioid sarcoma.

A pseudoalveolar pattern occasionally may present at the MRT periphery, and thus alveolar rhabdomyosarcoma may enter the differential diagnosis. The differential may be further complicated by positivity to desmin in MRT[64, 70] and to keratin in rhabdomyosarcoma.[73] Alveolar rhabdomyosarcoma, however, shows a greater cellular polymorphism, and thick and thin filaments or Z-band material are absent in MRT.

Prognosis

The outcome of MRT is poor. In about one-third of the cases, metastasis may be present at the time of diagnosis; disease course is rapid and fatal, usually within 6 months from diagno-

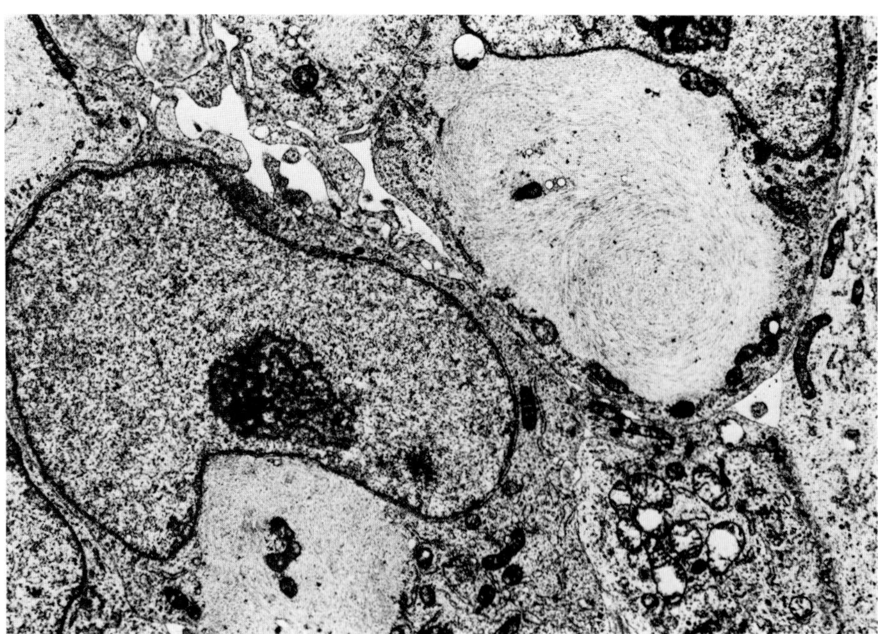

Fig. 12-18. Malignant rhabdoid tumor. Ultrastructurally the cytoplasmic inclusions are composed of whorls of intermediate filaments. ($\times$ 4000.)

sis. Principal sites of metastasis are lungs, lymph nodes, liver, and brain.[61]

REFERENCES

1. Lattes R: Tumors of the Soft Tissues (Revised). Atlas of Tumor Pathology. II Series. Fascicle I. Armed Forces Institute of Pathology. Washington, DC, 1982
2. Enzinger FM: Intramuscular myxoma. Am J Clin Pathol 43:104, 1965
3. Ireland D CR, Soule EH, Ivins JC: Myxoma of somatic soft tissues. A report of 58 patients, 3 with multiple tumors and fibrous dysplasia of bone. Mayo Clin Proc 48:401, 1973
4. Kindblom LG, Stener B, Angervall L: Intramuscular myxoma. Cancer 34:1737, 1974
5. Hashimoto H, Tsuneyoshi M, Daimaru Y, et al: Intramuscular myxoma. A clinicopathologic, immunohistochemical, and electron microscopic study. Cancer 58:740, 1986
6. Wirth WA, Leavitt D, Enzinger FM: Multiple intramuscular myxomas. Another extraskeletal manifestation of fibrous dysplasia. Cancer 27:1167, 1971
7. Sedmak DD, Hart WR, Belhobek GH, et al: Massive intramuscular myxoma associated with fibrous dysplasia of bone. Cleve Clin Q 50:469, 1983
8. Steeper TA, Rosai J: Aggressive angiomyxoma of the female pelvis and perineum. Report of nine cases of distinctive type of gynecologic soft tissue neoplasm. Am J Surg Pathol 7:463, 1983
9. Begin LR, Clement PB, Kirk ME, et al: Aggressive angiomyxoma of the pelvic soft parts: a clinicopathologic study of nine cases. Hum Pathol 16:621, 1985
10. Gonzalez-Crussi F, de Mello DE, Sotelo-Avila C: Omental-mesenteric myxoid hamartomas. Infantile lesions simulating malignant tumors. Am J Surg Pathol 7:567, 1983
11. Lyaskovsky J: Parachordoma. p. 262. In Eighth International Cancer Congress. Medgiz Publishing House, Moscow, 1962
12. Dabska M: Parachordoma. A new clinicopathologic entity. Cancer 40:1586, 1977
13. Povysil C, Matejovsky Z: A comparative ultrastructural study of chondrosarcoma, chordoid sarcoma, chordoma and chordoma periphericum. Pathol Res Pract 179:546, 1985
14. Christopherson WM, Foote FW Jr, Stewart FW: Alveolar soft-part sarcoma. Structurally characteristic tumors of uncertain histogenesis. Cancer 5:100, 1952
15. Horn RC, Stout AP: Granular cell myoblastoma. Surg Gynecol Obstet 76:315, 1943
16. Ackerman LV, Phelps CR: Malignant granular cell myoblastoma of the gluteal region. Surgery 20:511, 1946
17. Smetana HF, Scott WF Jr: Malignant tumors of nonchromaffin paraganglia. Milit Surg 109:330, 1951
18. Lieberman PH, Brennan MF, Kimmel M, et al: Alveolar soft-part sarcoma. A clinico-pathologic study of half a century. Cancer 63:1, 1989
19. Auerbach HE, Brooks JJ: Alveolar soft-part sarcoma. A clinicopathologic and immunohistochemical study. CAncer 60:66, 1987
20. Mukai M, Torikata C, Iri H, et al: Alveolar soft-part sarcoma. A review on its histogenesis and further studies based on electron microscopy, immunohistochemistry, and biochemistry. Am J Surg Pathol 7:679, 1983
21. Foschini MP, Ceccarelli C, Eusebi V, et al: Alveolar soft-part sarcoma: immunological evidence of rhabdomyoblastic differentiation. Histopathology 13:101, 1988
22. Hirose T, Kudo E, Hasegawa T, et al: Cytoskeletal properties of alveolar soft part sarcoma. Hum Pathol 21:204, 1990
23. Miettinen M, Ekfors T: Alveolar soft part sarcoma. Immunohistochemical evidence for muscle cell differentiation. Am J Clin Pathol 93:32, 1990
24. Persson S, Willems J-S, Kindblom L-G, Angervall L: Alveolar soft part sarcoma. An immunohistochemical, cytologic and electron-microscopic study and a quantitative DNA analysis. Virchows Arch [A] 412:499, 1988
25. Fisher ER, Reidbord H: Electron microscopic evidence suggesting the myogenous derivation of the so-called alveolar soft part sarcoma. Cancer 27:150, 1971
26. Enzinger FM, Weiss SW: p. 929. In Soft Tissue Tumors. 2nd Ed. CV Mosby, St. Louis, 1988
27. Evans HL: Alveolar soft-part sarcoma. A study of 13 typical examples and one with a histologically atypical component. Cancer 55:912, 1985
28. Font RL, Jurco S III, Zimmerman LE: Alveolar soft-part sarcoma of the orbit: a clinicopathologic analysis of seventeen cases and a review of the literature. Hum Pathol 13:569, 1982

29. Shipkey FH, Lieberman PH, Foote FW Jr, et al: Ultrastructure of alveolar soft part sarcoma. Cancer 17:821, 1964

30. Enzinger FM: Epitheliod sarcoma. A sarcoma simulating a granuloma or a carcinoma. Cancer 26:1029, 1970

31. Chase DR, Enzinger FM: Epitheliod sarcoma. Diagnosis, prognostic indicators, and treatment. Am J Surg Pathol 9:241, 1985

32. Manivel JC, Wick MR, Dehner LP, et al: Epitheliod sarcoma. An immunohistochemical study. Am J Clin Pathol 87:319, 1987

33. Schmidt D, Harms D: Epithelioid sarcoma in children and adolescents. An immunohistochemical study. Virchows Arch[A] 410:423, 1987

34. Persson S, Kindblom LG, Angervall L: Epitheliod sarcoma. An electron-microscopic and immunohistochemical study. Appl Pathol 6:1, 1988

35. Meis JM, Mackay B, Ordonez NG: Epitheliod sarcoma: An immunohistochemical and ultrastructural study. Surg Pathol 1:13, 1988

36. Prat J, Woodruff JM, Marcove RC: Epithelioid sarcoma. An analysis of 22 cases indicating the prognostic significance of vascular invasion and regional lymph node metastasis. Cancer 41:1472, 1978

37. Daimaru Y, Hashimoto H, Tsuneyoshi M, et al: Epithelial profile of epithelioid sarcoma. An immunohistochemical analysis of eight cases. Cancer 59:134, 1987

38. Tefft M, Vauter GF, Mitus A: Paravertebral "round cell" tumors in children. Radiology 92:1501, 1969

39. Angervall L, Enzinger FM; Extraskeletal neoplasm resembling Ewing's sarcoma. Cancer 36:240, 1975

40. Hashimoto H, Tsuneyoshi M, Daimaru Y, Enjoji M: Extraskeletal Ewing's sarcoma. A clinicopathologic and electron microscopic analysis of 8 cases. Acta Pathol Jpn 35:1087, 1985

41. Rud NP, Reiman HM, Pritchard DJ, et al: Extraosseous Ewing's sarcoma. A study of 42 cases. Cancer 64:1548, 1989

42. Lipinsky M, Braham K, Philip I, et al: Neuroectodermal-associated antigens on Ewing's sarcoma cell lines. Cancer Res 47:183, 1986

43. Jaffe R, Santamaria M, Yunis J, et al: The neuroectodermal tumor of bone. Am J Surg Pathol 8:885, 1984

44. Cavazzana AO, Miser JS, Jefferson J, Triche TJ: Experimental evidence of a neural origin of Ewing's sarcoma of bone. Am J Pathol 127:507, 1987

45. Dickman PS, Triche TJ: Extraosseous Ewing's sarcoma versus primitive rhabdomyosarcoma: diagnostic criteria and clinical correlation. Hum Pathol 17:881, 1986

46. Garvin AJ, Stanley WS, Bennett DD, et al: In vitro growth, heterotransplantation, and differentiation of a human rhabdomyosarcoma cell line. Am J Pathol 125:208, 1986

47. Moll R, Lee I, Gould VE, et al: Immunocytochemical analysis of Ewing's tumors. Patterns of expression of intermediate filaments and desmosomal proteins indicate cell type heterogeneity and pluripotential differentiation. Am J Pathol 127:288, 1987

48. Aurias A, Rimbaud C, Buffe D, et al: Chromosomal translocations in Ewing's sarcoma. N Engl J Med 309:496, 1983

49. Whang-Peng J, Triche TJ, Knutsen T, et al: Cytogenetic characterization of selected small round cell tumor of childhood. Cancer Genet Cytogenet 21:185, 1986

50. Casorso L, Pessia L, Satimo A, et al: Extraskeletal Ewing's tumor with translocation t(11;22) in a patient with Down syndrome. Cancer Genet Cytogenet 37:79, 1989

51. Mierau GW: Extraskeletal Ewing's sarcoma (peripheral neuroepithelioma). Ultrastruct Pathol 9:91, 1985

52. Shimada H, Newton WA, Soule EH, et al: Pathologic features of extraosseous Ewing's sarcoma: a report from the Intergroup Rhabdomyosarcoma Study. Hum Pathol 19:442, 1988

53. Yunis EJ: Ewing's sarcoma and related small round cell neoplasms in children. Am J Surg Pathol 10 (Suppl 1):54, 1986

54. Stout AP: Mesenchymoma, the mixed tumor of mesenchymal derivates. Ann Surg 127:278, 1948

55. Stout AP, Lattes R: Tumors of the soft tissues. Atlas of Tumor Pathology. II Series. Armed Forces Institute of Pathology, Washington DC, 1967

56. Enzinger FM, Weiss SW: p. 958. In Soft Tissue Tumors. 2nd Ed. CV Mosby, St. Louis, 1988

57. Klima M, Smith M, Spjut HJ, et al: Malignant mesenchymoma. Case report with electron microscopic study. Cancer 36:1086, 1975

58. Beckwith JB, Palmer NF: Histopathology and prognosis of Wilms' tumor. Results from the First National Wilms' Tumor Study. Cancer 41:1937, 1978

59. Haas JE, Palmer NF, Weinberg AG, et al: Ultrastructure of malignant rhabdoid tumor of the kidney. A distinctive renal tumor of children. Hum Pathol 12:646, 1981

60. Tsuneyoshi M, Daimaru Y, Hashimoto H, et al: Malignant soft tissue neoplasms with the histologic features of renal rhabdoid tumors: an ultrastructural and immunohistochemical study. Hum Pathol 16:1235, 1985

61. Sotelo-Avila C, Gonzalez-Crussi F, de Mello D, et al: Renal and extrarenal rhabdoid tumors in children: a clinicopathologic study of 14 patients. Semin Diagn Pathol 3:151, 1986

62. Dervan PA, Cahalane SF, Kneafsey P, et al: Malignant rhabdoid tumour of soft tissue. An ultrastructural and immunohistological study of a pelvic tumour. Histopathology 11:183, 1987

63. Balaton AJ, Vaury P, Videgrain M: Paravertebral malignant rhabdoid tumor in an adult. A case report with immunocytochemical study. Pathol Res Pract 182:713, 1987

64. Tsokos M, Kouraklis G, Chandra RS, et al: Malignant rhabdoid tumor of the kidney and soft tissues. Evidence for a diverse morphological and immunocytochemical phenotype. Arch Pathol Lab Med 113:115, 1989

65. Zanetti G, Giangaspero F: Rhabdomyoblastic nature of cytoplasmic inclusions in malignant rhabdoid tumor. Hum Pathol 13:410, 1982

66. Molenaar WM, DeJong B, Dam-Meiring A, et al: Epithelioid sarcoma or malignant rhabdoid tumor of soft tissue? Epithelioid immunophenotype and rhabdoid karyotype. Hum Pathol 20:347, 1989

67. Gonzalez-Crussi F, Goldschmidt RA, Hsueh W, et al: Infantile sarcoma with intracytoplasmic filamentous inclusions. Distinctive tumor of possible histiocytic origin. Cancer 49:2365, 1982

68. Vogel AM, Gown AM, Caughlan J, et al: Rhabdoid tumors of the kidney contain mesenchymal specific and epithelial intermediate filament proteins. Lab Invest 50:232, 1984

69. Schmidt D, Harms D, Zieger G: Malignant rhabdoid tumor of the kidney. Histopathology, ultrastructure and comments on differential diagnosis. Virchows Arch [A] 398:101, 1982

70. Schmidt D, Leuschner I, Harms D, et al: Malignant rhabdoid tumor. A morphological and flow cytometric study. Pathol Res Pract 184:202, 1989

71. Tsuneyoshi M, Daimaru Y, Hashimoto H, Enjoji M: The existence of rhabdoid cells in specified soft tissue sarcomas. Histopathological, ultrastructural and immunohistochemical evidence. Virchows Arch [A] 411:509, 1987

72. Ninfo V, Cavazzana AO: Congenital epithelioid neurofibroma with extensive tactile differentiation and rhabdoid-like inclusions. Surg Pathol 1:417, 1988

73. Miettinen M, Rapola J: Immunohistochemical spectrum of rhabdomyosarcoma and rhabdomyosarcoma-like tumors. Am J Surg Pathol 13:120, 1989

Index

Page numbers followed by f indicate figures; those followed by t indicate tables.